MEDICAL ABBREVIATIONS:

15,000 Conveniences at the Expense of Communications and Safety

Tenth Edition

Neil M Davis, MS, PharmD, FASHP

Professor Emeritus, Temple University
    School of Pharmacy, Philadelphia, PA,
Editor-in-Chief, Hospital Pharmacy
President, Safe Medication Practices
    Consulting, Inc.

D0400789

published by

Neil M Davis Associates
1143 Wright Drive
Huntingdon Valley, PA 19006-2721

Phone (215) 947-1752 (9 AM-6 PM EST, Mon-Fri)
FAX (215) 938-1937
Web site http://www.neilmdavis.com
E-mail med@neilmdavis.com

Contents

Dedication

This book is dedicated to Julie, my wife, for her support, patience, assistance, and love.

Acknowledgments

The assistance of Evelyn Canizares, Ann Sandt Kishbaugh, Matthew Davis, Robin Miller, Danial Baker, and Suzette Knight is gratefully acknowledged.

I would like to express my deep appreciation for the many contributions received from readers for their suggested additions and corrections. Please continue to send these to—

Dr. Neil M Davis
1143 Wright Drive
Huntingdon Valley PA 19006-2721
FAX (215) 938 1937
E-mail   med@neilmdavis.com

Preface

Website Version Access Information

Along with the purchase of each book, the book owner, at no extra cost, is entitled to a single-user access to the Internet version of the book. This license is valid for 24 months from the date of the initial log-in. Internet Explorer 4.0, Netscape 4.0, or AOL 5.0 can meet the minimum browser requirement.

Features of the Web-Version
- Will be updated monthly (suggestions from users are welcomed and will be incorporated).
- Can search for the meanings of abbreviations and acronyms.
- Will have a reverse-search feature, for example, looking for all the abbreviations that contain the word "laparoscopic."
- Can search for cross-referenced generic and brand names of drugs.
- Can search through the listings of symbols, lists, and normal laboratory values.
- Can read the full-text of the introductory chapters of the book.

Initial One-time Log-in for a Single-User Password
- Access the Website at *www.medabbrev.com*
- You will be asked for the 6-letter access code that appears on the front inside cover of the book. This will be the only time you are asked for this code.
- At this point just follow the directions.
- Note your sign-in name and your self-assigned password. This name/password will only permit one access at a time, so keep this information confidential to ensure your ready access to the book.

Searching for the Meaning of an Abbreviation
- Use upper OR lower case letters as the search engine is NOT case sensitive.

- Use normal upper OR lower case letters as the search engine is NOT sensitive to whether the letters are **bold-face** or *italicized*.
- Superscripts and subscripts are to be entered as regular text.
- For other details, just follow the simple instructions shown on the Website. The Web version of the book is the same as the print version except for the fact that it is searchable and is updated monthly.

Chapter 1
Introduction

Listed are 15,000 current acronyms, symbols, and other abbreviations and 22,000 of their possible meanings. This list has been compiled to assist individuals in reading and transcribing medical records, medically-related communications, and prescriptions. The list, although current and comprehensive, represents a portion of abbreviations in use and their many possible meanings as new ones are being coined every day.

WARNING

Abbreviations are a convenience, a time saver, a space saver, and a way of avoiding the possibility of misspelling words. However, a price can be paid for their use. Abbreviations are sometimes not understood, misread, or are interpreted incorrectly. Their use lengthens the time needed to train individuals in the health fields, wastes the time of healthcare workers in tracking down their meaning, at times delays the patient's care, and occasionally results in patient harm.

The publication of this list of abbreviations is not an endorsement of their legitimacy. It is not a guarantee that the intended meaning has been correctly captured, or an indication that they are in common use. Where uncertainty exists, the one who wrote the abbreviation must be contacted for clarification.

There are many variations in how an abbreviation can be expressed. Anterior-posterior has been written as AP, A.P., ap, and A/P. Since there are few standards and those who use abbreviations do not necessarily follow these standards, this book only shows anterior-posterior as AP. This is done to make it easier to find the meaning of an abbreviation as all the meanings of AP are listed together. This elimination of unnecessary duplication also keeps the book at a convenient size, thus enabling it to be sold at a reasonable price.

When an abbreviation is made up of a series of abbreviations, it may not be listed as such. In such instances, the meaning may be determined by looking up each set of abbreviations, as in the example of DTP$_a$-HIB-PNU-MEN, which means, diphtheria, tetanus toxoids, acellular pertussis; *Haemophilus influenzae* type b conjugate; pneumococcal (*Streptococcus pneumoniae*) conjugate; meningococcal (*Neisseria meningitidis*) conjugate (serogroups unspecified) vaccine.

Lower case letters are used when firm custom dictates as in Ag, Na, mCi, etc. The first letter of brand names are capitalized, whereas nonproprietary names appear in lower case.

The abbreviation AP is listed as meaning doxorubicin and cisplatin. The reason for this apparent disparity is that the official generic names (United States Adopted Names) are shown rather than the brand names Adriamycin® and Platinol AQ®. In the case of LSD, the official name, lysergide, is given, rather than the chemical name, lysergic acid diethylamide. The Latin derivations for older medical and pharmaceutical abbreviations (TID,*ter in die,* three times daily) may be found in *Remington.*[1]

Some abbreviations which have been encountered or that have been suggested for addition to the book have not been added. Some were obscene or completely insensitive. Others were so ambiguous as to be useless, such as LIDO, CORTI, and CEPH. Some served no real purpose as they were almost as long as the word they were abbreviating, such as DISCOMF for discomfort, FIOR for Fiorinal, FLEX for flexion, DEPO-M for Depo-Medrol, NEOSP for Neosporin, RMKBLE for remarkable.

Healthcare organizations are advised by the Joint Commission on Accreditation of Healthcare Organizations to formulate an approved list of abbreviations. Every attempt should be made to restrict this list to common abbreviations that are understood by all health professionals who must work with medical records. There are certain dangerous abbreviations that should not be approved, and a warning should be issued about their use (see Table 1 as well as

Table 1. Examples of dangerous abbreviations

Problem term	Reason	Suggested term
O.D. for once daily	Interpreted as right eye	Write "once daily"
q.o.d. for every other day	Interpreted as meaning "every once a day" or read as q.i.d.	Write "every other day"
q.d. for once daily	Read or interpreted as q.i.d.	Write "once daily"
q.n. for every night	Read as every hour	Write "every night," "HS" or nightly
q hs for every night	Read as every hour	Use "HS" or "at bedtime"
TIW for three times a week	Interpeted as T/W (Tuesday & Wednesday); as twice a week; as TID (three times daily)	Write "three times a week"
U for Unit	Read as 0, 4, 6, or cc	Write "unit"
O.J. for orange juice	Read as OD or OS	Write "orange juice"
µg (microgram)	When handwritten, misread as mg	Write "mcg"
sq or sub q for subcutaneous	The q is read as every	Use "subcut"
Chemical symbols	Not understood or misunderstood	Write full name
Lettered abbreviations for drug names or drug protocols	Not understood or misunderstood	Use generic or brand name(s)
Apothecary symbols or terms	Not understood or misunderstood	Use metric system
per os for by mouth	OS read as left eye	Use "by mouth," "orally," or "PO"
D/C for discharge	Interpreted as discontinue (orders for discharge medications result in premature discontinuance of current medication)	Write "discharge"
T/d for one per day	Read as T.I.D.	Use "once daily"
/ (a slash mark) for with, and, or per	Read as a one	Use, "and," "with," or "per"

3

notes in the text). A second list should be published by the healthcare organizations containing dangerous abbreviations that were purposely omitted from the approved list. The reasons for their omission should be stated.

Many inherent problems associated with abbreviations contribute to or cause errors. Reports of such errors have been published routinely.[2-5]

Abbreviations and symbols can easily be misread or interpreted in a unintended manner. For example:

(1) "HCT250 mg" was intended to mean hydrocortisone 250 mg but was interpreted as hydrochlorothiazide 50 mg (HCTZ50 mg).

(2) Flucytosine was improperly abbreviated as 5 FU, causing it to be read as fluorouracil. Flucytosine is abbreviated 5 FC and fluorouracil is 5 FU.

(3) Floxuridine was improperly abbreviated as 5 FU, causing it to be read as fluorouracil. Floxuridine is abbreviated FUDR and fluorouracil is 5 FU.

(4) MTX was thought to be mechlorethamine. MTX is methotrexate and mechlorethamine is abbreviated HN2.

(5) **The abbreviation "U" for unit is the most dangerous one in the book, having caused numerous tenfold insulin overdoses. The word unit should never be abbreviated.** The handwritten U for unit has been mistaken for a zero, causing tenfold errors. The handwritten U has also been read as the number four, six, and as "cc."

(6) OD, meant to signify once daily, has caused Lugol's solution to be given in the right eye.

(7) OJ meant to signify orange juice, looked like OS and caused saturated solution of potassium iodide to be given in the left eye.

(8) IVP, meant to signify intravenous push (Lasix 20 mg IVP), caused a patient to be given an intravenous pyelogram which is the usual meaning of this abbreviation.

(9) Na Warfarin (sodium warfarin) was read as "No Warfarin."

(10) The abbreviation "s̄" for "without" has been thought to mean "with" (c̄).

4

(11) The order for PT, intended to signify a laboratory test order for prothrombin time, resulted in the ordering of a physical therapy consultation.

(12) The abbreviation "TAB," meant to signify Triple Antibiotic (a coined name for a hospital sterile topical antibiotic mixture), caused patients to have their wounds irrigated with a diet soda. At another facility, with the same set of circumstances, they did not have TAB®, so they used Diet Shasta.®

(13) A slash mark (/) has been mistaken for a one, causing a patient to receive a 100 unit overdose of NPH insulin when the slash was used to separate an order for two insulin doses:

   6 units regular insulin/20 units NPH insulin

(14) Vidarabine, an antiviral agent, was ordered as ara-A; however, ara-C, which is cytarabine, an antineoplastic agent, was given.

(15) On several occasions, pediatric strength diphtheria-tetanus toxoids (DT) have been confused with adult strength tetanus-diphtheria toxoids (Td).

(16) DTP is commonly understood to refer to diphtheria-tetanus-pertussis vaccine, but in some hospitals it is also used as shorthand for a sedative cocktail of Demerol, Thorazine, and Phenergan. Several cases have occurred where a child was vaccinated rather than given the sedative mixture.

(17) What does the abbreviation MR mean? Some will guess measles-rubella vaccine (M-R-Vax II, Merck), while others will assume mumps-rubella vaccine (Biavax II, Merck).

(18) The abbreviation TIW (three times a week) was thought to mean Tuesday and Wednesday when the I was read as a slash mark. Due to confirmation bias (you see what you know), this uncommon abbreviation is seen as the more commonly used TID (three times a day).

(19) PCA, meant to be procainamide, was interpreted as patient-controlled analgesia.

(20) PGE_1 (alprostadil, Caverject) was read as P6 E1 (Alcon's ophthalmic pilocarpine and epinephrine solution).

(21) A nurse transcribed an oral order for the antibiotic

aztreonam as AZT, which was subsequently thought to be the antiviral drug zidovudine.

(22) An order for TAC 0.1%, intended to mean triamcinolone cream, was interpreted as tetracaine, Adrenalin, and cocaine solution.

(23) An order for SPA (salt poor albumin) was overlooked because it was not recognized as a drug order.

(24) Therapy was delayed and considerable professional time was wasted when an order for "Bactrim SS q 12 h on S/S" had to be clarified (Bactrim Single Strength every 12 hours on Saturday and Sunday).

(25) A physician wrote an order stating "may take own supply of EPO". The physician meant evening primrose oil, not Epogen (epoetin alfa).

(26) 4-MP was recommended to treat ethylene glycol poisoning. The medical resident mistakenly interpreted this as 6-MP (6-mercaptopurine). 4-MP is fomepizole (4 methylpyrazole) and 6-MP is mercaptopurine (6-mercaptopurine).

(27) An order for lomustine stated it was to be given at "hs". This was misinterpreted as to mean every night. After continuous administration, toxicity resulted in the patient's death. The drug is normally given once every 6 weeks. State complete orders such as "HS × 1 dose today," "HS nightly," or "HS nightly PRN for sleep."

(28) The directions for an order for Cortisporin Otic Solution indicated "Three drops in ® ear TID." The patient was given the drops in the rear rather than the right ear.

(29) There have been mix-ups between IL-2 and IL-11 when IL-2 is expressed as IL-II (Roman numeral 2). The II has been read as "IL eleven," and vice versa. IL-2 (interleukin 2) is aldesleukin (Proleukin) and IL-11 is oprelvekin (Neumega).

The author would appreciate receiving other examples of abbreviations that have been misinterpreted causing error or delays so that this section can be expanded.

A prescription could be written with directions as follows: "OD OD OD," to mean one drop in the right eye once daily!

Abbreviations should not be used for drug names as they are particularly dangerous. As previously illustrated, there is the possibility that the writer may, through mental error, confuse two abbreviations and use the wrong one. Similarly, the reader may attribute the wrong meaning to an abbreviation. To further confound the problem, some drug name abbreviations have multiple meanings (see ATR, CPM, CPZ, GEM, NITRO, and PBZ in Table 2). The abbreviation AC has been used for three different cancer chemotherapy combinations to mean Adriamycin and either cyclophosphamide, carmustine, or cisplatin.

Beside causing medication errors and incorrect interpretation of medical records, abbreviations can create problems because treatment is delayed while a health professional seeks clarification for the meaning of the abbreviation used. Abbreviations should not be used to designate drugs or combinations of drugs.

Certain abbreviations in the book are followed by a warning, "this is a dangerous abbreviation." This warning could be placed after many abbreviations, but was reserved for situations where errors have been published because these abbreviations were used or where the meaning is critical and not likely to be known. Such warning statements should also appear after every abbreviation for a drug or drug combination.

Abbreviations for medical facility names create problems as they are usually not recognized by the readers in other geographic areas. A clue to the fact that one is dealing with such an abbreviation is when it ends with MC, for Medical Center; HS, for Health System; MH, for Memorial Hospital; CH, for Community Hospital; UH, for University Hospital; and H, for Hospital.

When an abbreviation cannot be found in this book or when the listed meaning(s) do not make sense, there is a possibility that the abbreviation has been misread. As an example, a reader could not find the meaning of HHTS. On closer examination it really was +HTS, not HHTS. Also EWT could not be identified because it was really ENT.

Some common French and Spanish abbreviations are listed in the book. Because of language structure differences, abbreviations are often reversed, as in the case of HIV, which in Spanish and French is abbreviated as VIH.

7

Table 2. Examples of abbreviations that have contradictory or ambiguous meanings

ABP	= ambulatory blood pressure arterial blood pressure
ACU	= acute receiving unit ambulatory care unit
AMI	= amifostine amitriptyline
APC	= advanced pancreatic cancer advanced prostate cancer
ATR	= atropine atracurium
AZT	= zidovudine azathioprine
BO	= bowel open bowel obstruction
CF	= cystic fibrosis Caucasian female calcium leucovorin (citrovorum factor) complement fixation cancer-free cardiac failure coronary flow contractile force Christmas factor count fingers cisplatin and fluorouracil
CLD	= chronic liver disease chronic lung disease
CPM	= cyclophosphamide chlorpheniramine maleate
CPZ	= chlorpromazine Compazine
DW	= dextrose in water distilled water deionized water
DXM	= dexamethasone dextromethorphan
ESLD	= end-stage liver disease end-stage lung disease
FEC	= fluorouracil, epirubicin, and cyclophosphamide fluorouracil, etoposide, and cisplatin
GD	= Graves' disease Gaucher's disease

8

GEM	= gemfibrozil
	gemicitabine
HD	= Hansen's disease
	Hodgkin's disease
	Huntington's disease
ICA	= internal carotid artery
	intracranial abscess
	intracranial aneurysm
IT	= intrathecal
	intratracheal
	intratumoral
LFD	= lactose-free diet
	low fat diet
	low fiber diet
MS	= morphine sulfate
	multiple sclerosis
	mitral stenosis
	musculoskeletal
	medical student
	minimal support
	muscle strength
	mental status
	milk shake
	mitral sound
	morning stiffness
MTD	= maximum tolerated dose
	minimum toxic dose
MTZ	= mirtazapine
	mitoxantrone
NBM	= no bowel movement
	normal bowel movement
	nothing by mouth
NITRO	= nitroglycerin
	sodium nitroprusside
OLB	= open-liver biopsy
	open-lung biopsy
PBZ	= phenylbutazone
	pyribenzamine
	phenoxybenzamine
PORT	= postoperative radiotherapy
	postoperative respiratory therapy

PVO	= peripheral vascular occlusion
	portal vein occlusion
	pulmonary venous occlusion
RS	= Reiter's syndrome
	Reye's syndrome
	Raynaud's disease (syndrome)
	rumination syndrome
S & S	= swish and spit
	swish and swallow
SAD	= social anxiety disorder
	seasonal affective disorder
SDBP	= seated, standing, or supine diastolic blood pressure
SSE	= saline solution edema
	soapsuds edema
STF	= special tube feeding
	standard tube feeding
TICU	= thoracic intensive care unit
	transplant intensive care unit
	trauma intensive care unit
TMZ	= temazepam
	temozolomide
TS	= Tay-Sachs (disease)
	Tourette's syndrome
	Turner's syndrome
VAD	= vincristine, doxorubicin, (Adriamycin) and dexamethasone
	vincristine, doxorubicin (Adriamycin) and dactinomycin
VAP	= vincristine, Adriamycin, and prednisone
	vincristine, Adriamycin, and procarbazine
	vincristine, actinomycin D, and Platinol AQ
	vincristine, asparaginase, and prednisone

Chapter 5 contains a cross-referenced list of 3,300 generic and brand drug names. The list contains names of commonly prescribed and new drugs. Brand names have their first letter capitalized whereas generic names are in lower case. This list will enable readers to obtain the generic name for brand name products or brand names for generic names. It will also serve as a spelling check.

Coded drug names and abbreviations for drug names are found in the chapter on abbreviations (Chapter 3).

Chapter 6 is a table of normal laboratory values. Both the conventional and international values are listed. Each laboratory publishes a list of its normal values. These local lists should be reviewed to see if there are significant differences.

The Council of Biology Editors (CBE), in their 1983 edition of the *CBE Style Manual* listed about 600 abbreviations gathered from 15 internationally recognized authorities and organizations.[6] The majority of these symbols and abbreviations tend to be more scientifically oriented than those which would appear in medical records. In the few situations where the CBE abbreviations differ from what is presented in this book, the CBE abbreviation has been placed in parentheses after the meaning. As is the practice in the United States, mL has been used rather than ml and the spelling of liter, meter, etc. is used rather than litre and metre, even though ml, litre, and metre are listed in the *CBE Style Manual*. A new edition of the *CBE Style Manual* was published in 1995.[7] Again, in this edition, emphasis is placed on scientific abbreviations.

An examination of the 15,000 abbreviations and their 22,000 meanings is a testimonial to the problems and dangers associated with most undefined abbreviations.

References

1. Gennaro AR, ed. Remington's Pharmaceutical Sciences, 20th ed. Phila., PA: Lippincott Williams and Wilkins, 2000.

2. Davis NM, Cohen MR. Medication errors: causes and prevention. Huntingdon Valley, PA: Neil M Davis Associates; 1983.

3. Cohen MR. Medication error reports. Hosp Pharm (appears monthly from 1975 to the present).

4. Cohen MR. Medication errors. Nursing 2001 (appears monthly, starting in Nursing 77, to the present).

5. Davis NM. Med Errors. Am J Nursing (appears monthly from 1994 to 1995).

6. CBE Style Manual, 5th ed. Bethesda, MD: Council of Biology Editors; 1983.

7. Scientific Style and Format: The CBE Manual for Authors, Editors, and Publishers, 6th Ed. Council of Biological Editors-Cambridge University Press. Cambridge UK, New York, Victoria Australia: 1995.

Chapter 2

A Healthcare Controlled Vocabulary

Presently there are no standards for prescriber's orders, consultations, written prescriptions, standing orders, computer order sets, nurse's medication administration records, pharmacy profiles, hospital formularies, etc. Because in the healthcare field everyone does their own thing, there are many variations. These variations in the way abbreviations are expressed are not always understood and at times are misinterpreted. They cause delays in initiating therapy, cause accidents, waste time for everyone in clarifying these documents, lengthen the time it takes to train those working in the healthcare field, lengthen hospital stays, and waste money.

A controlled vocabulary similar to what is used in the aviation industry is needed. Everyone in the aviation industry "follows the book," and uses a controlled vocabulary. All pilots and air traffic controllers say, "alfa", "bravo", "charlie." See Table 1, the phonetic alphabet. They do not go off on their own and say "adam", "beef", "candy!" They say "one three," not thirteen, because thirteen sounds like thirty. Radio transmission in the aviation industry is not easy to decipher, yet because precision is critical everything possible is done to eliminate error. To prevent errors all radio transmissions are given only in English, every transmission is given in the same order and must be immediately repeated by the receiver to make sure it was heard correctly. Written and oral communication in the medical professions are just as critical and are also not easy to decipher, so establishing a controlled vocabulary is also necessary in this industry.

Listed below are three organizations that have ongoing projects related to standardizing medical terminology:

Computer-Based Patient Record Institute, Inc.
1000 East Woodfield Rd. Suite 102
Schuamburg, IL 60173

The United States Pharmacopeial Convention, Inc.
12601 Twinbrook Parkway
Rockville, MD, 20852

National Library of Medicine
Unified Medical Language Systems
8600 Rockville Pike
Bethesda, MD, 20894

Listed below (Table 2) is the start of a Healthcare Controlled Vocabulary. The basis for this controlled vocabulary is established standard terminology and the result of 35 years of studying medical errors by this author.

It is anticipated that a Healthcare Controlled Vocabulary, with professional organizations' input and backing, will grow and someday evolve into an "official standard." Your suggestions and comments are vital to this growth and eventual recognition. It is always safest to avoid the use of abbreviations unless a standard has been established and is well-publicized in your work environment.

Table 1. Phonetic Alphabet

The International Civil Aviation Organization phonetic alphabet is used by the aviation industry when communications conditions are such that the information cannot be readily received without their use. Health professionals also should use it when it is necessary to orally spell critical information.

Character	Telephony	Phonic
A	Alfa	(AL-FAH)
B	Bravo	(BRAH-VOH)
C	Charlie	(CHAR-LEE)
		or (SHAR-LEE)
D	Delta	(DELL-TA)
E	Echo	(ECK-OH)
F	Foxtrot	(FOKS-TROT)
G	Golf	(GOLF)
H	Hotel	(HOH-TEL)
I	India	(IN-DEE-AH)
J	Juliett	(JEW-LEE-ETT)
K	Kilo	(KEY-LOH)
L	Lima	(LEE-MAH)
M	Mike	(MIKE)
N	November	(NO-VEM-BER)
O	Oscar	(OSS-CAH)
P	Papa	(PAH-PAH)
Q	Quebec	(KEH-BECK)
R	Romeo	(ROW-ME-OH)
S	Sierra	(SEE-AIR-RAH)
T	Tango	(TANG-GO)
U	Uniform	(YOU-NEE-FORM)
		or (OO-NEE-FORM)
V	Victor	(VIK-TAH)
W	Whiskey	(WIS-KEY)
X	X-ray	(ECKS-RAY)
Y	Yankee	(YANG-KEY)
Z	Zulu	(ZOO-LOO)
1	One	(WUN)
2	Two	(TOO)
3	Three	(TREE)
4	Four	(FOW-ER)
5	Five	(FIFE)
6	Six	(SIX)
7	Seven	(SEV-EN)
8	Eight	(AIT)
9	Nine	(NIN-ER)
0	Zero	(ZEE-RO)

Table 2. Examples of a Controlled Vocabulary

Standard	What not to use or do	Comments
100 mg (100 space mg)	100mg (100 no space mg)	The USP* standard way of expressing a strength is to leave a space between the number and its units. Leaving this space makes it easier to read the number as can be seen below. 1mg 1 mg 10mg 10 mg 100mg 100 mg
1 mg	1.0 mg	This is a USP standard. When a trailing zero is used, the decimal point is sometimes not seen thus causing a tenfold overdose. These overdoses have caused injury and death.
0.1 mL	.1 mL	When the decimal point is not seen, this is read as 1 mL, causing a ten fold overdose.
once daily (Do not abbreviate.)	The abbreviation OD	The classic meaning for OD is right eye. Liquids intended to be given once daily are mistakenly given in the right eye.
	The abbreviation QD	When the Q is dotted too aggressively it looks like Q.I.D. and the medication is given four times daily. When a lower case q is used, the tail of the q has come up between the q and the d to make it look like qid. In the United Kingdom, Q.D. means four times daily
unit (Do not abbreviate. Write "unit" using a lower-case u)	The abbreviation U	The handwritten U is mistaken for a zero when poorly written causing a 10 fold overdose (i.e. 6 U regular insulin is read as 60). The poorly written U has also been read as a 4, 6, and cc. Write "unit," leaving a space between the number and the word unit.

16

Standard	What **not** to use or do	Comments
mg (Lower case mg with no period)	mg;, Mg;, Mg, MG, mgm, mgs	The USP standard expression is the mg
mL (lower case m with a capital L, no period)	mL;, ml, ml;, mls, mLs, cc	The USP standard expression is the mL
Use generic names or brand names	Do not abbreviate drug names or combinations of drugs, such as CPZ, PBZ, NTG, MS, 5FC, MTX, 6MP, MOPP, ASA, HCTZ, etc.	Abbreviated drug names and acronyms are not always known to the reader; at times they have more than one possible meaning, or are thought to be another drug.
		When the chemical name "6 mercaptopurine" has been used, six doses of mercaptopurine have been mistakenly administered. The generic name, mercaptopurine, should be used.
	Do not use shortened names or chemical names	When an unofficial shortened version of the name norfloxacin, norflox was used, Norflex was mistakenly given.
		An order for Aredia was read as Adriamycin, as some professionals abbreviated the name Adriamycin as "Adria" which looks like Aredia.
The metric system	The apothecary system (grains, drams, minims, ounces, etc.)	The Apothecary system is so rarely used it is not recognized or understood. The symbol for minim ($\mathfrak{m}$) is read as mL; the symbol for one dram (3 T) is read as 3 tablespoons, and gr (grain) is read as gram.
Use properly placed commas for numbers above 999, as in 10,000, or 5,000,000	5000000	Many people have difficulty in reading large numbers such as 5000000. The use of commas helps the reader to read these numbers correctly.

(continued)

17

Standard	What **not** to use or do	Comments
600 mg When possible, do not use decimal expressions. 25 mcg	0.6 g 0.025 mg	A USP standard. The elimination of decimals lessens the chance for error. Mistakes are made when reading numbers less than 1 with decimals.
Do not use the term "bolus" in conjunction with the administration of potassium chloride injection. Use specific concentrations and the time in which the drug should be administered.		Some physicians will erroneously indicate that potassium chloride injection should be "bolused" or be given "IV push," vaguely meaning that it should not be dripped in slowly. Many deaths have been reported when prescribers have been taken literally and the potassium chloride was given by bolus or IV push. Orders should be specific such as, "20 mEq of potassium chloride in 50 mL of 5% dextrose to run over 30 minutes."
use "and"	Do not use a slash mark or the symbol "&"	A slash mark looks like a one. An order written "6 units regular insulin/20 units NPH insulin," was read as 120 units of NPH insulin. The symbol "&" has been read as a 4.
Orally transmitted medical orders should be read back as heard for verification.	Do not assume that one has spoken or heard correctly.	During oral communications, speakers misspeak and/or transcribers mishear. To minimize these errors, the transmitter must repeat what was transcribed, and the transmitter must listen attentively when this is being done. Errors are less likely to occur when the prescription is complete. When spelling out words, use the phonetic alphabet shown in Table 1.

Standard	What **not** to use or do	Comments
When prescriptions are written or orally transmitted they must be complete. • dosage form must be specified • strength must be specified • directions must be specified • included in the directions must be the purpose or indication.	Incomplete orders	Prescribers on occasion think of one drug and mistakenly order another. Nurses and pharmacists on occasion misread prescriptions because of error, poor handwriting or poor oral communications, or look-alike or sound-alike drugs.[1] When the prescription is complete and the purpose or indication is included, these errors are less likely to occur. Listing the purpose or indication on the prescription label will assist in increasing patient adherence.
Written communications must be legible.	Illegible handwriting	Prescribers who cannot or will not write legibly must either print (if this would be legible), type, use a computer, or have an employee write for them and then immediately verify and sign the document.
Prescribe specific doses.	Do not prescribe 2 ampuls or 2 vials	There is often more than one size or concentration of drug available. Failing to be specific will lead to unintended doses being administered.
Establish a list of approved abbreviations with no abbreviation having more than one possible meaning within a context.	Everyone using their own abbreviations.	To understand the scope of this problem examine the contents of this book for abbreviations that have many meanings and for obscure abbreviations which would not generally be recognized.
Use h or hr for hour	°	An order written as q 4° has been read as q 40 or the symbol ° has not been understood.
Specify total amount of drug to be given in a single dose.[2]	Specify total amount of drug to be administered over a period of time.	Orders such as . . . . 1,600 mg over 4 days have caused death when mistakenly given as a single dose. Order should state . . . . 400 mg once daily for four days (2-1-99 to 2-4-99)

*USP = United States Pharmacopeia

1. Davis NM. Look-alike and sound alike drug names. Hosp Pharm 1999;34:1160–78
2. Kohler DR, Montello MJ, Green I, et al. Standardizing the expression and nomenclature of cancer treatment regimens. Am J Health-System Pharm. 1998;55:137–44

Chapter 3

Lettered Abbreviations and Acronyms

Where an abbreviation contains numbers, symbols, punctuation, spaces, etc., they are *not* considered during alphabetizing ["501 (k)" is listed under K]. Entries beginning with a *Greek letter* are alphabetized where the name of the letter would be found alphabetically.

The letter-by-letter (dictionary) system of alphabetizing is used ("*ad lib*" is listed under ADL).

Brand names (proprietary names) have their first letter capitalized, whereas nonproprietary (generic) names are in lower-case letters.

The listing of symbols, numbers, and Greek letters can be found in Chapter 4.

See WARNING in chapter 1.

A

			artery
			Asian
			assessment
			auscultation
		A+	blood type A positive
A	accommodation	A−	blood type A negative
	Acinetobacter	A′	ankle
	adenine	@	at
	age	(a)	axillary temperature
	alive	a	before
	ambulatory	A₁	aortic first heart sound
	angioplasty	A₂	aortic second sound
	anterior	A250	5% albumin 250 mL
	anxiety	A1000	5% albumin 1000 mL
	apical	A II	angiotensin II
	arterial	AA	acetic acid

achievement age
active assistive
acute asthma
African-American
Alcoholics Anonymous
alcohol abuse
alopecia areata
alveolar-arterial gradient
amino acid
anaplastic astrocytoma
anti-aerobic
antiarrhythmic agent
aortic aneurysm
aplastic anemia
arm ankle (pulse ratio)
ascending aorta
audiologic assessment
Australia antigen
authorized absence
automobile accident
cytarabine (ara-C) and doxorubicin (Adriamycin)

aa of each

A&A aid and attendance
arthroscopy and arthrotomy
awake and aware

A-a alveolar arterial (gradient)

a/A arterial-alveolar (gradient)

AIIA Angiotensin II antagonist

AAA abdominal aortic aneurysmectomy (aneurysm)
acute anxiety attack
Area Agenices on Aging
aromatic amino acids

A&AA active and active assistive

AAAASF American Association for Accreditation of Ambulatory Surgery Facilities

AAAE amino acid activating enzyme

AAAHC Accreditation Association of Ambulatory Health Care

AAC Adrenalin, atropine, and cocaine

advanced adrenocortical cancer
antimicrobial agent-associated colitis

AACG acute angle closure glaucoma

AACLR arthroscopic anterior cruciate ligament reconstruction

AAD acid-ash diet
antibiotic-associated diarrhea

A_1AD alpha$_1$-antitrypsin deficiency

AADA Abbreviated Antibiotic Drug Application

$[A\text{-}a]DO_2$ alveolar-arterial oxygen tension gradient

AAE active assistance exercise
acute allergic encephalitis

AAECS amino acid enriched cardioplegic solution

A/AEX active assistive exercise

AAF African-American female

AAFB alcohol acid-fast bacilli

AAG alpha-1-acid glycoprotein

AAH acute alcoholic hepatitis

AAI acute alcohol intoxication
arm-ankle index
atlantoaxial instability

AAK atlantoaxial kyphosis

AAL anterior axillary line

AAM African-American male
amino acid mixture

AAMI age associated memory impairment

AAMS acute aseptic meningitis syndrome

AAN AIDS-associated neutropenia
analgesic abuse nephropathy
analgesic-associated nephropathy
attending's admission notes

AANA American Association of Nurse Anesthetists

AAO	alert, awake, & oriented	AAU	acute anterior uveitis
AAO × 3	awake and oriented to time, place, and person	AAV	adeno-associated vector
			adeno-associated virus
		AAVV	accumulated alveolar ventilatory volume
AAOC	antacid of choice		
AAP	acute anterior poliomyelitis	AAWD	antiandrogen withdrawal
	assessment adjustment pass	AB	abortion
			Ace® bandage
AAPC	antibiotic-associated pseudomembranous colitis		antibiotic
			antibody
			Aphasia Battery
AAPMC	antibiotic-associated pseudomembranous colitis		apical beat
			armboard
			products meeting bioequivalence requirements for generic pharmaceuticals
a/ApO₂	arterial-alveolar oxygen tension ratio		
AAPSA	age-adjusted prostate-specific antigen		
		Aβ	beta-amyloid peptide
AAR	antigen-antiglobulin reaction	A/B	acid-base ratio
			apnea/bradycardia
	automated anesthesia record	A > B	air greater than bone (conduction)
AAROM	active-assistive range of motion	A & B	apnea and bradycardia
			assault and battery
AAS	acute abdominal series	AB+	AB positive blood type
	androgenic-anabolic steroid	AB−	AB negative blood type
		ABC	abacavir (Ziagen)
	Ann Arbor stage (Hodgkin's disease staging system)		abbreviated blood count
			absolute band counts
			absolute basophil count
	aortic arch syndrome		advanced breast cancer
	atlantoaxis subluxation		airway, breathing, and circulation
	atypical absence seizure		
AASCRN	amino acid screen		all but code (resuscitation order)
AASH	adrenal androgen-stimulating hormone		
			aneurysmal bone cyst
			antigen binding capacity
AAST	American Association for the Surgery of Trauma (trauma grading)		apnea, bradycardia, and cyanosis
			applesauce, bananas, and cereal (diet)
AAT	activity as tolerated		argon beam coagulator
	alpha-antitrypsin		aspiration, biopsy and cytology
	androgen ablation therapy		artificial beta cells
	at all times		automated blood count (no differential)
	atypical antibody titer		
A₁AT	alpha₁-antitrypsin		avidin-biotin complex
A₁AT-Pᵢ	alpha₁-antitrypsin (phenotyping)		

23

ABCD	amphotericin B cholesteryl sulfate complex (Amphotec; amphotericin B colloid dispersion)	ABI	ankle brachial index (ankle-to-arm systolic blood pressure ratio) atherothrombotic brain infarction
	asymmetry, **b**order irregularity, **c**olor variation, and **d**iameter more than 6 mm (melanoma warning signs in a mole)	ABID	antibody identification
		A Big	atrial bigeminy
		ABK	aphakic bullous keratopathy
	automated blood count (differential done manually)	ABL	abetalipoproteinemia allograft bound lymphocytes axiobuccolingual
ABCDE	botulism toxoid pentavalent	ABLB	alternate binaural loudness balance
ABCS	automated blood count, STKR (differential done by machine)	ABLC	amphotericin B lipid complex (Abelcet)
		A/B Mods	apnea/bradycardia moderate stimulation
ABD	after bronchodilator automated border detection type of plain gauze dressing	ABMS	autologous bone marrow support
		A/B MS	apnea/bradycardia mild stimulation
		ABMT	autologous bone marrow transplantation
Abd	abdomen abdominal abductor	ABN	abnormality(ies) advance beneficiary notice
ABDCT	atrial bolus dynamic computer tomography	abnl bld	abnormal bleeding
		ABNM	American Board of Nuclear Medicine
ABD GR	abdominal girth	abnor.	abnormal
ABD PB	abductor pollicis brevis	ABO	absent bed occupant blood group system (A, AB, B, and O)
ABD PL	abductor pollicis longus		
ABE	acute bacterial endocarditis adult basic education botulism equine trivalent antitoxin	ABP	ambulatory blood pressure androgen binding protein arterial blood pressure
		ABPA	allergic bronchopulmonary aspergillosis
ABECB	acute bacterial exacerbations of chronic bronchitis	ABPM	allergic bronchopulmonary mycosis ambulatory blood pressure monitoring
ABEP	auditory brain stem-evoked potentials		
ABF	aortobifemoral (bypass)	ABR	absolute bed rest auditory brain-stem response
ABG	air/bone gap aortoiliac bypass graft arterial blood gases axiobuccogingival		
		ABRS	acute bacterial rhinosinusitis
ABH	Ativan, Benadryl, and Haldol	ABS	absent

	absorbed		against clinical advice
	absorption		aminocaproic acid
	Accuchek® blood sugar		(Amicar)
	acute brain syndrome		anterior cerebral artery
	admitting blood sugar		anterior communicating
	Alterman-Bishop stent		artery
	antibody screen		anticanalicular antibodies
	at bedside	AC/A	accommodation
ABSS	Anderson Behavioral		convergence–
	State Scale		accommodation (ratio)
A/B SS	apnea/bradycardia self-	ACABS	acute community-acquired
	stimulation		bacterial sinusitis
ABT	aminopyrine breath test	ACAS	acute community-acquired
	antibiotic therapy		sinusitis
ABVD	Adriamycin®, bleomycin,	ACAT	acyl coenzyme A:
	vinblastine, and		cholesterol
	dacarbazine (DTIC)		acyltransferase
ABW	actual body weight	ACB	alveolar-capillary block
ABx	antibiotics		antibody-coated bacteria
AC	abdominal circumference		aortocoronary bypass
	acetate		before breakfast
	acromioclavicular	AcB	assist with bath
	activated charcoal	AC & BC	air and bone conduction
	acute	ACBE	air contrast barium enema
	air conditioned	ACC	acalculous cholecystitis
	air conduction		accident
	anchored catheter		accommodation
	antecubital		adenoid cystic carcinomas
	anticoagulant		administrative control
	arm circumference		center
	assist control		advanced colorectal
	before meals		cancer
	doxorubicin (Adriamycin)		ambulatory care center
	and cyclophosphamide		amylase creatinine
A-C	Astler-Coller (stages of		clearance
	colorectal cancer		anterior cingulate cortex
A/C	anterior chamber of the		automated cell count
	eye	ACCE	Academic Clinical
	assist/control		Coordinator Educator
A & C	alert and cooperative	AcCoA	acetyl-coenzyme A
A_{1C}	glycosylated hemoglobin	ACCR	amylase creatinine
	A_{1C}		clearance ratio
5-AC	azacitidine	ACCU	acute coronary care unit
9AC	rubitecan (9-aminocamp-	ACCU✔	Accucheck® (blood
	tothecin)		glucose monitoring)
ACA	acrodermatitis chronica	ACD	absolute cardiac dullness
	atrophicans		absorbent cover dressing
	acyclovir		acid-citrate-dextrose
	adenocarcinoma		allergic contact dermatitis

	anemia of chronic disease	ACHES	abdominal pain, chest pain, headache, eye problems, and severe leg pains (early danger signs of oral contraceptive adverse effects)
	anterior cervical diskectomy		
	anterior chamber diameter		
	anterior chest diameter		
	before dinner		
	dactinomycin (actinomycin D)	AC & HS	before meals and at bedtime
ACDC	antibody complement-dependent cytolysis	ACI	acceleration index
			adrenal cortical insufficiency
AC-DC	bisexual (homo- and heterosexual		aftercare instructions
ACDDS	Alcoholism/Chemical Dependency Detoxification Service		anabolic-catabolic index
			anemia of chronic illness
			autologous chondrocyte implantation
ACDF	anterior cervical diskectomy fusion	ACIOL	anterior chamber intraocular lens
ACDK	acquired cystic disease of the kidney	ACIP	Advisory Committee on Immunization Practices (of the Centers for Disease Control and Prevention)
ACDs	anticonvulsant drugs		
ACE	adrenocortical extract		
	adverse clinical event		
	aerosol cloud enhancer	ACJ	acromioclavicular joint
	angiotensin-converting enzyme	A/CK	Accuchek®
		ACL	accessory collateral ligament (hand)
	antegrade colonic enema		
	doxorubicin (Adriamycin), cyclophosphamide, and etoposide		anterior cruciate ligament (knee)
ACEI	angiotensin-converting enzyme inhibitor	aCL	anticardiolipin (antibody)
		ACLA	aclarubicin
ACF	aberrant crypt focus	ACLF	adult congregate living facility
	accessory clinical findings		
	acute care facility	ACLR	anterior cruciate ligament repair
	anterior cervical fusion		
ACG	accelerography	ACLS	advanced cardiac (cardiopulmonary) life support
	angiocardiography		
ACGME	Accreditation Council for Graduate Medical Education		Allen Cognitive Level Screen
		ACM	alternative/complementary medicine
ACH	adrenal cortical hormone		Arnold-Chiari malformation
	aftercoming head		
	arm girth, chest depth, and hip width	ACME	aphakic cystoid macular edema
ACh	acetylcholine		
ACHA	air-conduction hearing aid	ACMT	advanced combined modality therapy
AChE	acetylcholinesterase		
AChEIs	acetylcholinesterase inhibitors	ACMV	assist-controlled mechanical ventilation

26

ACN	acute conditioned neurosis		acute coronary syndromes
ACNP	Acute Care Nurse Practitioner		American Cancer Society anodal-closing sound
ACNU	nidran		before supper
ACOA	Adult Children of Alcoholics	ACSL	automatic computerized solvent litholysis
A COMM A	anterior communicating artery	ACSVBG	aortocoronary saphenous vein bypass graft
ACOS-OG	American College of Surgeons Oncology Group	ACSW	Academy of Certified Social Workers
ACP	accessory conduction pathway	ACT	activated clotting time aggressive comfort treatment
	acid phosphatase adamantinomatous craniopharyngioma		allergen challenge test anticoagulant therapy assertive community
	ambulatory care program antrochoanal polyp		treatment (program)
ACPA	anticytoplasmic antibodies	ACT-D	dactinomycin
AC-PC line	anterior commissure-posterior commissure line	Act Ex ACTG	active exercise AIDS Clinical Trial Group
AC-PH	acid phosphatase	ACTH	corticotropin
ACPO	acute colonic pseudo-obstruction		(adrenocorticotropic hormone)
ACPP	adrenocorticopolypeptide	ACT-Post	activated clotting time post-filter
ACPPD	average cost per patient day	ACT-Pre	activated clotting time pre-filter
ACPP PF	acid phosphatase prostatic fluid	ACTSEB	anterior chamber tube shunt encircling band
ACPS	anterior cervical plate stabilization	ACU	ambulatory care unit
ACQ	acquired Areas of Change Questionnaire	ACUP	adenocarcinoma of unknown primary (origin)
ACR	adenomatosis of the colon and rectum	ACV	acyclovir (Zovirax) amifostine, cisplatin, and vinblastine
	anterior chamber reformation		assist control ventilation atrial/carotid/ventricular
	anticonstipation regimen	A-C-V	A wave, C wave, and V
ACR20	American College of Rheumatology rating scale (20% or more improvement)	ACVD	wave acute cardiovascular disease
ACRC	advanced colorectal cancer	ACVP	doxorubicin (Adriamycin), cyclophosphamide, vincristine, and
ACS	abdominal compartment syndrome		prednisone
	acute confusional state	ACW	anterior chest wall apply to chest wall

27

acyl-CoA	acyl coenzyme A
AD	accident dispensary
	admitting diagnosis
	advance directive (living will)
	air dyne
	alternating days (this is a dangerous abbreviation)
	Alzheimer's disease
	androgen deprivation
	antidepressant
	assistive device
	atopic dermatitis
	axis deviation
	right ear
A&D	admission and discharge
	alcohol and drug
	ascending and descending
	vitamins A and D
ADA	adenosine deaminase
	American Dental Association
	American Diabetes Association
	Americans with Disabilities Act
	anterior descending artery
ADAM	adjustment disorder with anxious mood
ADAS	Alzheimer's Disease Assessment Scale
ADAS-COG	Alzheimer's Disease Assessment Scale-Cognitive Subscale
ADAT	advance diet as tolerated
ADAU	adolescent drug abuse unit
ADB	amorous disinhibited behavior
ADC	Aid to Dependent Children
	AIDS (acquired immune deficiency syndrome) dementia complex
	anxiety disorder clinic
	apparent diffusion coefficient
	average daily consumption
ADCA	autosomal dominant cerebellar ataxia
ADCC	antibody-dependent cellular cytotoxicity
A.D.C. VAAN DIML	mnemonic for formatting physician orders: Admit, Diagnosis, Condition, Vitals, Activity, Allergies, Nursing procedures, Diet, Ins and outs, Medication, Labs
ADD	adduction
	attention deficit disorder
	average daily dose
ADDH	attention-deficit disorder with hyperactivity
ADDL	additional
ADDM	adjustment disorder with depressed mood
ADDP	adductor pollicis
ADDs	AIDS (acquired immune deficiency syndrome)-defining diseases
ADDU	alcohol and drug dependence unit
ADE	acute disseminated encephalitis
	adverse drug event
ADEM	acute disseminating encephalomyelitis
ADE-NOCA	adenocarcinoma
ADEPT	antibody-directed enzyme prodrug therapy
AEDP	assisted end diastolic pressure
ADFU	agar diffusion for fungus
ADG	atrial diastolic gallop
	axiodistogingival
ADH	antidiuretic hormone
	atypical ductal hyperplasia
ADHD	attention-deficit hyperactivity disorder
ADI	allowable (acceptable) daily intake
	axiodistoincisal
A-DIC	doxorubicin and dacarbazine
Adj Dis	adjustment disorder

Adj D/O	adjustment disorder
ADL	activities of daily living
ad lib	as desired
	at liberty
ADM	administered (dose)
	admission
	adrenomedullin
	doxorubicin (Adriamycin)
ADME	absorption, distribution, metabolism, and excretion
ADO	axiodisto-occlusal
Ad-OAP	doxorubicin, vincristine, cytarabine, and prednisone
ADOL	adolescent
ADON	Assistant Director of Nursing
ADP	arterial demand pacing
	adenosine diphosphate
ADPKD	autosomal dominant polycystic kidney disease
ADPV	anomaly of drainage of pulmonary vein
ADQ	abductor digiti quinti
	adequate
ADR	acute dystonic reaction
	adverse drug reaction
	alternative dispute resolution
	doxorubicin (Adriamycin)
ADRIA	doxorubicin (Adriamycin)
ADS	admission day surgery
	anatomical dead space
	anonymous donor's sperm
	antibody deficiency syndrome
ADs	advance directives (living wills)
ADSU	ambulatory diagnostic surgery unit
ADT	admission, discharge, and transfer
	alternate-day therapy
	androgen deprivation treatment (therapy)
	anticipate discharge tomorrow

	any damn thing (a placebo)
	Auditory Discrimination Test
ADTP	Adolescent Day Treatment Program
	Alcohol Dependence Treatment Program
ADU	automated dispensing unit
ADV	adenovirus vaccine, not otherwise specified
ADV_4	adenovirus vaccine, type 4, live, oral
ADV_7	adenovirus vaccine, type 7, live, oral
A5D5W	alcohol 5%, dextrose 5% in water for injection
ADX	audiological diagnostic
AE	above elbow (amputation)
	accident and emergency (department)
	acute exacerbation
	adaptive equipment
	adverse event
	air entry
	antiembolitic
	arm ergometer
	aryepiglottic (fold)
A&E	accident and emergency (department)
AEA	above elbow amputation
	anti-endomysial antibody
AEB	as evidenced by
	atrial ectopic beat
AEC	at earliest convenience
AECB	acute exacerbations of chronic bronchitis
AECG	ambulatory electrocardiogram
AED	antiepileptic drug
	automated (automatic) external defibrillator
AEDD	anterior extradural defects
AEDF	absent end-diastolic flow (umbilical-artery Doppler ultrasonography)
AEDP	automated external defibrillator pacemaker

AEEU	admission entrance and evaluation unit
AEG	air encephalogram
	Alcohol Education Group
AEIOU TIPS	mnemonic for the diagnosis of coma: **A**lcohol, **E**ncephalopathy, **I**nsulin, **O**piates, **U**remia, **T**rauma, **I**nfection, **P**sychiatric, and **S**yncope
AELBM	after each loose bowel movement
AEM	active electrode monitor
	ambulatory electrogram monitor
	antiepileptic medication
AEP	auditory evoked potential
AEq	age equivalent
AER	acoustic evoked response
	albumin excretion rate
	auditory evoked response
Aer. M.	aerosol mask
AERS	adverse event reporting system
Aer. T.	aerosol tent
AES	adult emergency service
	anti-embolic stockings
AEs	adverse events
AET	alternating esotropia
	atrial ectopic tachycardia
AF	acid-fast
	afebrile
	amniotic fluid
	anterior fontanel
	antifibrinogen
	aortofemoral
	ascitic fluid
	atrial fibrillation
AFB	acid-fast bacilli
	aorto-femoral bypass
	aspirated foreign body
AFB$_1$	aflatoxin B$_1$
AFBG	aortofemoral bypass graft
AFBY	aortofemoral bypass (graft)
AFC	adult foster care
	air filled cushions

AFDC	Aid to Family and Dependent Children
AFE	amniotic fluid embolization
AFEB	afebrile
AFEU	ante partum fetal evaluation unit
AF/FL	atrial fibrillation/atrial flutter
aFGF	acidic fibroblast growth factor
AFH	angiomatoid fibrous histiocytoma
	anterior facial height
AFI	acute febrile illness
	amniotic fluid index
A fib	atrial fibrillation
AFIP	Armed Forces Institute of Pathology
AFKO	ankle-foot-knee orthosis
AFL	atrial flutter
AFLP	acute fatty liver of pregnancy
	amplified fragment length polymorphism
A Flu	atrial flutter
AFM	acute *Plasmodium falciparum* malaria
	atomic force microscopy
	doxorubicin (Adriamycin), fluorouracil, and methotrexate
AFM×2	double aerosol face mask
AFO	ankle fixation orthotic
	ankle-foot orthosis
AFOF	anterior fontanelõopen and flat
AFP	acute flaccid paralysis
	alpha-fetoprotein
	anterior faucial pillar
	ascending frontal parietal
AFQT	Armed Forces Qualification Test
AFRD	acute febrile respiratory disease
AFRIMS	Armed Forces Research Institute of Medical Sciences

AFS	allergic fungal sinusitis	A GLAC-TO-LK	alpha galactoside leukocytes
Aft/Dis	aftercare/discharge		
AFV	amniotic fluid volume	AGN	acute glomerulonephritis
AFVSS	afebrile, vital signs stable	$AgNO_3$	silver nitrate
AFX	air-fluid exchange	AgNORs	argyrophilic nucleolar organizer regions (staining)
AG	abdominal girth		
	adrenogenital		
	aminoglycoside	α_1-AGP	alpha$_1$-acid glycoprotein
	Amsler grid	AGPT	agar-gel precipitation test
	anion gap	AGS	adrenogenital syndrome
	antigen	AG SYND	adrenogenital syndrome
	anti-gravity	AGT	alanine-glyoxylate aminotransferase
	atrial gallop		
Ag	silver	AGTT	abnormal glucose tolerance test
A/G	albumin to globulin ratio		
AGA	accelerated growth area	AGU	aspartylglycosaminuria
	acute gonococcal arthritis	AGUS	atypical glandular cells of uncertain significance
	androgenetic alopecia	AGVHD	acute graft-versus-host disease
	antigliadin antibody		
	appropriate for gestational age	AGVI	Ahmed glaucoma valve implantation
	average gestational age	AH	abdominal hysterectomy
AGAS	accelerated graft atherosclerosis		amenorrhea and hirsutism
			amenorrhea-hyperprolac-tinemia
AG/BL	aminoglycoside/beta-lactam		antihyaluronidase
			auditory hallucinations
AGC	absolute granulocyte count	A&H	accident and health (insurance)
AGCUS	atypical glandular cells of undetermined significance	AHA	acetohydroxamic acid (Lithostat®)
			acquired hemolytic anemia
AGD	agar gel diffusion		autoimmune hemolytic anemia
AGE	acute gastroenteritis		
	advanced glycation end product(s)	AHAs	alpha hydroxy acids
	angle of greatest extension	AHase	antihyaluronidase
	anterior gastroenterostomy	AHB_c	hepatitis B core antibody
AGECAT	automatic geriatric examination for computer-assisted taxonomy	AHC	acute hemorrhagic conjunctivitis
			acute hemorrhagic cystitis
			Adolescent Health Center
AGF	angle of greatest flexion	AHCA	Agency for Healthcare Administration
AGG	agammaglobulinemia		American Healthcare Association
aggl.	agglutination		
AGI	alpha-glucosidase inhibitor	AHCPR	Agency for Health Care Policy and Research
AGL	acute granulocytic leukemia		

31

AHD	alien-hand syndrome	AHSCT	autologous hemopoietic stem-cell transplantation
	antecedent hematological disorder		
	arteriosclerotic heart disease	AHST	autologous hematopoietic stem cell transplantation
	autoimmune hemolytic disease	AHT	alternating hypertropia
AHE	acute hemorrhagic encephalomyelitis		autoantibodies to human thyroglobulin
AHEC	Area Health Education Center	AHTG	antihuman thymocyte globulin
AHF	antihemophilic factor	AI	accidentally incurred
	Argentine hemorrhagic fever (Junin virus) vaccine		apical impulse
			allergy index
			aortic insufficiency
AHF-M	antihemophilic factor (human), method M, (monoclonal purified)		artificial insemination
			artificial intelligence
		A & I	Allergy and Immunology (department)
AHFS	American Hospital Formulary Service		auscultation and inspection
AHG	antihemophilic globulin	AIA	Accommodation Independence Assessment
AHGS	acute herpetic gingival stomatitis		allergen-induced asthma
AHHD	arteriosclerotic hyper-tensive heart disease		allyl isopropyl acetamide
			anti-insulin antibody
AHI	apnea-hypopnea index		aspirin-induced asthma
AHJ	artificial hip joint	AI-Ab	anti-insulin antibody
AHL	apparent half-life	AIBF	anterior interbody fusion
AHM	ambulatory Holter monitoring	AICA	anterior inferior cerebellar artery
AHMO	anterior horizontal mandibular osteotomy		anterior inferior communicating artery
AHN	adenomatous hyperplastic nodule	AICBG	anterior interbody cervical bone graft
	Assistant Head Nurse	AICD	activation-induced cell death
AHP	acute hemorrhagic pancreatitis		automatic implantable cardioverter/defibrillator
	acute hepatic panel (see page 358)	AICS	acute ischemic coronary syndromes
	American Herbal Pharmacopeia and Therapeutic Compendium	AID	absolute iron deficiency
			acute infectious disease
AHS	adaptive hand skills		aortoiliac disease
	allopurinol hypersensitivity syndrome		artificial insemination donor
AHSA	Assistant Health Services Administrator		automatic implantable defibrillator

AIDH	artificial insemination donor husband	AIPC	androgen-independent prostate cancer
AIDKS	acquired immune deficiency syndrome with Kaposi's sarcoma	AIR	accelerated idioventricular rhythm
AIDS	acquired immunodeficiency syndrome	AIS	Abbreviated Injury Score adolescent idiopathic scoliosis anti-insulin serum
AIE	acute inclusion body encephalitis	AISA	acquired idiopathic sideroblastic anemia
AIF	aortic-iliac-femoral	AIS/ISS	Abbreviated Injury Scale/Injury Severity Score
AIH	artificial insemination with husband's sperm		
AIHA	autoimmune hemolytic anemia	AIT	auditory integration therapy
AIHD	acquired immune hemolytic disease	AITN	acute interstitial tubular nephritis
AIIS	anterior inferior iliac spine	AITP	autoimmune thrombocytopenia purpura
AILD	angioimmunoblastic lymphadenopathy with dysproteinemia	AIU	absolute iodine uptake adolescent inpatient unit
AIM	anti-inflammatory medication	AIVR	accelerated idioventricular rhythm
AIMS	Abnormal Involuntary Movement Scale Arthritis Impact Measurement Scales	AJ	ankle jerk
		AJCC	American Joint Committee on Cancer
		AJO	apple juice only
AIN	acute interstitial nephritis anal intraepithelial neoplasia anterior interosseous nerve	AJR	abnormal jugular reflex
		AK	above knee (amputation) actinic keratosis artificial kidney
AINS	anti-inflammatory non-steroidal	AKA	above-knee amputation alcoholic ketoacidosis all known allergies also known as
AIO	all-in-one (lipid emulsion, protein, carbohydrate, and electrolytes combined total parenteral nutrition)		
		AKS	alcoholic Korsakoff syndrome arthroscopic knee surgery
AIOD	aortoiliac occlusive disease	AKU	artificial kidney unit
		AL	acute leukemia argon laser arterial line assisted living axial length left ear
AION	anterior ischemic optic neuropathy		
AIP	acute infectious polyneuritis acute intermittent porphyria asymptomatic inflammatory prostatitis		
		Al	aluminum
		ALA	alpha-linolenic acid (α-linolenic acid)

alpha-lipoic acid
aminolevulinic acid (Levulan)
antileukotriene agent
antilymphocyte antibody
as long as

ALAC antibiotic-loaded acrylic cement

ALAD abnormal left axis deviation

ALA-GLN alanyl-glutamine

ALARA as low as reasonably achievable

ALAT alanine transaminase (alanine aminotransferase; SGPT)

ALAX apical long axis

ALB albumin
albuterol
anterior lenticular bevel

ALBUMS aldehyde linker-based ultrasensitive mismatch scanning

ALC acute lethal catatonia
alcohol
alcoholic liver cirrhosis
allogeneic lymphocyte cytotoxicity
alternate level of care
Alternate Lifestyle Checklist
axiolinguocervical

ALCA anomalous left coronary artery

ALCL anaplastic large-cell lymphoma

ALC R alcohol rub

ALD adrenoleukodystrophy
alcoholic liver disease
aldolase

ALDH aldehyde dehydrogenase

ALDOST aldosterone

ALF acute liver failure
arterial line filter
assisted living facility

ALFT abnormal liver function tests

ALG antilymphoblast globulin
antilymphocyte globulin

ALGB adjustable laparoscopic gastric banding

ALH atypical lobular hyperplasia

ALI acute lung injury
argon laser iridotomy

ALIF anterior lumbar intradiskal fusion

A-line arterial catheter

ALK alkaline
automated lamellar keratoplasty

ALK Ø alkaline phosphatase

ALK ISO alkaline phosphatase isoenzymes

ALK-P alkaline phosphatase

ALK PHOS ISO alkaline phosphatase isoenzyme

ALL acute lymphoblastic leukemia
acute lymphocytic leukemia
allergy

ALLD arthroscopic lumbar laser diskectomy

ALLO allogeneic

Allo-BMT allogenic bone marrow transplantation

ALM acral lentiginous melanoma
alveolar lining material
autoclave-killed *Leishmania major*

ALMI anterolateral myocardial infarction

ALN anterior lower neck
anterior lymph node
axillary lymph nodes

ALND axillary lymph node dissection

ALNM axillary lymph node metastasis

ALO axilinguo-occlusal

Al(OH)₃ aluminum hydroxide

ALOS average length of stay

ALP alkaline phosphatase
argon laser photocoagulation
Alupent

ALSG	Australian Leukemia Study Group	AM Care	brushing teeth, washing face and hands
ALTP	argon laser trabeculo-plasty	AMAD	morning admission
		AM/ADM	morning admission
ALPZ	alprazolam (Xanax)	AMAG	adrenal medullary autograft
ALR	adductor leg raise		
ALRI	acute lower-respiratory-tract infection	AMAL	amalgam
		AMAN	acute motor axonal neuropathy
	anterolateral rotary instability	AMAP	American Medical Accreditation Program
ALS	acute lateral sclerosis		
	advanced life support		as much as possible
	amyotrophic lateral sclerosis	Amask	aerosol mask
		AMAT	anti-malignant antibody test
ALT	alanine transaminase (SGPT)		
			Arm Motor Ability Test
	argon laser trabeculo-plasty	A-MAT	amorphous material
		AMB	ambulate
	autolymphocyte therapy		ambulatory
2 alt	every other day (this is a dangerous abbreviation)		amphotericin B
			as manifested by
ALTB	acute laryngotracheobron-chitis	AMBER	advanced multiple beam equalization radiography
ALTE	acute (aberrant, apparent) life threatening event		
		AMC	arm muscle circumference
alt hor	every other hour (this is a dangerous abbreviation)		arthrogryposis multiplex congenita
ALUP	Alupent	AM/CR	amylase to creatinine ratio
ALv	attachment level (dental)	AMD	age-related macular degeneration
ALVAD	abdominal left ventricular assist device		
			arthroscopic microdiskectomy
ALWMI	anterolateral wall myocardial infarct		axiomesiodistal
			dactinomycin (actinomycin D)
ALZ	Alzheimer's disease		
AM	adult male		methyldopa (alpha methyldopa)
	aerosol mask		
	amalgam	AME	agreed medical examination
	anovulatory menstruation		
	anterior midpapillary		anthrax meningoencephalitis
	morning (a.m.)		apparent mineralocorticoid excess (syndrome)
	myopic astigmatism		
AMA	against medical advice		Aviation Medical Examiner
	American Medical Association	AMegL	acute megokaryoblastic leukemia
	antimitochondrial antibody		
AMAC	adults molested as children	AMES-LAN	American sign language

35

AMF	aerobic metabolism facilitator	A-M pr	Austin-Moore prosthesis
	amifostine (Ethyol)	AMPT	metyrosine (alphameth-ylpara tyrosine)
	autocrine motility factor	AMR	acoustic muscle reflex
AMG	acoustic myography		alternating motion rates
	aminoglycoside	AMRI	anterior medial rotary instability
	axiomesiogingival		
	Federal Republic of German's equivalent to United States Food, Drug, and Cosmetic Act	AMS	acute maxillary sinusitis
			acute mountain sickness
			aggravated in military service
AMGA	American Medical Group Association		altered mental status
			amylase
AMI	acute myocardial infarction		aseptic meningitis syndrome
	amifostine (Ethyol)		atypical mole syndrome
	amitriptyline		auditory memory span
	axiomesioincisal	m-AMSA	amsacrine (acridinyl anisidide)
AMKL	acute megakaryocytic leukemia	AMSAN	acute motor sensory axonal neuropathy
AML	acute myelogenous leukemia	AMSIT	portion of the mental status examination: A—appearance, M—mood, S—sensorium, I—intelligence, T—thought process
	angiomyolipoma		
	anterior mitral leaflet		
AMLOS	arithmetic mean length of stay		
AMLR	auditory midlatency response		
		AMT	abbreviated mental test
	Marketing Authorization Application (French)		Adolph's Meat Tenderizer
AMM	agnogenic myeloid metaplasia		allogeneic (bone) marrow transplant
			aminopterin
AMML	acute myelomonocytic leukemia		amount
AMMOL	acute myelomonoblastic leukemia	AMTS	Abbreviated Mental Test Score
AMN	adrenomyeloneuropathy	AMU	accessory-muscle use
amnio	amniocentesis	AMV	alveolar minute ventilation
AMN SC	amniotic fluid scan		assisted mechanical ventilation
AMOL	acute monoblastic leukemia		
		AMY	amylase
AMP	adenosine monophosphate	AMY/CR	amylase/creatinine ratio
	ampere	AN	acoustic neuromas
	ampicillin		amyl nitrate
	ampul		anorexia nervosa
	amputation		anticipatory nausea
	antipressure mattress		Associate Nurse
AMPPE	acute multifocal placoid pigment epitheliopathy		avascular necrosis
		ANA	antinuclear antibody

ANAD	anorexia nervosa and associated disorders
ANADA	Abbreviated New Animal Drug Application
ANAG	acute narrow angle glaucoma
ANA SWAB	anaerobic swab
ANC	absolute neutrophil count
ANCA	antineutrophil cytoplasmic antibody
anch	anchored
ANCN	absolute neutrophil count nadir
ANCOVA	analysis of covariance
AND	anterior nasal discharge axillary node dissection
ANDA	Abbreviated New Drug Application
anes	anesthesia
ANF	antinuclear factor atrial natriuretic factor
ANG	angiogram
ANG II	angiotensin II
ANGIO	angiogram
ANH	acute normovolemic hemodilution artificial nutrition and hydration
ANISO	anisocytosis
ANK	ankle appointment not kept
ANLL	acute nonlymphoblastic leukemia
ANM	Assistant Nurse Manager
ANN	artificial neural network(s) axillary node̅negative
ANNA	artificial neural network analysis
ANOVA	analysis of variance
ANP	Adult Nurse Practitioner atrial natriuretic peptide (anaritide acetate) axillary node–positive
ANPR	advanced notice of proposed rule making
ANS	answer autonomic nervous system

ANSER	Aggregate Neurobehavioral Student Health and Education Review
ANT	anterior anthrax vaccine, not otherwise specified enpheptin (2-amino-5-nitrothiazol)
ANT_a	anthrax vaccine, absorbed
ante	before
ANTI A:AGT	anti–blood group A antiglobulin test
Anti bx	antibiotic
anti-D	anti-D immune globulin
anti-GAD	antibodies to glutamic acid decarboxylase
anti-HBc	antibody to hepatitis B core antigen (HBcAg)
anti-HBe	antibody to hepatitis B e antigen (HBeAg)
anti-HBs	antibody to hepatitis B surface antigen (HBsAg)
ant sag D	anterior sagittal diameter
ANTU	alpha naphthylthiourea
ANUG	acute necrotizing ulcerative gingivitis
ANV	acute nausea and vomiting
ANX	anxiety anxious
ANZDATA	Australia and New Zealand Dialysis and Transplant Registry
AO	abdominal obesity Agent Orange anterior oblique aorta aortic opening aortography axio-occlusal plate, screw (orthopedics) right ear
A-O	atlanto-occipital (joint)
A/O	alert and oriented
A & O	alert and oriented
A&O × 3	awake and oriented to person, place, and time

A&O × 4	awake and oriented to person, place, time, and object		anodal opening picture
			aortic pressure
			apnea of prematurity
AOAA	aminooxoacetic acid	AOR	adjusted odds ratio
AOAP	as often as possible		Alvarado Orthopedic Research
AOB	alcohol on breath		at own risk
AOBS	acute organic brain syndrome		auditory oculogyric reflex
AOC	abridged ocular chart	AORT REGURG	aortic regurgitation
	advanced ovarian cancer		
	amoxicillin, omeprazole, and clarithromycin	AORT STEN	aortic stenosis
	anode opening contraction	AOS	ambulatory outpatient surgery
	antacid of choice		anode opening sound
	area of concern		antibiotic order sheet
AOCD	anemia of chronic disease		aortic ostial stenoses
AOCL	anodal opening clonus		arrived on scene
AOD	adult onset diabetes	AOSC	acute obstructive suppurative cholangiotomy
	alcohol and (and/or) other drugs		
	alleged onset date	AOSD	adult-onset Still's disease
	arterial occlusive disease	AOTe	anodal opening tetanus
	Assistant-Officer-of-the-Day	AP	abdominoperineal
AODA	alcohol and other drug abuse		acute pancreatitis
			aerosol pentamidine
AODM	adult-onset diabetes mellitus		alkaline phosphatase
			angina pectoris
A of 1	assistance of one		antepartum
A of 2	assistance of two		anterior-posterior (x-ray)
AOI	area of induration		apical pulse
ao-il	aorta-iliac		appendectomy
AOIVM	angiographically occult intracranial vascular malformation		appendicitis
			arterial pressure
			arthritis panel (see page 358)
AOL	augmentation of labor		atrial pacing
AOLC	acridine-orange leukocyte cytospin		attending physician
AOLD	automated open lumbar diskectomy		doxorubicin (Adriamycin); cisplatin (Platinol AQ)
AOM	acute otitis media	A&P	active and present
	alternatives of management		anterior and posterior
			assessment and plans
AONAD	alert, oriented, and no acute distress		auscultation and percussion
AOO	anodal opening odor	A/P	ascites/plasma ratio
	continuous arterial asynchronous pacing	$A_2 > P_2$	second aortic sound greater than second pulmonic sound
AOP	anemia of prematurity		

APA	anticipatory postural adjustment		afferent pupillary defect
			anterior-posterior diameter
	antiphospholipid antibody		atrial premature depolarization
APAA	anterior parietal artery aneurysm		automated peritoneal dialysis
APACHE	Acute Physiology and Chronic Health Evaluation		pamidronate disodium (aminohydroxypropylidene diphosphate)
APAD	anterior-posterior abdominal diameter	APDC	Anxiety and Panic Disorder Clinic
APAG	antipseudomonal aminoglycosidic penicillin	APDT	acellular pertussis vaccine with diphtheria and tetanus toxoids
APAP	acetaminophen (N acetyl-para-aminophenol)	APE	absolute prediction error
APB	abductor pollicis brevis		acute psychotic episode
	atrial premature beat		acute pulmonary edema
APBSCT	autologous peripheral blood stem cell transplantation		Adriamycin, cisplatin (Platinol), and etoposide
APC	absolute phagocyte count		anterior pituitary extract
	activated protein C	APER	abdominoperineal excision of the rectum
	acute pharyngoconjunctiivitis (fever)	APG	ambulatory patient group
			Apgar (score)
	adenoidal-pharyngeal-conjunctival	APGAR	appearance (color), pulse (heart rate), grimace (reflex irritability), activity (muscle tone), and respiration (score reflecting condition of newborn)
	adenomatous polyposis of the colon and rectum		
	advanced pancreatic cancer		
	advanced prostate cancer		
	Ambulatory Payment Classification	APH	adult psychiatric hospital
			alcohol-positive history
	antigen-presenting cell		antepartum hemorrhage
	aspirin, phenacetin, and caffeine	APHIS	Animal and Plant Health Inspection Service
	asymptomatic prostate cancer	API	active pharmaceutical ingredients
			Asian-Pacific Islander
	atrial premature contraction	APIS	Acute Pain Intensity Scale
	autologous packed cells	APIVR	artificial pacemaker-induced ventricular rhythm
APCD	adult polycystic disease		
APCIs	atrial peptide clearance inhibitors	APKD	adult polycystic kidney disease
APCKD	adult polycystic kidney disease		adult-onset polycystic kidney disease
APD	acid peptic disease		
	action potential duration	APL	abductor pollicis longus

A

	accelerated painless labor
	acute promyelocytic leukemia
	anterior pituitary-like (hormone)
	chorionic gonadotropin
AP & L	anteroposterior and lateral
APLA	antiphospholipid antibody
APLD	automated percutaneous lumbar diskectomy
APLS	antiphospholipid syndrome
APMPPE	acute posterior multifocal placoid pigment epitheliopathy
APMS	acute pain management service
APN	acute panautonomic neuropathy
	acute pyelonephritis
APO	adverse patient occurrence
	apolipoprotein A-1
	doxorubicin (Adriamycin), prednisone, and vincristine (Oncovin)
APO(a)	apolipoprotein (A)
APOE	apolipoprotein E
APOE-4	apolipoprotein-E (gene)
APOLT	auxiliary partial orthotopic liver transplantation
APOPPS	adjustable postoperative protective prosthetic socket
APP	alternating pressure pad
	amyloid precursor protein
APPG	aqueous procaine penicillin G (dangerous terminology; since it is for intramuscular use only, write as penicillin G procaine)
appr.	approximate
appt.	appointment
APPY	appendectomy
APR	abdominoperineal resection
	acute radiation proctitis
AP & R	apical and radial (pulses)

APRN	Advanced Practice Registered Nurse
APRT	abdominopelvic radiotherapy
APRV	airway pressure release ventilation
APS	Acute Physiology Scoring (system)
	adult protective services
	Adult Psychiatric Service
	antiphospholipid syndrome
APSAC	anistreplase (anisoylated plasminogen streptokinase activator complex)
APSD	Alzheimer's presenile dementia
APSP	assisted peak systolic pressure
APSS	Associated Professional Sleep Societies
aPTT	activated partial thromboplastin time
APU	ambulatory procedure unit
	antepartum unit
APUD	amine precursor uptake and decarboxylation
APV	amprenavir (Agenerase)
APVC	partial anomalous pulmonary venous connection
APVR	aortic pulmonary valve replacement
APW	aortopulmonary window
aq	water
AQ	accomplishment quotient
aq dest	distilled water
AQLQ-J	Asthma Quality of Life Questionnaire—Juniper
AQLQ-M	Asthma Quality of Life Questionnaire—Marks
A quad	atrial quadrageminy
AR	Achilles reflex
	acoustic reflex
	active resistance
	airway resistance
	alcohol related
	allergic rhinitis

40

	androgen receptor	ARDS	adult respiratory distress syndrome
	ankle reflex		
	aortic regurgitation	ARE	active-resistive exercises
	Argyll Robertson (pupil)	ARF	acute renal failure
	assisted respiration		acute respiratory failure
	at risk		acute rheumatic fever
	aural rehabilitation	ARG	alkaline reflux gastritis
	autorefractor		arginine
Ar	argon	ARHL	age-related hearing loss
A&R	adenoidectomy with radium	ARHNC	advanced resected head and neck cancer
	advised and released	ARI	acute renal insufficiency
A-R	apical-radial (pulses)		acute respiratory infection
ARA	adenosine regulating agent		aldose reductase inhibitor
			arousal index
ara-A	vidarabine (Vira-A)	ARL	average remaining lifetime
ara-AC	fazarabine	ARLD	alcohol-related liver disease
ara-C	cytarabine		
ARAD	abnormal right axis deviation	ARM	anxiety reaction, mild
			artificial rupture of membranes
ARAS	ascending reticular activating system	ARMD	age-related macular degeneration
	atherosclerotic renal-artery stenosis	ARMS	alveolar rhabdomyosarcoma
ARB	angiotensin II receptor blocker		amplification refractory mutation system
	any reliable brand	ARN	acute retinal necrosis
ARBOR	arthropod-borne virus	AROM	active range of motion
ARBOW	artificial rupture of bag of water		artifical rupture of membranes
ARC	abnormal retinal correspondence	ARP	absolute refractory period
	AIDS-related complex		alcohol rehabilitation program
	Alcohol Rehabilitation Center	ARPF	anterior release posterior fusion
	anomalous retinal correspondence	ARPKS	autosomal recessive polycystic kidney disease
	American Red Cross		
ARCBS	American Red Cross Blood Services	ARPT	acid reflux provocation test
ARD	acute respiratory disease	ARR	absolue risk reduction
	adult respiratory distress		arrive
	antibiotic removal device	ARROM	active resistive range of motion
	antibiotic retrieval device		
	aphakic retinal detachment	ARRT	American Registry of Radiologic Technologists
ARDMS	American Registry of Diagnostic Medical Sonographers	ARS	antirabies serum

41

			atrial septal aneurysm
ART	Accredited Record Technician	ASA I	**American Society of anesthesiologists' classification**
	Achilles (tendon) reflex test		Healthy patient with localized pathological process
	acoustic reflex threshold(s)		
	antiretroviral therapy	ASA II	A patient with mild to moderate systemic disease
	arterial		
	assessment, review, and treatment	ASA III	A patient with severe systemic disease limiting activity but not incapacitating
	assisted reproductive technology		
	automated reagin test (for syphilis)	ASA IV	A patient with incapacitating systemic disease
ARTIC	articulation	ASA V	Moribund patient not expected to live.
Art T	art therapy		(These are American Society of Anesthesiologists' patient classifications. Emergency operations are designated by "E" after the classification.)
ARU	acute receiving unit		
	alcohol rehabilitation unit		
ARV	AIDS-related virus		
ARVC	arrhythmogenic right ventricular cardiomyopathy		
ARVD	arrhythmogenic right ventricular dysplasia	5-ASA	mesalamine (5-aminosalicylic acid) (this is a dangerous abbreviation as it is mistaken for five aspirin tablets)
ARVMB	anomalous right ventricular muscle bundles		
ARW	Accredited Rehabilitation Worker	ASAA	acquired severe aplastic anemia
ARWY	airway	ASACL	American Society of Anesthesiologists Classification
AS	activated sleep		
	anabolic steroid	ASAD	arthroscopic subacromial decompression
	anal sphincter		
	androgen suppression	AS/AI	aortic stenosis/aortic insufficiency
	ankylosing spondylitis		
	anterior synechia	A's & B's	apnea and bradycardia
	aortic stenosis	ASAP	Alcohol and Substance Abuse Program
	atherosclerosis		
	atropine sulfate		as soon as possible
	AutoSuture®	ASAT	aspartate transaminase (aspartate aminotransferase) (SGOT)
	doctor called through answering service		
	left ear		
ASA	American Society of Anesthesiologists	ASB	anesthesia standby
	argininosuccinate		
	aspirin (acetylsalicylic acid)		
	as soon as		

	asymptomatic bacteriuria	ASE	abstinence symptom evaluation
ASBO	adhesive small-bowel obstruction		acute stress erosion
ASC	altered state of consciousness	ASEX	Arizona Sexual Experiences (sexual dysfunction scale)
	ambulatory surgery center	ASF	anterior spinal fusion
	anterior subcapsular cataract		asymmetric screen film (radiology)
	antimony sulfur colloid	ASFR	age-specific fertility rate
	apocrine skin carcinoma	ASH	asymmetric septal hypertrophy
	ascorbic acid		
ASCAD	atherosclerotic coronary artery disease	AsH	hypermetropic astigmatism
ASCCC	advanced squamous cell cervical carcinoma	ASHD	arteriosclerotic heart disease
ASCCHN	advanced squamous cell carcinoma of the head and neck	ASI	active specific immunotherapy
ASCI	acute spinal cord injury		Anxiety Status Inventory
ASCO	American Society of Clinical Oncology	aSi	amorphous silicon
		ASIA	**American Spinal Injury Association (Score)**
ASCR	autologous stem cell rescue		A-Complete—No preservation of any motor and/or sensory function below the zone of injury
ASCS	autologous stem cell support		
ASCT	autologous stem cell transplantation		B-Incomplete—Preserved sensation
ASCUS	atypical squamous cell of undetermined significance		C-Incomplete—Preserved motor (non-functional)
ASCVD	arteriosclerotic cardiovascular disease		D-Incomplete—Preserved motor (functional)
ASCVR	arteriosclerotic cardiovascular renal disease		E-Complete Recovery
		ASIH	absent, sick in hospital
ASD	aldosterone secretion defect	ASIMC	absent, sick in medical center
	androstenedione	ASIS	anterior superior iliac spine
	annual summary dose (ionizing radiation)	ASK	antistreptokinase
	atrial septal defect	ASKase	antistreptokinase
	autism spectrum disorder(s)	ASL	American Sign Language
			antistreptolysin (titer)
ASD I	atrial septal defect, primum	ASLO	antistreptolysin-O
ASD II	atrial septal defect, secundum	ASLV	avian sarcoma and leukosis virus (Rous virus)
ASDH	acute subdural hematoma	AsM	myopic astigmatism

ASMA	antismooth-muscle antibody	ASVD	arteriosclerotic vessel disease
ASMI	anteroseptal myocardial infarction	ASYM	asymmetric(al)
		ASX	asymptomatic
ASO	aldicarb sulfoxide	AT	abdominothoracic
	allele-specific oligodeoxynucleotide (probes)		activity therapy (therapist)
			Addiction Therapist
			antithrombin
	antistreptolysin-O titer		applanation tonometry
	arterial switch operation		ataxia-telangiectasia
	arteriosclerosis obliterans		atraumatic
	automatic stop order		atrial tachycardia
As₂O₃	arsenic trioxide (Trisenox)	AT 10	dihydrotachysterol
ASOT	antistreptolysin-O titer	ATA	atmosphere absolute
ASP	acute suppurative parotitis	ATB	antibiotic
	acute symmetric polyarthritis		aquatic therapy bar
			atypical tuberculosis
	antisocial personality	ATC	acute toxic class
	asparaginase		aerosol treatment chamber
	aspartic acid		alcoholism therapy classes
ASPDV	anterior superior pancreaticoduodenal vein		all-terrain cycle
			antituberculous chemoprophylaxis
			around-the-clock
ASPVD	arteriosclerotic peripheral vascular disease		Arthritis Treatment Center
			Athletic Trainer, Certified
ASR	aldosterone secretion rate	ATCC	American Type Culture Collection
	automatic speech recognition		
		ATD	antithyroid drug(s)
ASS	anterior superior supine assessment		anticipated time of discharge
			asphyxiating thoracic dystrophy
asst	assistant		
AST	allergy skin test		autoimmune thyroid disease
	Aphasia Screening Test		
	aspartate transaminase (SGOT)	ATE	adipose tissue extraction
		ATEM	analytical transmission electron microscopy
	astemizole		
	astigmatism	ATF	Alcohol, Tobacco, and Firearms (Bureau)
AstdVe	assisted ventilation		
ASTH	asthenopia	At Fib	atrial fibrillation
ASTI	acute soft tissue injury	ATFL	anterior talofibular ligament
AS TOL	as tolerated		
ASTIG	astigmatism	AT III FUN	antithrombin III functional
ASTRO	astrocytoma	ATG	antithymocyte globulin
ASTM	American Society for Testing and Materials	ATHR	angina threshold heart rate
ASTZ	antistreptozyme test	ATI	Abdominal Trauma Index
ASU	acute stroke unit		acute traumatic ischemia
	ambulatory surgical unit		
ASV	antisnake venom		

44

ATL	Achilles tendon lengthening	ATSO	admit to (the) service of
	adult T-cell leukemia	ATSO4	atropine sulfate
	anterior temporal lobectomy	ATT	antitetanus toxoid
			arginine tolerance test
	anterior tricuspid leaflet	ATTN	attention
	antitension line	ATTR	amyloid transtyretin
	atypical lymphocytes	at. wt	atomic weight
ATLL	adult T-cell leukemia lymphoma	ATZ	anal transitional zone
		AU	allergenic (allergy) units
ATLS	acute tumor lysis syndrome		arbitrary units
			both ears
	advanced trauma life support	Au	gold
		A/U	at umbilicus
ATM	acute transverse myelitis	198Au	radioactive gold
	atmosphere	AUA score	American Urological Association—pertains to benign prostatic hypertrophy symptoms
At ma	atrial milliamp		
ATN	acute tubular necrosis		
ATNC	atraumatic normocephalic	AUB	abnormal uterine bleeding
aTNM	autopsy staging of cancer	AuBMT	autologous bone marrow transplant
ATNR	asymmetrical tonic neck reflex		
		AUC	area under the curve
ATO	arsenic trioxide (Trisenox)	AUCt	area under the curve to last time point
ATP	addiction treatment program		
		AUD	amplifiable units of DNA (deoxyribonucleic acid)
	adenosine triphosphate		
	anterior tonsillar pillar		arthritis of unknown diagnosis
	autoimmune thrombocytopenia purpura		
			auditory
		AUD COMP	auditory comprehension
ATPase	adenosine triphosphatase		
ATPS	ambient temperature & pressure, saturated with water vapor	AUDIT	Alcohol Use Disorders Identification Test
		AUG	acute ulcerative gingivitis
ATR	Achilles tendon reflex	AUGIB	acute upper gastrointestinal bleeding
	atracurium (Tracrium)		
	atrial	AUIC	area under the inhibitory curve
	atropine		
ATRA	all-trans retinoic acid (tretinoin-Vesanoid®)	AUL	acute undifferentiated leukemia
atr fib	atrial fibrillation	AUR	acute urinary retention
ATRO	atropine	AUS	acute urethral syndrome
ATRX	acute transfusion reaction		artificial urinary sphincter
ATU	alcohol treatment unit		auscultation
ATV	all-terrain vehicle	AUTO SP	automatic speech
ATS	antimony trisulfide	AV	anteverted
	antitetanic serum (tetanus antitoxin)		anticipatory vomiting
			arteriovenous
	anxiety tension state		atrioventricular

45

auditory visual

auriculoventricular

A:V — arterial-venous (ratio in fundi)

AVA — aortic valve atresia

arteriovenous anastomosis

AVB — atrioventricular block

AVC — acrylic veneer crown

atrioventricular conduction

AVD — aortic valve disease

apparent volume of distribution

arteriosclerotic vascular disease

atrioventricular delay

cerebrovascular accident (French, Spanish)

AVDP — asparaginase, vincristine, daunorubicin, and prednisone

avoirdupois

AVDO₂ — arteriovenous oxygen difference

AVE — aortic valve echocardiogram

atrioventricular extrasystole

AVED — ataxia with isolated vitamin E deficiency

AVF — arteriovenous fistula

augmented unipolar foot (left leg)

avg — average

AVGS — autologous vein graft stent

AVGs — ambulatory visit groups

AVH — acute viral hepatitis

AVHB — atrioventricular heart block

AVJR — atrioventricular junctional rhythm

AVL — augmented unipolar left (left arm)

AVLT — auditory verbal learning test

AVM — arteriovenous malformation

AVN — arteriovenous nicking

atrioventricular node

avascular necrosis

AVNR — atrioventricular nodal re-entry

AVNRT — atrioventricular node recovery time

atrioventricular nodal re-entry tachycardia

A-VO₂ — arteriovenous oxygen difference

AVOC — avocation

AVP — arginine vasopressin

AVPU — alert, (responds to) verbal (stimuli), (responds to) painful (stimuli), unresponsive (mnemonic used by EMTs to judge patients' level of consciousness)

AVR — aortic valve replacement

augmented unipolar right (right arm)

AVRP — atrioventricular refractory period

AVRT — atrioventricular reciprocating tachycardia

AVS — atriovenous shunt

AVSD — atrioventricular septal defect

AVSS — afebrile, vital signs stable

AVT — atrioventricular tachycardia

atypical ventricular tachycardia

AvWS — acquired von Willebrand's syndrome

AW — abdominal wall

abnormal wave

airway

A/W — able to work

A&W — alive and well

AWA — alcohol withdrawal assessment

as well as

A waves — atrial contraction wave

AWB — autologous whole blood

AWDW — assault with a deadly weapon

AWI	anterior wall infarct	
AWMI	anterior wall myocardial infarction	
AWO	airway obstruction	
AWOL	absent without leave	
AWP	airway pressure	
	average wholesale price	
AWRU	active wrist rotation unit	
AWS	alcohol withdrawal seizures (syndrome)	
AWU	alcohol withdrawal unit	
ax	axillary	
AXB	axillary block	
AXC	aortic cross clamp	
ax-fem.fem.	axilla-femoral-femoral (graft)	
AXND	axillary node dissection	
AXR	abdomen x-ray	
AxSYM®	immunodiagnostic testing equipment	
AXT	alternating exotropia	
AY	acrocyanotic (infant color)	
AZA	azathioprine (Imuran)	
AZA-CR	azacitidine	
5-AZC	azacitidine	
AzdU	azidouridine	
AZE	azelastine hydrochloride (Astelin)	
AZM	acquisition zoom magnification	
AZQ	diaziquone	
AZT	zidovudine (azidothymidine; Retrovir)	
A-Z test	Aschheim-Zondek test (diagnostic test for pregnancy)	

B

B	bacillus
	bands
	bilateral
	black
	bloody
	bolus
	both
	botulism (Vaccine B is botulism toxoid)
	brother
	buccal
	See "Plan B"
Ⓑ	both
B+	blood type B positive
B−	blood type B negative
B₁	thiamine HCl
B I	Billroth I (gastric surgery)
B II	Billroth II (gastric surgery)
B₂	riboflavin
B₃	nicotinic acid
b/4	before
B₅	pantothenic acid
B₆	pyridoxine HCl
B₇	biotin
B₈	adenosine phosphate
B₉	benign
B₁₂	cyanocobalamin
B19	parvovirus B19
Ba	barium
BA	backache
	Baptist
	benzyl alcohol
	bile acid
	biliary atresia
	blood agar
	blood alcohol
	bone age
	Bourns assist
	branchial artery
	broken appointment
	bronchial asthma
	buccoaxial
	butyric acid

47

B > A	bone greater than air	BAG	buccoaxiogingival
B < A	bone less than air	BAHA	bone-anchored hearing aid
B & A	brisk and active	BAI	breath-actuated inhalers
BAA	beta-adrenergic agonist		Brief Assessment
BAAM	Beck airway airflow		Interview
	monitor	BAL	balance
Bab	Babinski		blood alcohol level
BAC	benzalkonium chloride		British antilewisite
	blood alcohol		(dimercaprol)
	concentration		bronchoalveolar lavage
	bronchioloalveolar	BALB	binaural alternate loudness
	carcinoma		balance
	buccoaxiocervical	BALF	bronchoalveolar lavage
BACE	beta-site APP (amyloid		fluid
	precursor protein)-	B-ALL	B cell acute lymphoblastic
	cleaving enzyme		leukemia
BACI	bovine anti-	BALT	bronchus-associated
	cryptosporidium		lymphoid tissue
	immunoglobulin	BaM	barium meal
BACM	blocking agent	BAN	British Approved Name
	corticosteroid myopathy	BAND	band neutrophil (stab)
BACON	bleomycin, doxorubicin,	BANS	back, arm, neck and scalp
	lomustine, vincristine,	BAO	basal acid output
	and mechlorethamine	BAP	blood agar plate
BACOP	bleomycin,	BAPS	balance activation
	Adriamycin®,		proprioceptive system
	cyclophosphamide,		biomechanical ankle
	vincristine, and		platform system
	prednisone	BAPT	Baptist
BACPAC	Bulk Activities Post	Barb	barbiturate
	Approval Change	BARN	bilateral acute retinal
BACs	bacterial artificial		necrosis
	chromosomes	BAR	Benadryl, Ativan, and
BACT	bacteria	Troche	Reglan troche
	base-activated clotting	BAS	bile acid sequestrants
	time		boric acid solution
BAD	bipolar affective disorder	BaS	barium swallow
	blunt aortic disruption	BASA	baby aspirin (81 mg
BADL	basic activities of daily		chewable tablets of
	living		aspirin)
BaE	barium enema	BASIS	Basic Achievement Skills
BAE	bronchial artery		Individual Screener
	embolization	BASK	basket cells
BAEDP	balloon aortic end	baso.	basophil
	diastolic pressure	BASO	basophilic stippling
BAEP	brain stem auditory	STIP	
	evoked potential	BAT	Behavioral Avoidance Test
BAERs	brain stem auditory		blunt abdominal trauma
	evoked responses		borreliacidal-antibody test

	brightness acuity tester	BBM	banked breast milk
BATO	boronic acid adduct of technetium oxime	BBOW	bulging bag of water
batt	battery	BBP	blood-borne pathogen
BAVP	balloon aortic valvuloplasty		butyl benzyl phthalate
BAU	bioequivalent allergy units	BBR	bibasilar rales
BAV	bicuspid aortic valve	BBS	Berg Balance Scale
BAW	bronchoalveolar washing		bilateral breath sounds
BB	baby boy	BBSE	bilateral breath sounds equal
	backboard		
	back to back	BBSI	Brigance Basic Skills Inventory
	bad breath		
	bed bath	BBT	basal body temperature
	bed board		Buteyko breathing technique
	beta-blocker		
	blanket bath	BB to MM	belly button to medial malleolus
	blood bank		
	blow bottle	B Bx	breast biopsy
	blue bloaters	BC	back care
	body belts		basket catheter
	both bones		battered child
	breakthrough bleeding		bed and chair
	breast biopsy		beta carotene
	brush biopsy		bicycle
	buffer base		birth control
B&B	bismuth and bourbon		bladder cancer
	bowel and bladder		blood culture
B/B	backward bending		Blue Cross
BBA	born before arrival		bone conduction
BBB	baseball bat beating		Bourn control
	blood-brain barrier		breast cancer
	bundle branch block		buccocervical
BBBB	bilateral bundle branch block		buffalo cap (cap for intravenous line)
BBC	Brown-Buerger cystoscope	B/C	because
			blood urea nitrogen/creatinine ratio
BBD	baby born dead	B&C	bed and chair
	before bronchodilator		biopsy and curettage
	benign breast disease		board and care
BBE	biofield breast examination		breathed and cried
		BCA	balloon catheter angioplasty
BBFA	both bones forearm		basal cell atypia
BBFP	blood and body fluid precautions		bicinchoninic acid
			brachiocephalic artery
BBI	Bowman Birk inhibitor	BCAA	branched-chain amino acids
BBIC	Bowman Birk inhibitor concentrate		
BBL	bottle blood loss	BC < AC	bone conduction less than air conduction

BC > AC	bone conduction greater than air conduction	
B. cat	*Branhamella catarrhalis*	
B-CAVe	bleomycin, lomustine (CCNU), doxorubicin (Adriamycin), and vinblastine (Velban)	
BCB	Brilliant cresyl blue (stain)	
BCBR	bilateral carotid body resection	
BC/BS	Blue Cross/Blue Shield	
BCC	basal cell carcinoma	
	birth control clinic	
BCCa	basal cell carcinoma	
BCD	basal cell dysplasia	
	bleomycin, cyclophosphamide, and dactinomycin	
	borderline of cardial dullness	
BCDH	bilateral congenital dislocated hip	
BCE	basal cell epithelioma	
	beneficial clinical event	
B cell	B lymphocyte	
BCF	basic conditioning factor	
	Baylor core formula	
BCG	bacille Calmette-Guérin vaccine	
	bicolor guaiac	
BCH	benign coital headache	
BCHA	bone-conduction hearing aid	
BCI	blunt carotid injury	
BCIR	Barnett continent intestinal reservoir	
BCL	basic cycle length	
	bio-chemoluminescence	
B/C/L	BUN,(blood urea nitrogen),creatinine, lytes (electrolytes)	
BCLP	bilateral cleft lip and palate	
BCLS	basic cardiac life support	
BCM	below costal margin	
	birth control medication	
	birth control method	
	body cell mass	

BCME	bis (chloromethyl) ether
BCNP	Board Certified Nuclear Pharmacist
BCNU	carmustine
BCOC	bowel care of choice
	bowel cathartic of choice
BCP	biochemical profile
	birth control pills
	blood cell profile
	carmustine, cyclophosphamide, and prednisone
BCPAP	Broun's continuous positive airway pressure
BCQ	breast central quadrantectomy
BCR	breakpoint cluster region (gene)
	bulbocavernosus reflex
BCRE	black cohosh root extract
BCRS	Brief Cognitive Rate Scale
BCRT	breast conservation followed by radiation therapy
BCS	battered child syndrome
	breast conserving surgery
	Budd-Chiari syndrome
BCSF	bone cell stimulating factor
BCSS	bone cell stimulating substance
BCT	Bag Carrying Test
	breast-conserving therapy
	broad complex tachycardias
BCTP	bi-component triton tri-n-butyl phosphate
BCU	burn care unit
BCUG	bilateral cystourethrogram
BD	band neutrophil
	base deficit
	base down
	behavior disorder
	Behçet's disease
	bile duct
	birth date
	birth defect
	blood donor

	brain dead
	bronchial drainage
	bronchodilator
	buccodistal
	1,4-butanediol
	United Kingdom abbreviation for twice a day
B-D	Becton Dickinson and Company
BDAE	Boston Diagnostic Aphasia Examination
BDAS	balloon dilation atrial septostomy
BDBS	Bonnet-Dechaume-Blanc syndrome
BDC	burn-dressing change
BDD	body dysmorphic disorder
	bronchodilator drugs
BDE	bile duct exploration
BDF	bilateral distal femoral
	black divorced female
BDI	Beck Depression Inventory
BDI SF	Beck's Depression Inventory-Short Form
BDL	below detectable limits
	bile duct ligation
BDM	black divorced male
BDNF	brain-derived neurotrophic factor
B-DOPA	bleomycin, dacarbazine, vincristine (Oncovin), prednisone, and doxorubicin (Adriamycin)
BDP	beclomethasone dipropionate
	best demonstrated practice
BDR	background diabetic retinopathy
BDV	Borna disease virus
BE	bacterial endocarditis
	barium enema
	Barrett's esophagus
	base excess
	below elbow
	bread equivalent
	breast examination

B $\uparrow$ E	both upper extremities
B $\downarrow$ E	both lower extremities
B & E	brisk and equal
BEA	below elbow amputation
BEAC	carmustine (BiCNU), etoposide, cytarabine (ara-C), and cyclophosphamide
BEAM	brain electrical activity mapping
	carmustine BCNU), etoposide, cytarabine (ara-C), and methotrexate
BEAR	Bourn's electronic adult respirator
BEC	bacterial endocarditis
BED	binge-eating disorder
	biochemical evidence of disease
	biological equivalent dose
BEE	basal energy expenditure
BEF	bronchoesophageal fistula
BEGA	best estimate of gestational age
BEH	behavior
	benign essential hypertension
Beh Sp	behavior specialist
BEI	bioelectric impedance
	butanol-extractable iodine
BEL	blood ethanol level
BEP	bleomycin, etoposide, and cisplatin (Platinol)
	brain stem evoked potentials
BE-PEG	balanced electrolyte with polyethylene glycol
BEV	billion electron volts
	bleeding esophageal varices
BF	black female
	bone fragment
	boyfriend
	breakfast fed
	breast-feed
B/F	bound-to-free ratio
B & F	back and forth
%BF	percentage of body fat

51

BFA	baby for adoption		Braxton Hicks contractions
	basilic forearm	bHCG	beta human chorionic
	bifemoral arteriogram		gonadotropin
BFC	benign febrile convulsion	BHD	carmustine, hydroxyurea,
bFGF	basic fibroblast growth		and dacarbazine
	factor	B-HEXOS-	beta hexosaminidase A
BFL	breast firm and lactating	A-LK	leukocytes
B-FLY	butterfly	BHI	biosynthetic human
BFM	black married female		insulin
BFNC	benign familial neonatal		brain-heart infusion
	convulsions	BHN	bridging hepatic necrosis
BFP	biologic false positive	BHR	bronchial hyperrespon-
	blue fluorescent protein		siveness (hyperactivity)
BFR	blood filtration rate	BHP	boarding home
	blood flow rate		placement
B. frag	*Bacillus fragilis*		British Herbal
BFT	bentonite flocculation test		Pharmacopeia
	biofeedback training	BHS	Beck Hopelessness Scale
BFU$_e$	erythroid burst-forming		beta-hemolytic
	unit		streptococci
BG	baby girl		breath-holding spell
	basal ganglia	BHT	borderline hypertensive
	blood glucose		breath hydrogen test
	bone graft		butylated hydroxytoluene
B-G	Bender-Gestalt (test)	BI	Barthel Index
BGA	Bundesgesundheitsamt		base in
	(German drug		Boehringer Ingelheim
	regulatory agency)		Pharmaceuticals, Inc.
B-GA-	beta galactosidase		bowel impaction
LACTO			brain injury
BGC	basal-ganglion	Bi	bismuth
	calcification	BIA	bioelectrical impedance
BGCT	benign glandular cell		analysis
	tumor		biospecific interaction
BGDC	Bartholin gland duct cyst		analysis
BGDR	background diabetic	BIB	brought in by
	retinopathy	BIBA	brought in by ambulance
BGL	blood glucose level	BIC	brain injury center
BGM	blood glucose	BICAP	bipolar electrocoagulation
	monitoring		therapy
bGS	biopsy Gleason score	Bicarb	bicarbonate
BGT	Bender-Gestalt test	BiCNU®	carmustine
	blood glucose testing	BICROS	bilateral contralateral
BGTT	borderline glucose		routing of signals
	tolerance test	BICU	burn intensive care unit
BH	bowel habits	BID	brought in dead
	breath holding	*BID*	twice daily
BHA	butylated hydroxyanisole	BIDA	amonafide
BHC	benzene hexachloride		

BIDS	bedtime insulin, daytime sulfonylurea		biceps jerk
			body jacket
BIF	bifocal		bone and joint
BIG	botulism immune globulin	BJE	bone and joint examination
BIGEM	bigeminal		
BIH	benign intracranial hypertension		bones, joints, and extremities
	bilateral inguinal hernia	BJI	bone and joint infection
BIL	bilateral	BJM	bones, joints, and muscles
	brother-in-law	BJOA	basal joint osteoarthritis
BILAT SLC	bilateral short leg case	BJP	Bence Jones protein
		BK	below knee (amputation)
BILAT SXO	bilateral salpingo-oophorectomy		bradykinin
			bullous keratopathy
Bili	bilirubin	BKA	below knee amputation
BILI-C	conjugated bilirubin	BKC	blepharokerato-conjunctivitis
BIL MRY	bilateral myringotomy		
BIMA	bilateral internal mammary arteries	bkft	breakfast
		Bkg	background
BIN	twice a night (this is a dangerous abbreviation)	BKTT	below knee to toe (cast)
		BKWC	below knee walking cast
BIND	Biological Investigational New Drug	BKWP	below-knee walking plaster (cast)
BIO	binocular indirect ophthalmoscopy	BL	baseline (fetal heart rate)
			bioluminescence
BIOF	biofeedback		bland
BIP	bipolar affective disorder		blast cells
	bleomycin, ifosfamide, and cisplatin (Platinol)		blood level
			blood loss
	brain injury program		blue
BiPAP	bilevel (biphasic) positive airway pressure		bronchial lavage
			Burkitt's lymphoma
BiPD	biparietal diameter	B/L	brother-in-law
BIPP	bismuth iodoform paraffin paste	BLA	Biological License Application
BIR	back internal rotation	BLB	Boothby-Lovelace-Bulbulian (oxygen mask)
BIRB	Biomedical Institutional Review Board		
			bronchoscopic lung biopsy
BIS	Bispectral Index		
Bi-SLT	bilateral, sequential single lung transplantation	BLBK	blood bank
		BLBS	bilateral breath sounds
bisp	bispinous diameter	BL = BS	bilateral equal breath sounds
BIT	behavioral inattention test		
BIVAD	bilateral ventricular assist device	bl cult	blood culture
		B-L-D	breakfast, lunch, and dinner
BIW	twice a week (this is a dangerous abbreviation)		
		bldg	bleeding
BIZ-PLT	bizarre platelets	bld tm	bleeding time
BJ	Bence Jones (protein)		

BLE	both lower extremities	BMAT	basic motor ability test(s)
BLEED	ongoing *b*leeding, *l*ow blood pressure, *e*levated prothrombin time, *e*rratic mental status, and unstable comorbid *d*isease (risk factors for continued gastrointestinal bleeding)	BMB	bone marrow biopsy
		BMBF	German Ministry of Education and Research
		BMC	bone marrow cells
			bone marrow culture
			bone mineral content
		BMD	Becker muscular dystrophy
BLEO	bleomycin sulfate		bone marrow depression
BLESS	bath, laxative, enema, shampoo, and shower		bone mineral density
		BME	basal medium Eagle (diploid cell culture)
BLG	bovine beta-lactoglobulin		biomedical engineering
BLIC	beta-lactamase inhibitor combination		brief maximal effort
		BMET	basic metabolic panel (see page 358)
BLIP	beta-lactamase inhibiting protein	BMF	between meal feedings
			black married female
BLL	bilateral lower lobe	BMFDS	Burke-Marsden-Fahn's dystonia rating scale
	blood lead level		
	brows, lids, and lashes	BMG	benign monoclonal gammopathy
BLLS	bilateral leg strength		
BLM	bleomycin sulfate	BMI	body mass index
BLN	bronchial lymph nodes	BMJ	bones, muscles, joints
BLOBS	bladder obstruction	BMK	birthmark
BLOC	brief loss of consciousness	BMM	black married male
			bone marrow micrometastases
BLPB	beta-lactamase-producing bacteria	BMMC	bone marrow mononuclear T cells
BLPO	beta-lactamase-producing organism	BMMM	bone marrow micrometastases
BLQ	both lower quadrants	B-MODE	brightness modulation
BLR	blood flow rate	BMP	basic metabolic profile (panel) (see page 358)
BLS	basic life support		
BLT	blood-clot lysis time		behavior management plan
	brow left transverse		
B.L. unit	Bessey-Lowry units	BMPs	bone-morphogenic proteins
BLV	bovine leukemia virus		
BM	bacterial meningitis	BMR	basal metabolic rate
	black male		best motor response
	bone marrow	BMRM	bilateral modified radical mastectomy
	bone metastases		
	bowel movement	BMS	Bristol-Myers Squibb Company
	breast milk		
BMA	biomedical application	BMT	bilateral myringotomy and tubes
	bismuth subsalicylate, metronidazole, and amoxicillin		
	bone marrow aspirate		

	bismuth subsalicylate, metronidazole, and tetracycline	BOB	born on arrival born out of asepsis ball on back
BMTH	bismuth, metronidazole, tetracycline, and a histamine H$_2$-receptor antagonist	BOC BOD	beats of clonus bilateral orbital decompression burden of disease
		Bod Units	Bodansky units
BMTN	bone marrow transplant neutropenia	BOE BOH	bilateral otitis externa bundle of His
BMTT	bilateral myringotomy with tympanic tubes	BOLD	bleomycin, vincristine (Oncovin®), lomustine, and dacarbazine
BMTU	bone marrow transplant unit		blood oxygenation level dependent
BMU	basic multicellular unit	BOM	benign ovarian mass
BN	bladder neck bulimia nervosa	BOMA	bilateral otitis media bilateral otitis media, acute
BNBAS	Brazelton Neonatal Behavioral Assessment	BOME	bilateral otitis media with effusion
BNC	binasal cannula bladder neck contracture	BOMP	bleomycin, vincristine (Oncovin), mitomycin, and cisplatin (Platinol AQ)
BNCT	boron neutron capture therapy		
BNE	but not exceeding	BOO	bladder outlet obstruction
BNF	British National Formulary	BOOP	bronchitis obliterans with organized pneumonia
BNI	blind nasal intubation	BOP	bleeding on probing
BNL	below normal limits breast needle localization	BOR	bowels open regularly bronchia-oto-renal (syndrome)
Bn M	bone marrow		
BNO	bladder neck obstruction bowels not open	BORN	State Board of Registration in Nursing
BNP	brain natriuretic peptide	BOS	base of support
BNPA	binasal pharyngeal airway	BOSS	Becker orthopedic spinal system
BNR	bladder neck retraction		
BNS	benign nephrosclerosis	BOT	base of tongue
BNT	back to normal Boston Naming Test	BOU BOUGIE	burning on urination bougienage
BO	base out because of	BOVR	Bureau of Vocational Rehabilitation
	behavior objective body odor	BOW BOW-I	bag of water bag of water-intact
	bowel obstruction bowel open	BOW-R	bag of water-ruptured
	bucco-occlusal	BP	bathroom privileges
B & O	belladonna & opium (suppositories)		bed pan bench press
BOA	behavioral observation audiometry		benzoyl peroxide

	bipolar	BPPP	bilateral pedal pulses present
	birthplace		
	blood pressure	BP,P,R,T,	blood pressure, pulse, respiration, and temperature
	body powder		
	British Pharmacopeia		
	bullous pemphigoid	BPPV	benign paroxysmal positional vertigo
	bypass		
BP-200	Bourn's Infant Pressure Ventilator	BPR	blood per rectum blood pressure recorder
BPA	birch pollen allergy	BPRS	Brief Psychiatric Rating Scale
BPAD	bipolar affective disorder		
BPb	whole blood lead concentration	BPS	bilateral partial salpingectomy blood pump speed
BPCF	bronchopleural cutaneous fistula	BPs	systolic blood pressure
BPI	bipolar disorder, Type I	BPSD	bronchopulmonary segmental drainage
BPII	bipolar type II disorder		
BPD	benzoporphyrin derivative biparietal diameter borderline personality disorder bronchopulmonary dysplasia	BPV	benign paroxysmal vertigo benign positional vertigo bovine papilloma virus
		Bq	becquerel
		BQL	below quantifiable levels
BPd	diastolic blood pressure	BQR	brequinar sodium
BPF	bronchopleural fistula	BR	bathroom
BPH	benign prostatic hypertrophy		bedrest Benzing retrograde birthing room
BPG	bypass graft penicillin G benzathine (Bicillin L-A; Permapen) for IM use only		blink reflex bowel rest brachioradialis breech bridge
BPI	bactericidal/permeability increasing (protein)		bright red brown
	Brief Pain Inventory	Br	bromide
BPIG	bacterial polysaccharide immune globulin		bromine
		BRA	bananas, rice (rice cereal), and applesauce (diet)
BPL	benzylpenicilloylpolylysine		
BPLA	blood pressure, left arm		brain
BPLND	bilateral pelvic lymph node dissection	BRADY	bradycardia
		BRANCH	branch chain amino acids
BPM	beats per minute breaths per minute	BRAO	branch retinal artery occlusion
BPN	bacitracin, polymyxin B, and neomycin sulfate	BRAS	bilateral renal artery stenosis
BPO	benzoyl peroxide bilateral partial oophorectomy	BRAT	bananas, rice (rice cereal), applesauce, and toast Baylor rapid autologous transfuser
BPP	biophysical profile		

	blunt thoracic abdominal		breath sounds
	trauma	B & S	Bartholin and Skene
BRATT	bananas, rice (rice cereal),		(glands)
	applesauce, tea, and		bending and stooping
	toast		Brown and Sharp (suture
BRB	blood-retinal barrier		sizes)
	bright red blood	BS×4	bowel sounds in all four
BRBR	bright red blood per		quadrants
	rectum	BSA	body surface area
BRBPR	bright red blood per		bowel sounds active
	rectum	BSAB	Balthazar Scales of
BRC	bladder reconstruction		Adaptive Behavior
BRCM	below right costal margin	BSAb	broad-spectrum antibiotics
BrdU	bromodeoxyuridine	BSAP	bone-specific alkaline
BRex	breathing exercise		phosphatase
Br Fdg	breast-feeding	BSB	bedside bag
BRJ	brachial radialis jerk		body surface burned
BRM	biological response	BSC	basosquamous (cell)
	modifiers		carcinoma
BRN	brown		bedside care
BRO	brother		bedside commode
BROM	back range of motion		biological safety cabinet
BRONK	bronchoscopy		burn scar contracture
BRP	bathroom privileges	BSCC	bedside commode chair
BR RAO	branch retinal artery		Bjork-Shiley
	occlusion		convexoconcave
BR RVO	branch retinal vein		(valves)
	occlusion	BSD	baby soft diet
BRS	baroreceptor reflex		bedside drainage
	sensitivity	BSE	bovine spongiform
BrS	breath sounds		encephalopathy
BRSV	bovine respiratory		breast self-examination
	syncytial virus	BSEC	bedside easy chair
BRU	basic remodeling unit	BSepF	black separated female
	(osteon)	BSepM	black separated male
	brucellosis (Brucella	BSER	brain stem evoked
	melitensis) vaccine		responses
BRVO	branch retinal vein	BSF	black single female
	occlusion		busulfan
BS	barium swallow	BSG	Bagolini striated glasses
	bedside		brain stem gliomas
	before sleep	BSGA	beta streptococcus group
	Behçet's syndrome		A
	Bennett seal	BSI	bloodstream infection
	blind spot		body substance isolation
	blood sugar		brain stem injury
	Blue Shield	BSL	Biological Safety Level
	bone scan		blood sugar level
	bowel sounds	BSL-1	Biosafety Level 1

B

BS L base	breath sounds diminished, left base	BSU	Bartholin, Skene's, urethra (glands)
BSM	black single male		behavioral science unit
	blood safety module	BSu	blood sugar
BSN	Bachelor of Science in Nursing	BSUTD	baby shots up to date
			Base Service Unit
	bowel sounds normal	BSW	Bachelor of Social Work
BSNA	bowel sounds normal and active		bedscale weight
		BT	bedtime
BSNMT	Bachelor of Science in Nuclear Medicine Technology		behavioral therapy
			bituberous
			bladder tumor
BSNT	breast soft and nontender		Blalock-Taussig (shunt)
BSNUTD	baby shots not up to date		bleeding time
			blood transfusion
BSO	bilateral salpingo-oophorectomy		blood type
			blunt trauma
	l-buthionine sulfoximine		brain tumor
bSOD	bovine superoxide dismutase		breast tumor
			bowel tones
BSOM	bilateral serous otitis media	Bt	*Bacillus thuringiensis*
		B-T	Blalock-Taussig (shunt)
BSP	body substance precautions	B/T	between
		Bt#	bottle number
	bone sialoprotein	BTA	below the ankle
	Bromsulphalein®		bladder tumor antigen
BSPA	bowel sounds present and active		bladder tumor-associated analytes
BSPM	body surface potential mapping	BTA-A	botulinum toxin A (Botox)
BSR	bowels sounds regular	BTB	back to bed
BSRI	Bem Sex Role Inventory		beat-to-beat (variability)
BSRT (R)	Bachelor of Science in Radiologic Technology (Registered)		breakthrough bleeding
		BTBV	beat-to-beat variability
		BTC	bilateral tubal cautery
BSS	Baltimore Sepsis Scale		biliary tree cancer
	bedside scale		bladder tumor check
	bismuth subsalicylate		by the clock
	black silk sutures	BTE	Baltimore Therapeutic Equipment
BSS®	balanced salt solution		behind-the-ear (hearing aid)
BSSG	sitogluside		
BSSO	bilateral sagittal split osteotomy		bisected, totally embedded
BSSS	benign sporadic sleep spikes	BTF	blenderized tube feeding
		BTFS	breast tumor frozen section
BSST	breast self-stimulation test	BTG	beta thromboglobulin
BST	bedside testing	B-Thal	beta thalassemia
	bovine somatotropin		
	brief stimulus therapy		

58

BTHOOM	beats the hell out of me (better stated as "differed diagnosis")	BUS	Bartholin, urethral, and Skene's glands
			bulbourethral sling
BTI	biliary tract infection	BUSV	Bartholin urethral Skeins vagina
	bitubal interruption		
BTKA	bilateral total knee arthroplasty	BUT	biopsy urease test
			break up time
BTL	bilateral tubal ligation	BV	bacterial vaginitis
BTM	bilateral tympanic membranes		biological value
			blood volume
	bismuth subcitrate, tetracycline, and metronidazole	BVAD	biventricular assist device
		BVD	bovine viral diarrhea
		BVE	blood volume expander
BTMEAL	between meals	BVF	bulboventricular foramen
BTO	bilateral tubal occlusion	BVH	biventricular hypertrophy
BTP	bismuth tribromophenate	BVL	bilateral vas ligation
		BVM	bag valve mask
	breakthrough pain	BVMG	Bender Visual-Motor Gestalt (test)
BTPABA	bentiromide		
BTPS	body temperature pressure saturated	BVO	branch vein occlusion
		BVR	Bureau of Vocational Rehabilitation
BTR	bladder tumor recheck		
BTS	Blalock-Taussig shunt	BVRO	bilateral vertical ramus osteotomy
BTSH	bovine thyrotropin		
BTU	behavior therapy unit	BVRT	Benton Visual Retention Test
BTW	back to work		
	between	BVT	bilateral ventilation tubes
BTW M	between meals	BW	birth weight
BTX	Botulinum toxin type A (Botox)		bite-wing (radiograph)
			body water
BU	base up (prism)		body weight
	below umbilicus	B & W	Black and White (milk of magnesia & aromatic cascara fluidextract)
	Bodansky units		
	burn unit		
	busulfan	BWA	bed wetter admission
BUA	broadband ultrasound attenuation	BWCS	bagged white cell study
		BWF	Blackwater fever
BuCy	busulfan and cyclophosphamide	BWFI	bacteriostatic water for injection
BUD	budesonide (Rhinocort)	BWidF	black widowed female
BUdR	bromodeoxyuridine	BWidM	black widowed male
BUE	both upper extremities	BWS	battered woman syndrome
BUFA	baby up for adoption		Beckwith-Wiedemann syndrome
BUN	blood urea nitrogen		
	bunion	BWs	bite-wing (x-rays)
BUO	bleeding of undetermined origin	BWT	bowel wall thickness
		BWX	bite-wing x-ray
BUR	back-up rate (ventilator)	Bx	biopsy
Burd	Burdick suction	B × B	back to back

BX BS	Blue Cross and Blue Shield
BXM	B cell crossmatch
ΦBZ	phenylbutazone
BZD	benzodiazepine
BZDZ	benzodiazepine

C

C	ascorbic acid
	carbohydrate
	Catholic
	Caucasian
	Celsius
	centigrade
	chlamydia
	clubbing
	conjunctiva
	constricted
	cyanosis
	cytosine
	hundred
c	with
C'	cervical spine
C+	with contrast
C−	without contrast
C 1	cyclopentolate 1% ophthalmic solution (Cyclogyl)
C_1–C_7	cervical vertebra 1 through 7
C_1–C_8	cervical nerves 1 through 8
C_1 to C_9	precursor molecules of the complement system
C_1 .... C_{12}	cranial nerves 1 to 12
C3	complement C3
C4	complement C4
CI-CV	Drug Enforcement Agency scheduled substances class one through five
C_{II}	second cranial nerve
CA	cancelled appointment
	Candida albicans
	carcinoma
	cardiac arrest
	carotid artery
	celiac artery
	cellulose acetate (filter)
	Certified Acupuncturist
	chronologic age

	Cocaine Anonymous
	community-acquired
	compressed air
	continuous aerosol
	coronary angioplasty
	coronary artery
Ca	calcium
C/A	conscious, alert
Ca++	calcification
CA 125	cancer antigen 125
C&A	Clinitest® and Acetest®
CAA	coloanal anastamosis
	crystalline amino acids
CAB	catheter-associated bacteriuria
	cellulose acetate butyrate
	combined androgen blockade
	complete atrioventricular block
	coronary artery bypass
CAB-BAGE	coronary artery bypass graft
CABG	coronary artery bypass graft
CaBI	calcium bone index
CaBP	calcium-binding protein
CABS	coronary artery bypass surgery
CAC	cardioacceleratory center
	Certified Alcohol Counselor
	Community Action Center
	coronary artery calcification
CACI	computer-assisted continuous infusion
CaCl₂	calcium chloride
CaCO₃	calcium carbonate
CACP	cisplatin
CACS	cancer-related anorexia/cachexia
CAD	cadaver (kidney donor)
	calcium alginate dressing
	computer-aided diagnosis
	computer-aided dispatch
	coronary artery disease
CADAC	Certified Alcohol and Drug Abuse Counselor

CADASIL	cerebral autosomal dominant arteriopathy with subcortical infarcts and leukoencephalopathy
CADD®	Computerized Ambulatory Drug Delivery (pump)
CADP	computer-assisted design of prosthesis
CADRF	coronary artery disease risk factors
CADXPL	cadaver transplant
CAE	cellulose acetate electrophoresis
	coronary artery endarterectomy
	cyclophosphamide, doxorubicin (Adriamycin), and etoposide
CAEC	cardiac arrhythmia evaluation center
CaEDTA	calcium disodium edetate
CAF	chronic atrial fibrillation
	controlled atrial flutter/fibrillation
	cyclophosphamide, doxorubicin (Adriamycin), and fluorouracil
CAFF	controlled atrial fibrillation/flutter
CAFT	Clinitron® air fluidized therapy
CAG	chronic atrophic gastritis
	closed angle glaucoma
	continuous ambulatory gamma globin (infusion)
	coronary arteriography
CaG	calcium gluconate
CAGE	a questionnaire for alcoholism evaluation (JAMA 1984; 252: 1905-7) C Have you ever felt the need to cut down on your drinking? A Have you ever felt annoyed by criticism of

C

your drinking? <u>G</u> Have you ever felt guilty abut your drinking? <u>E</u> Have you ever taken a drink (<u>eye</u> opener) first thing in the morning?

CAH	chronic active hepatitis
	chronic aggressive hepatitis
	congenital adrenal hyperplasia
CAHB	chronic active hepatitis B
CAI	carbonic anhydrase inhibitors
	carboxyamide aminoimidazoles
	computer-assisted instructions
'caid	Medicaid
CAIV	cold-adapted influenza virus vaccine
CAL	callus
	calories (cal)
	chronic airflow limitation
C_{alb}	albumin clearance
cal ct	calorie count
CALD	chronic active liver disease
CALGB	Cancer and Leukemia Group B
CALLA	common acute lympho-blastic leukemia antigen
CAM	campylobacter vaccine
	Caucasian adult male
	cell adhesion molecules
	child abuse management
	complementary and alternative medicine
	confusion assessment method
	cystic adenomatoid malformation
CAMCOG	Cambridge Cognitive Examination
CAMD	computer-aided molecular design
CAMF	cyclophosphamide, Adriamycin, methotrexate, and fluorouracil
CAMP	cyclophosphamide, doxorubicin (Adriamycin), methotrexate, and procarbazine
cAMP	cyclic adenosine monophosphate
CAMs	cell adhesion molecules
CAN	contrast-associated nephropathy
	cord around neck
CA/N	child abuse and neglect
CANC	cancelled
c-ANCA	antineutrophil cytoplasmic antibody
CANDA	computer-assisted new drug application
CAN-KLB	*Candida albicans, Klebsiella pneumoniae* vaccine
CANP	Certified Adult Nurse Practitioner
CAO	chronic airway (airflow) obstruction
CaO_2	arterial oxygen concentration
CaOx	calcium oxalate
CAP	cancer of the prostate
	capsule
	cellulose acetate phthalate
	chaotic atrial tachycardia
	chemistry admission profile
	chloramphenicol
	community-acquired pneumonia
	compound action potentials
	cyclophosphamide, doxorubicin (Adria-mycin), and cisplatin
CaP	cancer of the prostate
Ca/P	calcium to phosphorus ratio
CAPB	central auditory processing battery
CAPD	continuous ambulatory peritoneal dialysis

C

CAPLA	computer-assisted product license application		combined androgen suppression
CAPS	aspects of **c**ognition, **a**ffective state, **p**hysical condition, and **s**ocial factors (patient assessment; parameters)	CASA	computer-assisted surgery cancer-associated serum antigen
			Center on Addiction and Substance Abuse
	caffeine, alcohol, pepper, and spicy food (dietary restrictions)		computer-assisted semen analysis
CAPWA	computerized arterial pulse waveform analysis	CaSC	carcinoma of the sigmoid colon
		CASHD	coronary arteriosclerotic heart disease
CAR	cardiac ambulation routine carotid artery repair	CASP	Child Analytic Study Program
	coronary artery revascularization	CASS	computer-aided sleep system
	Coxsackie adenovirus receptor	CAST®	color allergy screening test
CA-RA	common adductor-rectus abdominis	CAT	Cardiac Arrest Team carnitine acetyl transferase
CARB	carbohydrate		
CARBO	Carbocaine® carboplatin		cataract Children's Apperception Test
CARD	Cardiac Automatic Resuscitative Device		coital alignment technique computed axial tomography
CARES	Cancer Rehabilitation Evaluation System		methcatinone
CARF	Commission on Accreditation of Rehabilitation Facilities	CATH	catheter catheterization Catholic
CARM	Centre for Adverse Reactions Monitoring (New Zealand)	CATS	catecholamines
		CATT	card agglutination test with stained trypanosomes
C-arm	fluoroscopy image intensifier	CAU	Caucasian
CARN	Certified Addiction Registered Nurse	CAUTI	catheter-associated urinary tract infection
CART	classification and regression tree	CAV	computer-aided ventilation congenital absence of vagina
CARTI	community-acquired respiratory tract infection(s)		cyclophosphamide, doxorubicin (Adriamycin), and vincristine
CAS	carotid artery stenosis cerebral arteriosclerosis	CAV-1	canine adenovirus type 1
	Chemical Abstracts Service	CAVB	complete atrioventricular block
	Clinical Asthma Score		

C

CAVC	common artrioventricular canal	CBCT	community based clinical trials
CAVE	Content Analysis of Verbatim Explanation	CBD	closed bladder drainage common bile duct corticobasal degeneration
	cyclophosphamide, doxorubicin, (Adriamycin) vincristine, and etoposide	CBDE	common bile duct exploration
		CBE	charting by exception child birth education
CAVH	continuous arteriovenous hemofiltration	CBER	Center for Biologics Evaluation and Research (FDA)
CAVHD	continuous arteriovenous hemodialysis		
CAVM	cerebral arteriovenous malformation	CBF	cerebral blood flow
		CBFS	cerebral blood flow studies
CAV-P-VP	cyclophosphamide, doxorubicin (Adriamycin), vincristine, cisplatin, and etoposide	CBFV	cerebral blood flow velocity
		CBG	capillary blood glucose
		CBGM	capillary blood glucose monitor
CAVR	continuous arteriovenous rewarming	CBI	continuous bladder irrigation
CAVS	calcific valve stenosis	CBM	cryopreserved bone marrow
CAVU	continuous arteriovenous ultrafiltration	CBN	chronic benign neutropenia
CAW	carbonaceous-activated water (Willard Water)		collected by nurse
CAX	central axis	CBP	chronic benign pain copper-binding protein
CB	cesarean birth chronic bronchitis code blue conjugated bilirubin (direct)	CBPP	contagious bovine pleuropneumonia
		CBPS	congential bilateral perisylvian syndrome coronary bypass surgery
c/b	complicated by	CBR	carotid bodies resected chronic bedrest clinical benefit responders complete bedrest
C & B	chair and bed crown and bridge		
CBA	chronic bronchitis and asthma cost-benefit analysis County Board of Assistance	CBRAM	controlled partial rebreathing-anesthesia method
		CB RRR s M/R/G	cardiac beat, regular rhythm and rate without murmurs, rubs, or gallops
CBAVD	congenital bilateral absence of the vas deferens		
		CBrS	clear breath sounds
CBC	carbenicillin complete blood count contralateral breast cancer	CBS	Caregiver Burden Screen Charles Bonnet's syndrome
CBCDA	carboplatin		
CBCL	Child Behavior Checklist		

	chronic brain syndrome		critical care area
	coarse breath sounds	CCAM	congential cystic
	Cruveilhier-Baumgarten		adenomatoid
	syndrome		malformation (of the
CBT	cognitive behavioral		lung)
	therapy	CCAP	capsule cartilage articular
CBU	cumulative breath units		preservation
CBV	central blood volume	CCAT	common carotid artery
	cyclophosphamide,		thrombosis
	carmustine (BiCNu),	CCB	calcium channel
	and etoposide (VePesid)		blocker(s)
CBZ	carbamazepine (Tegretol)		Community Care Board
CBZE	carbamazepine epoxide		corn, callus, and bunion
CC	cardiac catheterization	CCC	Cancer Care Center
	Catholic		central corneal clouding
	cerebral concussion		(Grade 0+ to 4+)
	chief complaint		Certificate of Clinical
	choriocarcinoma		Competency
	chronic complainer		child care clinic
	circulatory collapse		Comprehensive Cancer
	clean catch (urine)		Center
	comfort care	C/cc	colonies per cubic
	complications and		centimeter
	comorbidity	CC & C	colony count and culture
	coracoclavicular	CCC-A	Certificate of Clinical
	cord compression		Competence in
	corpus callosum		Audiology
	creatinine clearance	CCCE	Clinical Center
	critical condition		Coordinator Educator
	cubic centimeter (cc),	CCC-SP	Certificate of Clinical
	(mL)		Competence in Speech-
	with correction (with		Language Pathology
	glasses)	CCD	charged-coupled device
C_c	concentration of drug in		childhood celiac
	the central compartment		disease
C/C	cholecystectomy and		chin-chest distance
	operative	CCDC	Certified Chemical
	cholangiogram		Dependency Counselor
	complete upper and lower	CCDS	color-coded duplex
	dentures		sonography
CCII	Clinical Clerk–2nd year	CCE	clubbing, cyanosis, and
C & C	cold and clammy		edema
CCA	calcium-channel		countercurrent
	antagonist		electrophoresis
	circumflex coronary artery	CCF	cephalin cholesterol
	common carotid artery		flocculation
	concentrated care area		compound comminuted
	countercurrent		fracture
	chromatography		congestive cardiac failure

C

	crystal-induced chemotactic factor	C-collar	cervical collar
		CCP	crystalloid cardioplegia
CCFE	cyclophosphamide, cisplatin, fluorouracil, and estramustine	CCPD	continuous cycling (cyclical) peritoneal dialysis
CCFs	chronic-care facilities	CCR	cardiac catheterization recovery
CCG	Children's Cancer Group		continuous complete remission
CCH	community care home Cook County Hospital		counterclockwise rotation
CCHD	complex congenital heart disease	C_{cr}	creatinine clearance
		CCRC	Certified Clinical Research Coordinator
	cyanotic congenital heart disease		continuing care residential community
CCHF	Congo-Crimean hemorrhagic fever	CCRN	Certified Critical Care Registered Nurse
CCHS	congenital central hypoventilation syndrome	CCRT	combined chemo-radiotherapy
CCI	chronic coronary insufficiency corrected count increment	CCRU	critical care recovery unit
		CCS	cell cycle-specific certified coding specialist
CCK	cholecystokinin	CC & S	cornea, conjunctiva, and sclera
CCK-OP	cholecystokinin octapeptide	CCSA	Canadian Cardiovascular Society Angina (score)
CCK-PZ	cholecystokinin pancreozymin	CCSK	clear cell sarcoma of the kidney
CCL	cardiac catheterization laboratory critical condition list	CCSP	Certified Chiropractic Sports Physician
CCl_4	carbon tetrachloride	CCS-P	Certified Coding Specialist, Physician-Based
CCLE	chronic cutaneous lupus erythematosus		
CCM	calcium citrate malate cerebral cavernous malformation	CCT	calcitriol carotid compression tomography
	Certified Care Manager children's case management		Certified Cardiographic Technician
	cyclophosphamide, lomustine (CCNU; CeeNU), and methotrexate		closed cerebral trauma closed cranial trauma congenitally corrected transposition (of the great vessels)
CCMSU	clean catch midstream urine		Critical Care Technician
CCMU	critical care medicine unit		crude coal tar
CCN	continuing care nursery	CCTGA	congenitally corrected transposition of the great arteries
CCNS	cell cycle-nonspecific		
CCNU	lomustine		
CCO	continuous cardiac output		

CCT in PET	crude coal tar in petroleum	CD8	antigenic marker on suppressor/cytotoxic T cells (also called OKT 8, T8, and Leu 8)
CCTV	closed circuit television		
CCU	coronary care unit		
	critical care unit	C&D	curettage and desiccation
CCUA	clean catch urinalysis		cystectomy and diversion
CCUP	colpocystourethropexy		cytoscopy and dilatation
CCV	Critical Care Ventilator (Ohio)	CDA	Certified Dental Assistant chenodeoxycholic acid (chenodiol)
	critical closing volume		congenital dyserythro-poietic anemia
CCW	childcare worker		
	counterclockwise		
CCWR	counterclockwise rotation	2-CDA	cladribine (Leustatin; chlorodeoxyadenosine)
CCX	complications		
CCY	cholecystectomy	CDAD	Clostridium difficile-associated diarrhea
CD	cadaver donor		
	candela	CDAI	Crohn's Disease Activity Index
	Castleman's disease		
	celiac disease	CDAK	Cordis Dow Artificial Kidney
	cervical dystonia		
	cesarean delivery	CDAP	continuous distended airway pressure
	character disorder		
	chemical dependency	CDB	cough and deep breath
	childhood disease	CDC	calculated day of confinement
	chronic dialysis		
	closed drainage		cancer detection center
	clusters of differentiation		carboplatin, doxorubicin, and cyclophosphamide
	common duct		
	communication disorders		Centers for Disease Control and Prevention
	complementarity-determining		
			Certified Drug Counselor
	complicated delivery		chenodeoxycholic acid (chenodiol)
	conjugate diameter		
	continuous drainage		Clostridium difficile colitis
	convulsive disorder		
	cortical dysplasia	CDCA	chenodeoxycholic acid (chenodiol)
	Crohn's disease		
	cumulative doses	CDCP	Centers for Disease Control and Prevention (CDC is official abbreviation)
	cyclodextran		
	cytarabine and daunorubicin		
Cd	cadmium	CDD	Certificate of Disability for Discharge
	concentration of drug		
C/D	cigarettes per day		Clostridium difficile disease
	cup to disk ratio		
CD4	antigenic marker on helper/inducer T cells (also called OKT 4, T4, and Leu3)		cytidine deaminase
		CDDP	cisplatin
		CDE	canine distemper encephalitis

C

67

	Certified Diabetes Educator			complete decongestive physiotherapy
	common duct exploration			crystalline degradation product
CDER	Center for Drug Evaluation and Research (FDA)		CDQ	cytidine diphosphate corrected development quotient
CDFI	color Doppler flow imaging		CDR	clinical data repository Clinical Dementia Rating
CDG	carbohydrate-deficient glycoprotein			continuing disability review
CDGE	constant denaturant gel electrophoresis		CDRH	Center for Devices and Radiological Health
CDGP	constitutional delay of growth and puberty		CDR(H)	cup-to-disk ratio horizontal
CDH	chronic daily headache congenital diaphragmatic		CDRs	complementary determining regions
	hernia		CDR(V)	cup-to-disk ratio vertical
	congenital dislocation of hip		CDS	closed door seclusion color Doppler sonography
	congenital dysplasia of the hip		CDSC	Communicable Disease Surveillance Centre (United Kingdom)
CDHP	5-chloro-2 4-dihydroxypyridine		CDSPIES	congestive heart failure, drugs, spasm,
CDI	Children's Depression Inventory			pneumothorax, infection, embolism,
	clean, dry, and intact color Doppler imaging			and secretions (differential diagnosis
	Cotrel Duobosset Instrumentation			mnemonic)
CDIC	*Clostridium difficile*-induced colitis		CDT	carbohydrate-deficient transferrin
C Dif	*Clostridium difficile*			Chemical Dependency Technician
CDK	climatic droplet keratopathy			connecting discourse tracking (measure of
	cyclin-dependent kinase			speech perception)
CDKI	cyclin-dependent kinase inhibitor			cystic dysplasia of the testis
CDK2	cyclin-depenent kinases 2		CDTA	cyclohexane-1,2-diaminetetraacetic acid
CDLC	continuous double-loop closure		CDTM	collaborative drug therapy management
CDLE	chronic discoid lupus erythematosus		CDU	chemical dependency unit
CdLS	Cornelia de Lange's syndrome		CDV	canine distemper virus cardiovascular
CDP	chemical dependence profile		CDX	chlordiazepoxide
	Child Development Program		cdyn	dynamic compliance
			CE	California encephalitis

	capillary electrophoresis	CEI	continuous extravascular infusion
	carboplatin and etoposide		
	cardiac enlargement		converting enzyme inhibitor
	cardiac enzymes		
	cardioesophageal	CEL	cardiac exercise laboratory
	cataract extraction	CELP	chronic erosive lichen planus
	central episiotomy		
	chemoembolization	CEM	Clinical Event Manager
	chest expansion	CEMD	consultative examination by physician
	cholesterol ester		
	community education	CEN	Certified (Nurse)– Emergency Room
	consultative examination		
	continuing education	CENOG	computerized electroneuro-ophthalmogram
	contrast echocardiology		
C&E	consultation and examination		
		CEO	chief executive officer
	cough and exercise	CEP	cardiac enzyme panel
	curettage and electrodesiccation		cognitive evoked potential
CEA	carcinoembryonic antigen		congenital erythropoietic porphyria
	carotid endarterectomy		countercurrent electrophoresis
	cost-effectiveness analysis		
CEB	calcium entry blocker		cyclophosphamide, etoposide, and cisplatin (Platinol)
	carboplatin, etoposide, and bleomycin		
CEBV	chronic Epstein-Barr virus	CEPH	cephalic
CEC	capillary electrochromatography		cephalosporin
	Council for Exceptional Children	CEPH FLOC	cephalin flocculation
CECD	congenital endothelial corneal dystrophy	CEPP (B)	cyclophosphamide, etopside, procarbazine, prednisone, and bleomycin
CEc̄/IOL	cataract extraction with intraocular lens		
CECT	contrast-enhanced computed tomography	CER	conditioned emotional response
CED	cystoscopy-endoscopy dilation	CE&R	central episiotomy and repair
CEE	conjugated equine estrogen (Premarin; conjugated estrogen)	CERA	cortical evoked response audiometry
		CERAD	Consortium to Establish a Registry for Alzheimer's Disease
CEF	chick embryo fibroblast	CERD	chronic end-stage renal disease
	cyclophosphamide, epirubicin, and fluorouracil		
CEFOT	cefotaxime	CERULO	ceruloplasmin
CEFOX	cefoxitin	CERV	cervical
CEFTAZ	ceftazidime	CES	Cauda equina syndrome
CEFUR	cefuroxime		central excitatory state

C

69

	cognitive environmental stimulation	
	estrogen, conjugated (conjugated estrogen substance)	
CESB	chronic electrical stimulation of the brain	
CES-D	Center for Epidemiologic Studies – Depression	
CESI	cervical epidural steroid injection	
CET	common extensor tendon	
CETP	cholesterol ester transfer protein	
CEV	cyclophosphamide, etoposide, and vincristine	
CE w/IOL	cataract extraction with intraocular lens	
CF	calcium leucovorin (citrovorum factor)	
	cancer-free	
	cardiac failure	
	Caucasian female	
	Christmas factor	
	cisplatin and fluorouracil	
	complement fixation	
	contractile force	
	count fingers	
	cystic fibrosis	
C&F	cell and flare	
	chills and fever	
CFA	common femoral artery	
	complete Freund's adjuvant	
	cryptogenic fibrosing alveolitis	
	cystic fibrosis anthropathy	
CFAC	complement-fixing antibody consumption	
C-factor	cleverness factor	
CFCs	chlorofluorocarbons	
CFD	color-flow Doppler	
	computational fluid dynamics	
CFF	critical fusion (flicker) frequency	

CFFT	critical flicker fusion threshold
CFH	chemical fume hood
CFI	confrontation fields intact
CFIDS	chronic fatigue immune dysfunction syndrome
CFL	calcaneofibular ligament
	cisplatin, fluorouracil, and leucovorin calcium
CFLX	ciprofloxacin
	circumflex
CFM	cerebral function monitor
	close fitting mask
	craniofacial microsomia
	cyclophosphamide, fluorouracil, and mitoxantrone
CFNS	chills, fever, and night sweats
CFP	cystic fibrosis protein
CFPT	cyclophosphamide, fluorouracil, prednisone, and tamoxifen
CFR	case-fatality rates
	Code of Federal Regulations
	coronary flow reserve
CFS	cancer family syndrome
	Child and Family Service
	childhood febrile seizures
	chronic fatigue syndrome
	congenital fibrosarcoma
CFSAN	Center for Food Safety and Applied Nutrition (NIH)
CFT	chronic follicular tonsillitis
	complement fixation test
CFTR	cystic fibrosis transmembrane (conductance) regulator
	cystic fibrosis transmembrane receptor
CFU	colony-forming units
CFU-E	colony-forming unit–erythroid
CFU-G	colony-forming unit–granulocyte

CFU-G/M   colony-forming unit–granulocyte/macrophage

CFU-M   colony-forming unit–macrophage

CFU-S   colony-forming unit–spleen

CFV   common femoral vein

CFVR   coronary flow velocity reserve

CG   cardiogreen (dye)
caregiver
cholecystogram
contact guarding
contralateral groin

CGA   comprehensive geriatric assessment
contact guard assist

CGB   chronic gastrointestinal (tract) bleeding

CGD   chronic granulomatous disease
cobalt gray equivalent

CGF   continuous gavage feeding (infant feeding)

CGI   Clinical Global Impressions (scale)

CGIC   Clinical Global Impression of Change

CGI-S   Clinical Global Impressions, Severity of Illness

CGL   chronic granulocytic leukemia
with correction/with glasses

CGM   central gray matter

CGMP   Current Good Manufacturing Practices

cGMP   cyclic guanine monophosphate

CGN   chronic glomerulonephritis

C-GRD   coffee-ground

CGRP   calcitonin gene-related peptide

CGS   cardiogenic shock
catgut suture

   centimeter-gram-second system

CGTT   cortisol glucose tolerance test

cGy   centigray

CH   chest
chief
child (children)
chronic
cluster headache
concentric hypertrophy
congenital hypothyroidism
convalescent hospital
crown-heal

C_h hepatic clearance

ch^1 Christ Church chromosone

CH_{50} total hemolytic complement

C&H   cocaine and heroin

CHA   compound hypermetropic astigmatism
congenital hypoplastic anemia

CHAD   cyclophosphamide, altretamine, (hexamethylmelamine), doxorubicin (Adriamycin), and cisplatin (DDP)

CHAI   continuous hepatic artery infusion

CHAM-OCA   cyclophosphamide, hydroxyurea, dactinomycin, methotrexate, vincristine, leucovorin, and doxorubicin

CHAM-PUS   Civilian Health and Medical Program of the Uniformed Services

CHAP   child health associate practitioner
cyclophosphamide, altretamine, (hexamethylmelamine), doxorubicin (Adriamycin), and cisplatin (Platinol AQ)

C

71

CHARGE	coloboma (of eyes), hearing deficit, choanal atresia, retardation of growth, genital defects (males only), and endocardial cushion defect	CHG	change
		CHI	chikungunya virus vaccine
			closed head injury
			contrast harmonic imaging
CHART	complaint, history, assessment, Rx (treatment), transport		creatinine-height index
		CHILD	congenital hemidysplasia with ichthyosiform nevus and limb defects (syndrome)
	continuous hyperfractionated accelerated radiotherapy		
		CHIN	community health information network
CHB	chronic hepatitis B	CHIP	comprehensive health insurance plan
	complete heart block		
	congenital heart block		iproplatin
CHBHA	congenital Heinz body hemolytic anemia	Chix	chickenpox
		CHL	conductive hearing loss
CHC	concentric hypertrophic cardiomyopathy	ChloMP	chlorambucil, mitoxantrone, and prednisolone
CH₃– CCNU	semustine		
		ChlVPP	chlorambucil, vinblastine, procarbazine, and prednisone
CHCT	caffeine-halothane contracture test		
cHct	central hematocrit	CHN	central hemorrhagic necrosis
CHD	center hemodialysis		Chinese herb nephropathy
	changed diaper		community nursing home
	childhood diseases	CHO	carbohydrate
	chronic hemodialysis		Chemical Hygiene Officer
	common hepatic duct		Chinese hamster ovary
	congenital heart disease	C_{H_2O}	free-water clearance
	coordinate home care	CHO_a	cholera vaccine, attenuated live (oral)
CHE	chronic hepatic encephalopathy		
		CHO_{cn^-} LPS	cholera vaccine, lipopolysaccharide-toxin conjugate
CHEF	clamped homogeneous electric field		
		C_2H_5OH	alcohol (ethyl alcohol)
CHEM 7	see page 358	CHO_{i-w}	cholera vaccine, inactivated whole cell
CHEMO	chemotherapy		
ChemoRx	chemotherapy	CHO_{i-w-BS}	cholera vaccine, inactivated whole cell, B subunit
CHEOPS	Children's Hospital of Eastern Ontario Pain Scale		
		chol	cholesterol
		c̄ hold	withhold
CHESS	chemical shift suppression	CHO_o	cholera, oral vaccine
CHF	congestive heart failure	CHOP	cyclophosphamide, doxorubicin, vincristine (Oncovin), prednisone
	Crimean hemorrhagic fever		
CHFV	combined high frequency of ventilation		

C

72

CHOP-Bleo — cyclophosphamide, doxorubicin (hydroxydaunorubicin), vincristine (Oncovin), prednisone, and bleomycin

CHO$_{tox}$ — cholera toxin/toxoid vaccine

CHPB — Canadian Health Protection Branch (the equivalent of the U.S. Food and Drug Administration)

CHPX — chickenpox

CHR — Cercaria-Hullen reaction
chronic
complete hematological response

CHRPE — congenital hypertrophy of the retinal pigment epithelium

CHRS — congenital hereditary retinoschisis

CHS — Chediak-Higashi syndrome
contact hypersensitivity

CHT — Certified Hand Therapist
Certified Hyperbaric Technician
closed head trauma

CHTN — chronic hypertension

CHU — closed head unit

CHUC — Certified Health Unit Coordinator

CHVP — cyclophosphamide, doxorubicin (hydroxydaunorubicin), teniposide (VM26), and prednisone

CHW — community health workers

CHWG — chewing gum

CI — cardiac index
cesium implant
Clinical Instructor
cochlear implant
cognitively impaired
commercial insurance
complete iridectomy
confidence interval
continuous infusion
coronary insufficiency

Ci — curie(s)

CIA — calcaneal insufficiency avulsion
chronic idiopathic anhidrosis

CIAA — competitive insulin autoantibodies

CIAED — collagen-induced autoimmune ear disease

CIB — Carnation Instant Breakfast®
crying-induced bronchospasm
cytomegalic inclusion bodies

CIBD — chronic inflammatory bowel disease

CIBI — Clinician Interview Based Impression (of change)

CIBIC — Clinician Interview-Based Impression of Change

CIBIC-plus — Clinician's Interview-Based Impression of Change with Caregiver Input

CIBP — chronic intractable benign pain

C-IBS — constipated predominant irritable bowel syndrome

CIC — cardioinhibitory center
circulating immune complexes
clean intermittent catheterization
completely in the canal (hearing aid)
coronary intensive care

CICE — combined intracapsular cataract extraction

CICU — cardiac intensive care unit

CICVC — centrally inserted central venous catheter

CID — cervical immobilization device
chemotherapy-induced diarrhea

C

	combined immunodeficiency	CIN	cervical intraepithelial neoplasia
	cytomegalic inclusion disease		chemotherapy induced neutropenia
CIDP	chronic inflammatory demyelinating		chronic interstitial nephritis
	polyradiculoneuropathy (polyneuropathy)	C_{IN}	insulin clearance
		CIND	cognitive impairment, no dementia
CIDS	cellular immunodeficiency syndrome	CINE	chemotherapy-induced nausea and emesis
	continuous insulin delivery system		cineangiogram
CIE	capillary immunoelectrophoresis	CINV	chemotherapy-induced nausea and vomiting
	chemotherapy induced emesis	CIO	corticosteroid-induced osteoporosis
	congenital ichthyosiform erythroderma	CIOMS	The Council for International Organization of Medical Sciences
	counterimmuno-electrophoresis		
	crossed immunoelectrophoresis	CIP	Cardiac Injury Panel
CIEA	continuous infusion epidural analgesia		critical illness polyneuropathy
CIEP	counterimmuno-electrophoresis	CIPD	chronic intermittent peritoneal dialysis
	crossed immunoelectrophoresis	CIR	continent intestinal reservior
CIFN	chemotherapy-induced fever and neutropenia	Circ	circulation
			circumcision
CIG	cigarettes		circumference
CIH	continuous infusion haloperidol	circ. & sen.	circulation and sensation
CIHD	chronic ischemic heart disease	CIS	Cancer Information Service (National Cancer Institute)
CII	continuous insulin infusion		carcinoma in situ
CIIA	common internal iliac artery		Commonwealth of Independent States
CIL	carbamazepine-induced lupus		continuous interleaved sampling
CIM	change in menses	CI&S	conjunctival irritation and swelling
	chemotherapy-induced mucositis	CISC	clean intermittent self-catheterization
	convective interaction media	CISCA	cisplatin, cyclophosphamide, and doxorubicin (Adriamycin)
	corticosteroid-induced myopathy		
CIMCU	cardiac intermediate care unit	CISD	critical incident stress debriefing (used by EMTs)

Cis-DDP	cisplatin		clear liquid
CISM	critical incident stress management (debriefing used by EMTs)		cleft lip
			cloudy
			critical list
CIS-R	Clinical Interview Schedule, Revised		cycle length
			lung compliance
CI-Stim	cochlear implant stimulation	C_L	compliance of the lungs
CIT	conventional immunosuppressive therapy	CLA	community living arrangements
			congenital lactic acidosis
			congenital laryngeal atresia
	conventional insulin therapy		conjugated linoleic acid
CIT IDS	citation identifiers (National Library of Medicine)	CLAMSS	cleavage- and ligation-associated mutation-specific sequencing
CITP	capillary isotachophoresis	CLAP	contact laser ablation of prostate
CIU	chronic idiopathic urticaria	CLAS	congenital localized absence of skin
CIV	common iliac vein	CLASS	computer laser assisted surgical system
	continuous intravenous (infusion)	CLASS I	congestive heart failure with no limitation with ordinary activity, (New York Heart Association Classification)
CIVI	continuous intravenous infusion		
CIXU	constant infusion excretory urogram		
CIWA-Ar	Clinical Institute Withdrawal Assessment for Alcohol–revised	CLASS II	congestive heart failure with slight limitation of physical activity
CJD	Creutzfeldt-Jakob disease		
cJET	congenital junctional ectopic tachycardia	CLASS III	congestive heart failure with marked limitation of physical activity
CJR	centric jaw relation		
CK	check	CLASS IV	congestive heart failure with inability to engage in any physical activity without symptoms
	creatine kinase		
CK-BB	creatine kinase BB band (primarily in brain)		
CKC	cold knife conization	Clav	clavicle
CK-ISO	creatine kinase isoenzyme	CLB	chlorambucil
CK-MB	creatine kinase MB fraction (primarily in cardiac muscle)		coccidian-like body
		CLB_{atx}	*Clostridium botulinum* antitoxin
CK MM	creatine kinase MM fraction (primarily in skeletal muscle)	CLBBB	complete left bundle branch block
		CLBD	cortical Lewy body disease
CKW	clockwise		
Cl	chloride	CLBP	chronic low back pain
CL	central line	CLB_{tox}	*Clostridium botulinum* toxoid vaccine
	chemoluminescence		

C

75

CLC	cork leather and celastic (orthotic)		community living skills
		CLSE	calf lung surfactant extract (Infasurf)
CL/CP	cleft lip and cleft palate		
CLD	chronic liver disease	CLT	chronic lymphocytic thyroiditis
	chronic lung disease		complex lymphedema therapy
	Clostridium difficile vaccine		
			cool lace tent
Cl_d	dialysis clearance	Cl_T	total body clearance
CLE	centrilobular emphysema	CLV	cutaneous leukocytoclastic vasculitis
	congenital lobar emphysema		
		CL VOID	clean voided specimen
	continuous lumbar epidural (anesthetic)	CLW_c	*Clostridium welchii* type C (Pigbel) toxoid vaccine
CLED	cysteine lactose electrolyte-deficient (agar)		
		clysis	hypodermoclysis
		cm	centimeter
CLEIA	chemiluminescent enzyme immunoassay	CM	capreomycin
			cardiac monitor
CLEP	college level examination program		case management
			case manager
CLF	cholesterol-lecithin flocculation		Caucasian male
			centimeter (cm)
CLG	clorgyline		chondromalacia
CLH	chronic lobular hepatitis		cochlear microphonics
C_h	hepatic clearance		common migraine
CLI	central lymphatic irradiation		continuous microwave
			continuous murmur
	clomipramine		contrast media
	critical leg ischemia		costal margin
CLIA	Clinical Laboratory Improvement Act		cow's milk
			culture media
Cl_{int}	intrinsic clearance		cutaneous melanoma
CLL	chronic lymphocytic leukemia		cystic mesothelioma
			tomorrow morning (this is a dangerous abbreviation)
CLLE	columnar-lined lower esophagus		
cl liq	clear liquid	cm1	circumflex marginal 1
Cl_{nr}	nonrenal clearance	cm2	circumflex marginal 2
CLO	Campylobacter-like organism	cm^2	square centimeters
		cm^3	cubic centimeter
	close	CMA	Certified Medical Assistant
	cod liver oil		compound myopic astigmatism
CL & P	cleft lip and palate		
CL PSY	closed psychiatry		cost-minimization analysis
Cl_r	renal clearance		cow's milk allergy
Cl Red	closed reduction	CMAF	centrifuged microaggregate filter
CLRO	community leave for reorientation		
CLS	capillary leak syndrome		

CMAI	Cohen-Mansfield Agitation inventory	CMGN	chronic membranous glomerulonephritis
CMAPs	compound muscle action potentials	CMH	current medical history
		CMHC	community mental health center
C_{max}	maximum concentration of drug	CMHN	Community Mental Health Nurse
CMB	carbolic methylene blue	CMI	case mix index
CMBBT	cervical mucous basal body temperature		cell-mediated immunity
			clomipramine
CMC	carboxymethylcellulose		Cornell Medical Index
	carpal metacarpal (joint)	CMID	cytomegalic inclusion disease
	chloramphenicol		
	chronic mucocutaneous candidosis	C_{min}	minimum concentration of drug
	closed mitral commissurotomy	CMIR	cell-mediated immune response
CMD	congenital muscular dystrophy	CMJ	carpometacarpal joint
		CMK	congenital multicystic kidney
	cytomegalic disease	CML	cell-mediated lympholysis
CMDRH	Center for Medical Devices and Radiological Health (of the Food and Drug Administration)		chronic myelogenous leukemia
			chronic myeloid leukemia
		CMM	Comprehensive Major Medical (insurance)
CME	cervicomediastinal exploration (examination)		cutaneous malignant melanoma
		CMME	chloromethyl methyl ether
	continuing medical education	CMML	chronic myelomacrocytic leukemia
	cystoid macular edema	CMMS	Columbia Mental Maturity Scale
CMER	current medical evidence of record	CMN	congenital mesoblastic nephroma
CMF	cyclophosphamide, methotrexate and fluorouracil	CMO	cardiac minute output
			cetyl myristoleate
CMFP	cyclophosphamide, methotrexate, fluorouracil, and prednisone		Chief Medical Officer
			comfort measures only (resuscitation order)
CMFT	same as CMF with tamoxifen		consult made out
		CMO 1	corticosterone methyl oxidase type 1
CMFVP	cyclophosphamide, methotrexate, fluorouracil, vincristine, and prednisone	CMOP	cardiomyopathy
		C-MOPP	cyclophosphamide, mechlorethamine, vincristine (Oncovin), procarbazine, and prednisone
CMG	cystometrogram		
CMGM	chronic megakaryocytic granulocytic myelosis		

CMP	cardiomyopathy	CMTX	chemotherapy treatment
	chondromalacia patellae	CMUA	continuous motor unit activity
	comprehensive (complete) metabolic profile (see page 358)	CMV	cisplatin, methotrexate, and vinblastine
	cushion mouthpiece		controlled mechanical ventilation
CMPF	cow's milk, protein-free		conventional mechanical ventilation
CMPT	cervical mucous penetration test		cool mist vaporizer
CMR	cerebral metabolic rate		cytomegalovirus
	child (1–4 years) mortality rates		cytomegalovirus vaccine
CMRI	cardiac magnetic resonance imaging	CMVIG	cytomegalovirus immune globulin
CMRNG	chromosomally mediated resistant *Neisseria gonorrhoeae*	CMVS	culture midvoid specimen
		CN	congenital nystagmus
CMRO	chronic multifocal recurrent osteomyelitis		cranial nerve
CMRO$_2$	cerebral metabolic rate for oxygen		tomorrow night (this is a dangerous abbreviation)
		Cn	cyanide
CMS	children's medical services	C/N	contrast-to-noise ratio
	circulation motion sensation	CN II–XII	cranial nerves 2 through 12
	chocolate milkshake	CNA	Certified Nurse Aide
	constant moderate suction		chart not available
CMSC	Certified Medical Staff Coordinator	C_{Na}	sodium clearance
		CNAG	chronic narrow angle glaucoma
CMSUA	clean midstream urinalysis	CNAP	continuous negative airway pressure
CMT	carpometatarsal (joint)	CNB	core-needle biopsy
	Certified Massage Therapist	CNC	clinical nurse coordinator
	Certified Medical Transcriptionist		Community Nursing Center
	Certified Music Therapist	CNCbl	cyanocobalamin
	cervical motion tenderness	CND	canned
	Charot-Marie-Tooth (phenotype)		cannot determine
	Chiropractic manipulative treatment		chronic nausea and dyspepsia
	choline magnesium trisalicylate (Trilisate)	CNDC	chronic nonspecific diarrhea of childhood
	combined modality therapy	CNE	chronic nervous exhaustion
			could not establish
	continuing medication and treatment	CNEP	continuous negative extrathoracic pressure
	cutis marmorata telangiectasia	C-NES	conversion nonepileptic seizures

CNF	cyclophosphamide, mitoxantrone (Novatantrone), and fluorouracil		CNTA	combined neurosurgical and transfacial approach
CNH	central neurogenic hypernea		CNTF	ciliary neurotrophic factor
	contract nursing home		CNV	choroidal neovascularization
CNHC	chronodermatitis nodularis helicis chronicus		CNVM	choroidal neovascular membrane
	community nursing home care		CO	carbon monoxide
CNL	chemonucleolysis			cardiac output
CNLD	chronic neonatal lung disease			castor oil
				centric occlusion
CNM	certified nurse midwife			Certified Orthoptist
CNMT	Certified Nuclear Medicine Technologist			cervical orthosis
				corn oil
CNN	congenital nevocytic nevus		Co	court order
				cobalt
CNO	Chief Nursing Officer		C/O	check out
	community nursing organization			complained of
				complaints
CNOP	cyclophosphamide, mitoxantrone (Novantrone), vincristine (Oncovin), and prednisone		^{60}Co	under care of radioactive isotope of cobalt
			CO_2	carbon dioxide
			CO_3	carbonate
			COA	children of alcoholic
CNOR	Certified Nurse, Operating Room		CoA	coenzyme A
CNP	capillary nonprofusion			coarctation of the aorta
CNPB	continuous negative pressure breathing		COAD	chronic obstructive airway disease
				chronic obstructive arterial disease
CNPS	cardiac nuclear probe scan		COAG	chronic open angle glaucoma
CNR	contrast-to-noise ratio			
CNRN	Certified Neurosurgical Registered Nurse		COAGSC	coagulation screen
			COAP	cyclophosphamide, vincristine (Oncovin), cytarabine (ara-C), and prednisone
CNS	central nervous system			
	Certified Nutrition Specialist			
	Clinical Nurse Specialist		COAR	coarctation
	coagulase-negative staphylococci		COARCT	coarctation
			COB	cisplatin, vincristine (Oncovin), and bleomycin
	Crigler-Najjar syndrome			
CNSD	Certified Nutrition Support Dietitian			coordination of benefits
CNSHA	congenital nonspherocytic hemolytic anemia		COBE	chronic obstructive bullous emphysema
CNT	could not tell		COBS	chronic organic brain syndrome
	could not test			

C

COBT	chronic obstruction of biliary tract		Computer Output to Laser Disk
COC	calcifying odontogenic cyst	COLD A	cold agglutin titer
		Collyr	eye wash
	chain of custody	col/ml	colonies per milliliter
	combination oral contraceptive	colp	colporrhaphy
		COLTRU	*colletotrichum truncatum*
	continuity of care	COM	center of mass
COCCIO	coccidioidomycosis		chronic otitis media
COCM	congestive cardiomyopathy	COMBO	combination ultrasound with electrical stimulation
COD	cataract, right eye		
	cause of death	COMF	comfortable
	chronic oxygen dependency	COMLA	cyclophosphamide, vincristine (Oncovin), methotrexate, calcium leucovorin, and cytarabine (ara-C)
	codeine		
	coefficient of oxygen delivery		
	condition on discharge	COMM E	Committee E, a German Federal Health Agency committee for the evaluation of herbal remedies
CODE 99	patient in cardiac or respiratory arrest		
COD-MD	cerebro-oculardysplasia muscular dystrophy		
CODO	codocytes	COMP	compensation
COE	court-ordered examination		complications
COEPS	cortically originating extrapyramidal symptoms		composite
			compound
			compress
COER-24	24-hour controlled-onset, extended-release (dosage form)		cyclophosphamide, vincristine (Oncovin), methotrexate, and prednisone
COFS	cerebro-oculo-facio-skeletal	COMS	clinical outcomes management system
COG	center of gravity	COMT	catechol-*O*-methyl-transferase
	Central Oncology Group		
	cognitive function tests	CON	catheter over a needle
COGN	cognition		certificate of need
COGTT	cortisone-primed oral glucose tolerance test		conservatorship
		CON A	concanavalin A
		conc.	concentrated
COH	carbohydrate	CONG	congenital
	controlled ovarian hyperstimulation		gallon
		CONJ	conjunctiva
COHb	carboxyhemoglobin	CONPA-DRI I	cyclophosphamide, vincristine, doxorubicin, and melphalan
Coke	Coca-Cola®		
	cocaine		
COL	colonoscopy	CONPA-DRI II	conpadri I plus high-dose methotrexate
COLD	chronic obstructive lung disease		

CONPA-DRI III	conpadri I plus intensified doxorubicin		coronary
		CORA	conditioned orientation reflex audiometry
CoNS	coagulase-negative staphylococci	CORBA	Common-Object Request Broker Architecture
CONT	continuous contusions	CORE	cardiac or respiratory emergency
CON-TRAL	contralateral	CORF	Comprehensive Outpatient Rehabilitation Facility
CONTU	contusion		
CONV	conversation	COR P	cor pulmonale
Conv. ex.	convergence excess	CORT	Certified Operating Room Technician
CO-Ox	Co-oximetry		
COP	center of pressure	COS	cataract, left eye
	change of plaster		change of shift
	cicatricial ocular pemphigoid		Chief of Staff
	Colibacilosis porcina vaccine		clinically observed seizure
			controlled ovarian stimulation
	colloid osmotic pressure		Crisis Outpatient Services
	complaint of pain	C_{osm}	osmolal clearance
	cycophosphamide, vincristine (Oncovin), and prednisone	COSTART	Coding symbols for a thesaurus of adverse reaction terms
COP 1	copolymer 1	COT	content of thought
COPA	cuffed oropharyngeal airway	COTA	Certified Occupational Therapy Assistant
COP-BLAM	cyclophosphamide, vincristine (Oncovin), prednisone, bleomycin, doxorubicin (Adriamycin), and procarbazine (Matulane)	COTE	comprehensive occupational therapy evaluation
		COTT CH	cottage cheese
		COTX	cast off to x-ray
		COU	cardiac observation unit
			cataracts, both eyes
COPD	chronic obstructive pulmonary disease	COV	coefficient of variation
		COWA	controlled oral word association
COPE	chronic obstructive pulmonary emphysema	COWS	cold to the opposite and warm to the same
COPP	cyclophosphamide, vincristine, procarbazine, and prednisone	COX	Coxsackie virus
			cyclo-oxygenase
			cytochrome C oxidase
COPS	community outpatient service	COX-2	cyclo-oxygenase-2
		CP	centric position
COPT	circumoval precipitin test		cerebral palsy
CoQ10	coenzyme Q_{10}		Certified Paramedic
COR	coefficient of reproducibility		chemical peel
			chemistry profiles
	conditioned orientation response		chest pain
			chloroquine-primaquine

chondromalacia patella
chronic pain
chronic pancreatitis
cleft palate
clinical pathway
closing pressure
convenience package
cor pulmonale
creatine phosphokinase
cyclophosphamide and cisplatin (Platinol)
cystopanendoscopy

C_p concentration of drug plasma
phosphate clearance

Cp *Chlamydia pneumoniae*

C/P carbohydrate-to-protein ratio

C&P compensation and pension
complete and pushing
cystoscopy and pyelography

CPA cardiopulmonary arrest
carotid photoangiography
cerebellar pontile angle
chest pain alert
color power angiography
conditioned play audiometry
costophrenic angle
cyclophosphamide
cyproterone acetate

CPAF chlorpropamide-alcohol flush

C_{PAH} para-amino hippurate clearance

CPAP continuous positive airway pressure

CPB cardiopulmonary bypass
cisplatin, cyclophosphamide, and carmustine (BiCNU)
competitive protein binding

CPBA competitive protein-binding assay

CPBP cardiopulmonary bypass

CPC cancer prevention clinic
cerebral palsy clinic
Certified Procedural Coder
chronic passive congestion
clinicopathologic conference
coil planet centrifuge
continue plan of care

CPC-H Certified Procedural Coder, Hospital-Based

CPCR cardiopulmonary-cerebral resuscitation

CPCS clinical pharmacokinetics consulting service

CPD cephalopelvic disproportion
chorioretinopathy and pituitary dysfunction
chronic peritoneal dialysis
citrate-phosphate-dextrose

CPDA-1 citrate-phosphate-dextrose-adenine-one

CPDA-2 citrate phosphate dextrose adenine-two

CPDD calcium pyrophosphate deposition disease

CPDG2 carboxypeptidase-G2

CPE cardiogenic pulmonary edema
chronic pulmonary emphysema
Clinical Pastoral Education
clubbing, pitting, or edema
complete physical examination

CPE-C cyclopentenylcytosine

CPEO chronic progressive external ophthalmoplegia

CPER chest pain emergency room

CPET cardiopulmonary exercise testing

CPETU chest pain evaluation and treatment unit

CPF cerebral perfusion pressure

C

CPFT	Certified Pulmonary Function Technologist	CPMP	Committee for Proprietary Medicinal Products (of the European Union)
CPG	clinical practice guidelines		
CPG2	carboxypeptidase G2	CPN	chronic pyelonephritis
CPGN	chronic progressive glomerulonephritis	CPO	continue present orders
		CPOE	computerized physician (prescriber) order entry
CPH	chronic persistent hepatitis		
CPhT	Certified Pharmacy Technician	CPOX	chicken pox
		CPP	central precocious puberty
CPI	constitutionally psychopathia inferior		cerebral perfusion pressure
			chronic pelvic pain
CPID	chronic pelvic inflammatory disease		coronary perfusion pressure
			cryo-poor plasma
CPIP	chronic pulmonary insufficiency of prematurity	CPPB	continuous positive pressure breathing
		CPPD	calcium pyrophosphate dihydrate
CPK	creatine phosphokinase (BB, MB, MM are isoenzymes)		cisplatin
		CP & PD	chest percussion and postural drainage
CPK-1	creatine phosphokinase MM fraction	CPPS	chronic pelvice pain syndrome
CPK-2	creatine phosphokinase MB fraction	CPPV	continuous positive pressure ventilation
CPK-BB	creatine phosphokinase BB fraction	CPQ	Conner's Parent Questionnaire
CPKD	childhood polycystic kidney disease	CPR	cardiopulmonary resuscitation
CPK-MB	creatine phosphokinase of muscle band		computer-based patient records
CPL	criminal procedure law		computerized patient record
CPM	cancer pain management		tablet (French)
	central pontine myelinolysis	CPR-1	all measures except cardiopulmonary resuscitation
	chlorpheniramine maleate		
	Clinical Practice Model		
	continue present management		
	continuous passive motion	CPR-2	no extraordinary measures (to resuscitate)
	counts per minute		
	cycles per minute	CPR-3	comfort measures only
	cyclophosphamide	CPRAM	controlled partial rebreathing anesthesia method
CPmax	peak serum concentration		
CPMDI	computerized pharmacokinetic model-driven drug infusion		
		CP/ROMI	chest pain, rule out myocardial infarction
CPmin	trough serum concentration	CPRS-OCS	Comprehensive Psychiatric Rating Scale, Obsessive-Compulsive Subscale
CPMM	constant passive motion machine		

C

CPS	carbamyl phosphate synthetase
	cardiopulmonary support
	chest pain syndrome
	child protective services
	Chinese paralytic syndrome
	chloroquine-pyrimethamine sulfadoxine
	clinical performance score
	clinical pharmacokinetic service
	coagulase-positive staphylococci
	complex partial seizures
	counts per second
	cumulative probability of success
CPs	clinical pathways
CPS I	carbamyl phosphate synthetase I
cPSA	complexed prostate-specific antigen
CPSC	Consumer Product Safety Commission
CPSI	Chronic Prostatitis Symptom Index
CPT	camptothecin
	carnitine palmitoyl transferase
	chest physiotherapy
	child protection team
	chromo-perturbation
	cold pressor test
	Continuous Performance Test
	current perception threshold
	Current Procedural Terminology (coding system)
CPT-2000	Current Procedural Terminology, 2000 Edition
CPT-11	irinotecan hydrochloride (Camptosar)
CPTA	Certified Physical Therapy Assistant

CPT/C	current perception threshold, computerized
CPTH	chronic post-traumatic headache
CPU	children's psychiatric unit
	clinical pharmacology unit
CPUE	chest pain of unknown etiology
CPUM	Certified Professional in Utilization Management
CPV	cowpox virus
CPX	complete physical examination
CPZ	chlorpromazine Compazine® (CPZ is a dangerous abbreviation as it could be either)
CQDS	cumulative quality disruption score
CQI	continuous quality improvement
CR	cardiac rehabilitation
	cardiorespiratory
	case reports
	chief resident
	chorioretinal
	clockwise rotation
	closed reduction
	colon resection
	complete remission
	contact record
	controlled release
	cosmetic rhinoplasty
	creamed
	crutches
	cycloplegia retinoscopy
Cr	chromium
C/R	conscious, rational
C & R	convalescence and rehabilitation
	cystoscopy and retrograde
CR$_1$	first cranial nerve
CRA	central retinal artery
	chronic rheumatoid arthritis
	cis-retinoic acid (isotretinion, Accutane®)

	Clinical Research Associate	
	colorectal anastomosis	
	corticosteroid-resistant asthma	
CRABP	cellular retinoic acid binding protein	
CRAbs	chelating recombinant antibodies	
CRADA	Cooperative Research and Development Agreement (with NIH)	
CRAG	cerebral radionuclide angiography	
CrAg	cryptococcal antigen	
CRAMS	circulation, respiration, abdomen, motor, and speech	
CRAN	craniotomy	
CRAO	central retinal artery occlusion	
CRAX	crackers	
CRBBB	complete right bundle branch block	
CRBP	cellular retinol-binding protein	
CRBSI	vascular-catheter-related bloodstream infections	
CRC	case review committee	
	child-resistant container	
	clinical research center	
	Clinical Research Coordinator	
	colorectal cancer	
CR & C	closed reduction and cast	
CrCl	creatinine clearance	
CRD	childhood rheumatic disease	
	chronic renal disease	
	chronic respiratory disease	
	colorectal distension	
	cone-rod dystrophy	
	congenital rubella deafness	
	crown-rump distance	
CRE	cumulative radiation effect	
CREAT	serum creatinine	
CREF	cycloplegic refraction	

CRELM	screening tests for Congo-Crimean, Rift Valley, Ebola, Lassa, and Marburg fevers
CREP	crepitation
CREST	calcinosis, Raynaud's disease, esophageal dysmotility, sclerodactyly, and telangiectasia
CRF	cardiac risk factors
	case report form
	chronic renal failure factor
CRH	corticotropic releasing hormone
CRFZ	closed reduction of fractured zygoma
CRH	corticotropin-releasing hormone
CRHCa	cancer-related hypercalcemia
CRI	Cardiac Risk Index
	catheter-related infection
	chronic renal insufficiency
CRIB	Clinical Risk Index for Babies
CRIE	crossed radioimmuno-electrophoresis
CRIF	closed reduction and internal fixation
CRIMF	closed reduction/intermaxillary fixation
CRIS	controlled-release infusion system
crit	hematocrit
CRKL	crackles
CRL	crown rump length
CRM	continual reassessment method
	cream
	cross-reacting mutant
CRM +	cross-reacting material positive
CRMD	children with retarded mental development
CRN	crown

CRNA	Certified Registered Nurse Anesthetist		congenital rubella syndrome
CRNH	Certified Registered Nurse in Hospice		continuous running suture cryoreductive surgery
CRNI	Certified Registered Nurse Intravenous	CRST	cytokine-release syndrome calcification, Raynaud's
CRNP	Certified Registered Nurse Practitioner		phenomenom, scleroderma, and telangiectasia
CRO	cathode ray oscilloscope contract research organization(s)	CRT	cadaver renal transplant capillary refill time Cardiac Rescue
CROM	cervical range of motion		Technician
CROS	contralateral routing of signals		cathode ray tube central reaction time Certified Rehabilitation
CRP	canalith repositioning procedure		Therapist copper reduction test
	chronic relapsing pancreatitis		cranial radiation therapy crutch training
	coronary rehabilitation program	Cr Tr CRTs	case report tabulations
	C-reactive protein	CRTT	Certified Respiratory
C&RP	curettage and root planning		Therapy Technician
CRPA	C-reactive protein agglutinins	CRTX CRU	cast removed take x-ray cardiac rehabilitation unit
CRPD	chronic restrictive pulmonary disease		clinical research unit
CRPF	chloroquine-resistant *Plasmodium falciparum*	CRV CRVF	central retinal vein congestive right ventricular failure
CRPS I	complex regional pain syndrome type I	CRVO	central retinal vein occlusion
CRQ	Chronic Respiratory (Disease) Questionnaire	CRx CIIRx	chemotherapy Century II Bicarbonate
CRR	community rehabilitation residence		Dialysis Machine
CRRT	continuous renal replacement therapy	CRYO	cryoablation cryosurgery
CRS	Carroll Self-Rating Scale	CRYST CS	crystals cardioplegia solution
	catheter-related sepsis		cat scratch
	Center for Scientific Review (NIH)		cervical spine cesarean section
	Chemical Reference Substances		chest strap cholesterol stone
	child restraint system(s)		chlorobenzylidene
	Chinese restaurant syndrome		malononitrile cigarette smoker
	chronic rhinosinusitis		clinically significant
	cocaine-related seizure(s)		clinical stage
	colon-rectal surgery		close supervision

	conditionally susceptible	C S&D	cleaned, sutured, and dressed
	congenital syphilis	CSDD	Center for the Study of Drug Development
	conjunctiva-sclera		
	consciousness	CSE	combined spinal/epidurals
	conscious sedation		cross-section
	consultation		echocardiography
	consultation service	C sect.	cesarean section
	coronary sinus	CSF	cerebrospinal fluid
	corticosteroid(s)		colony-stimulating factors
	cranial setting	CSFELP	cerebrospinal fluid electrophoresis
	Cushing's syndrome		
	cycloserine	CSFP	cerebrospinal fluid pressure
	o-chlorobenzylidene malononitrile		
C&S	conjunctiva and sclera	CSGIT	continuous-suture graft-inclusion technique
	cough and sneeze		
	culture and sensitivity	C-Sh	chair shower
C/S	cesarean section	CSH	carotid sinus hypersensitivity
	consultation		
	culture and sensitivity		chronic subdural hematoma
CSA	central sleep apnea	CSI	Computerized Severity Index
	compressed spectral activity		
			continuous subcutaneous infusion
	controlled substance analogue		coronary stent implantation
	corticosteroid-sensitive asthma		craniospinal irradiation
CsA	cyclosporine (cyclosporin A)	CsI	cesium iodide
CsA-ME	cyclosporine microemulsion (Neoral)	CSICU	cardiac surgery intensive care unit
CSAP	cryosurgical ablation of the prostate	CSID	congenital sucrase-isomaltase deficiency
CSB	caffeine sodium benzoate	CSII	continuous subcutaneous insulin infusion
	Cheyne-Stokes breathing	CS IV	clinical stage 4
	Children's Services Board	CSL	chemical safety level
CSBF	coronary sinus blood flow	CSLU	chronic status leg ulcer
CSBO	complete small bowel obstruction	CSM	carotid sinus massage
			cerebrospinal meningitis
CSC	cornea, sclera, and conjunctiva		cervical spondylotic myelopathy
	cryopreserved stem cells		circulation, sensation, and movement
CSCI	continuous subcutaneous infusion		Committee on Safety of Medicines (United Kingdom)
CSCR	central serous chorioretinopathy		
CSD	cat scratch disease	CSME	cotton-spot macular edema
	celiac sprue disease		

CSMN	chronic sensorimotor neuropathy	
CSN	cystic suppurative necrosis	
CSNB	congenital stationary night blindness	
CSNRT	corrected sinus node recovery time	
CSNS	carotid sinus nerve stimulation	
CSO	Consumer Safety Officer (FDA)	
	copied standing orders	
CSOM	chronic serous otitis media	
	chronic suppurative otitis media	
CSP	cellulose sodium phosphate	
	chiral stationary phase	
C-spine	cervical spine	
CSR	central supply room	
	Cheyne-Stokes respiration	
	corrected sedimentation rate	
	corrective septorhinoplasty	
C-S RT	craniospinal radiotherapy	
CSS	Canadian Stroke Scale (score)	
	carotid sinus stimulation	
	Central Sterile Services	
	chemical sensitivity syndrome	
	chewing, sucking, and swallowing	
	child safety seats	
	Churg-Strauss syndrome	
C_{SS}	concentration of drug at steady-state	
CSSD	closed system sterile drainage	
CST	cardiac stress test	
	castration	
	central sensory conducting time	
	cerebroside sulfotransferase	
	Certified Surgical Technologist	

	contraction stress test
	convulsive shock therapy
	cosyntropin stimulation test
	static compliance
C_{STAT}	static lung compliance
CSU	cardiac surgery unit
	cardiac surveillance unit
	cardiovascular surgery unit
	casualty staging unit
	catheter specimen of urine
CSW	Clinical Social Worker
CSWSS	continuous spike-waves during slow sleep
CT	calcitonin
	cardiothoracic
	carpal tunnel
	cellulose triacetate (filter)
	cervical traction
	chemotherapy
	chest tube
	circulation time
	client
	clinical trial
	clotting time
	coagulation time
	coated tablet
	compressed tablet
	computed tomography
	Coomb's test
	corneal thickness
	corneal transplant
	corrective therapy
	cytarabine and thioguanine
	cytoxic drug
C_t	concentration of drug in tissue
C/T	compared to
CTA	catamenia (menses)
	clear to auscultation
C-TAB	cyanide tablet
CTAP	clear to auscultation and percussion
	computed tomography during arterial portography
CTB	ceased to breathe

	cholera toxin B	CTM	Chlor-Trimeton®
CTC	Cancer Treatment Center		clinical trials materials
	circular tear capsulotomy		computed tomographic
	clinical trial certificate		myelography
	(United Kingdom's	CT/MPR	computed tomography
	equivalent to the		with multiplanar
	Investigational New		reconstructions
	Drug Application)	CTN	calcitonin
	Common Toxicity Criteria	C & T N,	color and temperature
	cyclophosphamide,	BLE	normal, both lower
	thiotepa, and		extremities
	carboplatin	cTnI	cardiac troponin I
CTCL	cutaneous T-cell	cTNM	clinical-diagnostic staging
	lymphoma (mycosis		of cancer
	fungoides)	CTP	comprehensive treatment
CT & DB	cough, turn & deep breath		plan
CTD	carpal tunnel	CTPA	clear to percussion and
	decompression		auscultation
	chest tube drainage	CTPN	central total parenteral
	connective tissue disease		nutrition
	corneal thickness depth	CTR	carpal tunnel release
	cumulative trauma		carpal tunnel repair
	disorder		Certified Tumor Registrar
CTDW	continues to do well		cosmetic transdermal
CTEP	Cancer Therapy		reconstruction
	Evaluation Program	CTRS	Certified Therapeutic
CTF	Colorado tick fever		Recreation Specialist
	continuous tube feeding		Conners Teachers Rating
C/TG	cholesterol to triglyceride		Scale
	ratio	CT-RT	chemo-radiotherapy
CTGA	complete transposition of	CTS	cardiothoracic surgeon
	the great arteries		carpal tunnel syndrome
	corrected transposition of	CTSP	called to see patient
	the great arteries	CTW	central terminal of Wilson
CTH	clot to hold	CTX	cerebrotendinous
CTHA	computed tomography		xanthomatosis
	hepatic arteriography		cervical traction
CTI	certification of terminal		chemotherapy
	illness		cyclophosphamide
CTICU	cardiothoracic intensive		(Cytoxan®)
	care unit	CTXN	contraction
CTID	chemotherapy-induced	CTZ	chemoreceptor trigger
	diarrhea		zone
CTL	cervical, thoracic, and		co-trimoxazole
	lumbar		(sulfamethoxazole and
	chronic tonsillitis		trimethoprin)
	cytotoxic T-lymphocytes	CU	cause undetermined
CTLSO	cervicothoracic-		cause unknown
	lumbosacral orthosis		chronic undifferentiated

C

	color unit	CVAT	costovertebral angle tenderness
	convalescent unit		
	Cuprophan (filter)	CVB	chronic villi biopsy
Cu	copper		group B coxsackievirus
C$_u$	urea clear clearance	CVC	central venous catheter
C/U	checkup		chief visual complaint
CUA	clean urinalysis		consonant vowel
	cost-utility analysis		consonant
CUC	chronic ulcerative colitis	CVD	cardiovascular disease
	Clinical Unit Clerk		collagen vascular disease
CUD	cause undetermined	CVDU	chronic ventilator-dependent unit
	controlled unsterile delivery		
		CVEB	cisplatin, vinblastine, etoposide, and bleomycin
CUFCM	Century Ultrafiltration Control Machine		
CUG	cystourethrogram	CVENT	controlled ventilation
Cu-IUD	copper intrauterine device	CVF	cardiovascular failure
CUP	carcinoma of unknown primary (site)		central visual field
			cervicovaginal fluid
CUPS	carcinoma of unknown primary site	CVG	coronary vein graft
		CVHD	chronic valvular heart disease
CUR	curettage		
	cystourethrorectocele	CVI	carboplatin, etoposide, ifosfamide, and mesna uroprotection
CUS	carotid ultrasound		
	chronic undifferentiated schizophrenia		cerebrovascular insufficiency
	contact urticaria syndrome		common variable immunodeficiency (disease)
CUSA	Cavitron ultrasonic suction aspirator		
CUT	chronic undifferentiated type (schizophrenia)		continuous venous infusion
CUTA	congenital urinary tract anomaly	CVICU	cardiovascular intensive care unit
CV	cardiovascular	CVID	common variable immune deficiency
	cell volume		
	cisplatin and etoposide	CVINT	cardiovascular intermediate
	coefficient of variation		
	color vision	CVL	central venous line
	common ventricle		clinical vascular laboratory
	consonant vowel		
	contrast venography	CVM	Center for Veterinary Medicine (NIH)
	curriculum vitae		
C/V	cervical/vaginal	CVMT	cervical-vaginal, motion tenderness
CVA	cerebrovascular accident		
	costovertebral angle	CVN	central venous nutrient
CVAD	central venous access device	CVNSR	cardiovascular normal sinus rhythm
CVAH	congenital virilizing adrenal hyperplasia	CVO	central vein occlusion

	conjugate diameter of pelvic inlet	CWA	chemical warfare agents
CvO_2	mixed venous oxygen content	CWAF	Chemical Withdrawal Assessment Flowsheet
CVOD	cerebrovascular obstructive disease	CWAP	continuous wave arthroscopy pump
CVOR	cardiovascular operating room	CWD	cell wall defective
		CWE	cotton-wool exudates
CVP	central venous pressure cyclophosphamide, vincristine, and prednisone	CWL	Caldwell-Luc
		CWMS	color, warmth, movement, and sensation
CVPP	lomustine, vinblastine, procarbazine, and prednisone	CWP	centimeters of water pressure childbirth without pain coal worker's pneumoconiosis cold wet packs
CVR	cerebral vascular resistance cerebrovascular resuscitation coronary vascular reserve	cWPW	concealed Wolff-Parkinson-White syndrome
CVRI	coronary vascular resistance index	CWR	clockwise rotation
CVS	cardiovascular surgery cardiovascular system challenge virus standard chorionic villi sampling clean voided specimen continuing vegetative state	CWS	Certified Wound Care Specialist comfortable walking speed cotton-wool spots
		CWT	compensated work training
CVSCU	cardiovascular special care unit	CWV	closed wound vacuum
		CX	cancel cervix chronic circumflex artery culture cylinder axis cystectomy
CVST	cardiovascular stress test cerebral venous sinus thrombosis		
CVSU	cardiovascular specialty unit		
CVT	calf vein thrombosis	CXA	circumflex artery
CVTC	central venous tunneled catheter	CxBx	cervical biopsy
		CxMT	cervical motion tenderness
CVU	clean voided urine	CXR	chest x-ray
CVUG	cysto-void urethrogram	CXTX	cervical traction
CVVH	continuous venovenous hemofiltration	CY	cyclophosphamide
		C&Y	Children with Youth (program)
CW	careful watch case worker chest wall clockwise compare with	CYA	cover your ass
		CyA	cyclosporine
C/W	consistent with crutch walking	CyADIC	cyclophosphamide, doxorubicin (Adriamycin), and dacarbazine

CYC	cyclophosphamide
Cyclo C	cyclocytidine HCl
CYL	cylinder
CYP	cytochrome P-450
CYP450	cytochrome P450 system
CYRO	cryoprecipitate
CYSTA	cystathionine
CYSTO	cystogram
	cystoscopy
CYT	cyclophosphamide
CYTA	cytotoxic agent
CYVA DIC	cyclophosphamide, vincristine, Adriamycin®, and dacarbazine
CZE	capillary zone electrophoresis
CZI	crystalline zinc insulin (regular insulin)
CZP	clonazepam (Klonopin)

D

D	daughter
	day
	dead
	decay
	depression
	dextrose
	dextro
	diarrhea
	diastole
	dilated
	diminished
	Dinamap (blood pressure monitor)
	diopter
	distal
	distance
	divorced
D+	note has been dictated/ look for report
D−	note not dictated, save chart for doctor
$D_{0(2/7/00)}$	Day zero (the day treatment begins, February 7th, 2000)
D_1	day one (first day of treatment)
D-1 . . . . D-12	dorsal vertebrae 1 to 12 dorsal nerves 1-12
D_1	first diagonal branch (coronary artery)
D_2	second diagonal branch (coronary artery) ergocalciferol
2/d	twice a day (this is a dangerous abbreviation)
2-D	two-dimensional
3-D	three-dimensional
D_3	cholecalciferol
D-3+7	cytarabine and daunorubicin
4D	4 prism diopters
4-D	four-dimensional
D5	dextrose 5% injection

5xD	five times a day (this is a dangerous abbreviation)	DAE	diving air embolism
		DAF	decay-accelerating factor
D-15	Farnsworth panel D-15 color vision test		delayed auditory feedback
		DAFE	Dial-A-Flow Extension®
D50	50% dextrose injection	DAFM	double aerosol face mask
D$_{5/.45}$	dextrose 5% in 0.45% sodium chloride injection	DAG	diacylglyerol dianhydrogalactitol
		DAH	diffuse alveolar hemorrhage
DA	dark adaptation (test)		
	Debtors Anonymous		disordered action of the heart
	degenerative arthritis		
	delivery awareness	DAI	diffuse axonal injury
	Dental Assistant	DAL	diffuse aggressive lymphomas
	diagnostic arthroscopy		
	diastolic augmentation		drug analysis laboratory
	direct admission	DALE	disability-adjusted life expectancy
	direct agglutination		
	diversional activity	DALM	dysplasia-associated lesion or mass
	dopamine		
	drug addict	DALY	disability-adjusted life year(s)
	drug aerosol		
Da	daltons	DAM	diacetylmonoxine
D/A	discharge and advise	DAMA	discharged against medical advice
DAA	dead after arrival		
	dissection aortic aneurysm	DANA	drug induced antinuclear antibodies
DA/A	drug/alcohol addiction		
DAB	days after birth	DAo	descending aorta
	diamino benzidine	DAOM	depressor anguli oris muscle
DABA	Diplomate of the American Board of Anesthesiology		
		DAP	dapsone
			diabetes-associated peptide
DAC	day activity center		
	disabled adult child		diastolic augmentation pressure
	Division of Ambulatory Care		
			distending airway pressure
DACL	Depression Adjective Checklists		
			Draw-A-Person
DACS	density-adjusted cell sorting	DAPT	Draw-A-Person Test
		DAR	daily affective rhythm
DACT	dactinomycin (Cosmegen)		data, action, response
DAD	diffuse alveolar damage	DARE	data, action, response, and evaluation
	diode array detector		
	dispense as directed	DARP	drug abuse rehabilitation program
	drug administration device		
	father		drug abuse reporting program
DADS	distal acquired demyelinating symmetrical (neuropathy)	D/ART	depression/awareness, recognition and treatment

D

DAS	day of admission surgery	DBED	penicillin G benzathine
	developmental apraxia of speech	dBEMCL	decibel effective masking contralateral
	died at scene	D₅BES	dextrose in balanced
DAs	daily activities		electrolyte solution
DASE	dobutamine-atropine stress echocardiography	DBI®	phenformin HCl
		DBIL	direct bilirubin
DASH	Dietary Approaches to Stop Hypertension (diet)	DBKT	Diabetes: Basic Knowledge Test
		DBL	double beta-lactam
DAST	Drug Abuse Screening Test	DBM	dibenzoylmethane
		DBMT	displacement bone marrow transplantation
DAT	daunorubicin, cytarabine, (ara-C), and thioguanine	DBP	D-binding protein
	definitely abnormal tracing (electrocardiogram)		diastolic blood pressure dibutyl phthalate
	dementia of the Alzheimer type	DBPCFC	double-blind, placebo-controlled food challenge
	diet as tolerated		
	diphtheria antitoxin	DBPT	dacarbazine (DTIC),
	direct agglutination test		carmustine (BCNU),
	direct amplification test		cisplatin (Platinol), and
	direct antiglobulin test		tamoxifen
DAU	daughter	DBQ	debrisoquin
	drug abuse urine	DBS	deep brain stimulation
DAUNO	daunorubicin		desirable body weight
DAVA	vindesine sulfate (Eldisine; desacetyl vinblastine amide sulfate)		diminished breath sounds
			dried blood stain
		DBW	dry body weight
		DBZ	dibenzamine
DAV SEP	deviated septum	DC	daunorubicin and cytarabine
DAW	dispense as written		daycare
DAWN	Drug Abuse Warning Network		decrease
dB	decibel		dextrocardia
DB	database		diagonal conjugate
	date of birth		direct Coombs (test)
	deep breathe		discharge
	demonstration bath		discomfort
	dermabrasion		Doctor of Chiropractic
	diaphragmatic breathing	D&C	dilation and curettage
	difficulty breathing		direct and consensual
	direct bilirubin	D/C	disconnect
	double blind		discontinue
DB & C	deep breathing and coughing	DCA	directional coronary atherectomy
DBD	milolactol (dibromodulicitol)		disk/condyle adhesion double cup arthroplasty
DBE	deep breathing exercise		sodium dichloroacetate

94

DCAG	double coronary artery graft	DCMXT	dichloromethotrexate
		DCN	Darvocet N®
DCAP-BTLS	deformities, contusions, abrasions, and punctures/penetrations, burns, tenderness, lacerations, and swelling (an assessment mnemonic used by EMTs)	DCNU	chlorozotocin
		DCO	diffusing capacity of carbon monoxide
		DCP	dynamic compression plate
		DCP®	calcium phosphate, dibasic
		DCPM	daunorubicin, cytarabine, prednisolone, and mercaptopurine
DC-ART	disease controlling anti-rheumatic therapy		
DC&B	dilation, currettage, and biopsy	DCPN	direction-changing positional nystagmus
DCBE	double contrast barium enema	DCR	dacryocystorhinostomy delayed cutaneous reaction
DCC	day care center diabetes care clinic direct current cardioversion	DCRF	data case report forms
		3DCRT	three-dimensional conformal radiation therapy
DCCF	dural carotid-cavernous fistula	DCS	decompression sickness dorsal column stimulator
DCCT	Diabetes Control and Complications Trial (questionnaire)	DCSA	double contrast shoulder arthrography
DC'd	discontinued	DCT	daunorubicin, cytarabine, and thioguanine deep chest therapy direct (antiglobulin) Coombs test
DCE	delayed contrast-enhancement designated compensable event		
		DCTM	delay computer tomographic myelography
DCF	data collection form Denomination Commune Francaise (French-approved nonproprietary name) pentostatin (Nipent; 2′ deoxycoformycin)	DCU	day care unit
		DCUS	duplex color ultrasonography
		DCW	direct care worker
DCFS	Department of Children and Family Services	DCYS	Department of Children and Youth Services
DCG	diagnostic cardiogram	DD	delayed diarrhea delivery date dependent drainage Descemet's detachment detrusor dyssynergia developmentally delayed developmental disabilities developmentally disabled dialysis dementia died of the disease
DCH	delayed cutaneous hypersensitivity		
DCIA	deep circumflex iliac artery (flap)		
DCIS	ductal carcinoma *in situ*		
DCLHb	diaspirin cross-linked hemoglobin		
DCM	dementia care mapping dilated cardiomyopathy		

D

	differential diagnosis	DDRA	dead despite resuscitation attempt
	discharge diagnosis		
	disk diameter	DDS	dialysis disequilibrium syndrome
	Doctor of Divinity		
	double dose (used by Radiology)		Doctor of Dental Surgery
	down drain		double decidual sac (sign)
	dry dressing		4, 4-diaminodiphenyl-sulfone (dapsone)
	dual disorder		
	Duchenne's dystrophy	DDST	Denver Development Screening Test
	due date		
D/D	diarrhea/dehydration	DDT	chlorophenothane
D → D	discharge to duty	DDTP	drug dependence treatment program
D & D	debridement and dressing		
	diarrhea and dehydration	DDx	differential diagnosis
	drilling and drainage	DE	dermal epidermal (junction)
DDA	dideoxyadenosine		
DDAVP®	desmopressin acetate		digitalis effect
DDC	zalcitabine (dideoxy-cytidine; Hivid)	D_5E_{48}	5% Dextrose and Electrolyte 48
DDD	defined daily doses	D_5E_{75}	5% Dextrose and Electrolyte 75
	degenerative disk disease		
	dense deposit disease	2-DE	two-dimensional echocardiography
	fully automatic pacing		
DDDR	pacemaker code (D = chamber paced-**d**ual, D = chamber sensed-**d**ual, D = response to sensing-**d**ual, R = programmability-**r**ate modulation)	3-DE	three-dimensional echocardiography
		D&E	dilation and evacuation
		DEA#	Drug Enforcement Administration number (physician's federal narcotic number)
DDE	dichlorodiphenylethylene	DEAE	diethylaminoethyl
DDGB	double-dose gallbladder (test)	DEB	diepoxybutane (test)
			dystrophic epidermolysis bullosa
DDH	developmental dysplasia of the hip	DEC	deciduous (primary teeth)
			decrease
DDHT	double dissociated hypertropia		diethylcarbamazine (Hetrazan)
DDI	didanosine (dideoxyinosine; Videx)		Drug Evaluation and Classification (a standardized curriculum to train police officers)
	dressing dry, intact		
DDIs	drug-drug interactions		
DDis	developmental disorder	DECA	nandrolone decanoate
DDMC	diabetes disease management clinic	DECAFS	Department of Children and Family Services
DDNS	digestive disease and nutrition service	DECEL	deceleration
		decub	decubitus
DDP	cisplatin	DED	diabetic eye disease

	died in emergency department	DEVR	duck embryo vaccine dominant exudative vitreoretinopathy
DEEDS	drugs, exercise, education, diet, and self-monitoring	DEX	dexamethasone
DEEG	depth electroencephalogram		dexter (right)
	deteriorating electroencephalogram		dexverapamil
DEET	diethyltoluamide	DEXA	dual-energy x-ray absorptiometry
DEF	decayed, extracted, or filled	DF	day frequency (of voiding)
	defecation		decayed and filled
	deficiency		deferred
2-DEF	two-dimensional echo-derived ejection fraction		defibrotide
DEFT	defendant		degree of freedom
	driven equilibrium Fourier transform (technique)		dengue fever
			dexfenfluramine
DEG	diethylene glycol		diabetic father
degen	degenerative		diastolic filling
DEHP	diethylhexyl phthalate		dietary fiber
DEL	delivered		dorsiflexion
	delivery		drug free
	deltoid		dye free
DEM	drug evaluation matrix	DFA	delayed feedback audiometry
DEMRI	dynamic enhanced magnetic resonance imaging		diet for age
			difficulty falling asleep
DEP ST SEG	depressed ST segment		direct fluorescent antibody
			distal forearm
DER	disulfiram-ethanol reaction	DFD	defined formula diets
			degenerative facet disease
DERM	dermatology	DFE	dilated fundus examination
DES	desflurane (Supreme)		distal femoral epiphysis
	diethylstilbestrol	DFG	direct forward gaze
	diffuse esophageal spasm	DFI	disease-free interval
	disequilibrium syndrome	DFLE	disability-free life expectancy
	Dissociative Experience Scale	DFM	decreased fetal movement
	dry eye syndrome		deep finger massage
DESAT	desaturation		deep friction massage
DESF	desflurane (Suprane)	DFMC	daily fetal movement count
DESI	Drug Efficacy Study Implementation	DFMO	eflornithine (difluoro-methylornithine)
DET	diethyltryptamine	DFMR	daily fetal movement record
	dipyridamole echocardiography test		
DETOX	detoxification	DFO	deferoxamine (Desferal)
DEV	deviation	DFOM	deferoxamine (Desferal)

DFP	diastolic filling period isofluorophate (diisopropyl fluorophosphate)	DHANP	Diplomate of the Homeopathic Academy of Naturopathic Physicians
DFR	diabetic floor routine		
DFRC	deglycerolized frozen red cells	DHAP	dexamethasone, high-dose cytarabine, (ara-A) cisplatin (Platinol AQ)
DFS	disease-free survival		
	Division of Family Services	DHBV	duck hepatitis B virus
		DHCA	deep hypothermia circulatory arrest
	Doppler flow studies		
DFSP	dermatofibrosarcoma protuberans	DHCC	dihydroxycholecalciferol
		DHD	dissociated horizontal deviation
DFU	dead fetus in uterus		
	diabetic foot ulcer	DHE 45®	dihydroergotamine mesylate
DFV	D'Aoust Fineman virus		
	dengue fever vaccine	DHEA	dehydroepiandrosterone
	diarrhea, fever, and vomiting	DHEAS	dehydroepiandrosterone sulfate
DFW	Dexide face wash	DHF	dengue hemorrhagic fever
DFWO	dorsiflexory wedge osteotomy		
		DHFR	dihydrofolate reductase
DG	diagnosis	DHHS	Department of Health and Human Services
	dorsal glides		
	downward gaze	DHI	Dizziness Handicap Inventory
DGA	DiGeorge anomaly		
DGE	delayed gastric emptying		dynamic hyperinflation
DGF	delayed graft function	DHIC	detrusor hyperactivity with impaired contractility
DGGE	denaturing gradient gel electrophoresis		
DGI	disseminated gonococcal infection	DHL	diffuse histocytic lymphoma
DGL	deglycyrrhizinated licorice	DHP	dihydropyridine
DGR	duodenogastric reflux	DHP-1	dehydropeptidase-1
DGM	ductal glandular mastectomy	DHPG	ganciclovir
		DHPLC	denaturing high-performance liquid chromatography
DH	delayed hypersensitivity		
	Dental Hygienist		
	dermatitis herpetiformis	DHPR	dihydropteridine reductase
	developmental history	DHPS	dihydopteroate synthase
	diaphragmatic hernia	DHR	delayed hypersensitivity reaction
D+H	delusions and hallucinations		
		DHS	Department of Human Services
D-H	Dimon-Hughston (intertrochanteric osteotomy technique)		
			duration of hospital stay
			dynamic hip screw
DHA	dihydroxyacetone	DHST	delayed hypersensitivity test
	docosahexaenoic acid		
DHAC	dihydro-5-azacytidine	DHT	dihydrotachysterol
DHAD	mitoxanthrone HCl		dihydrotestosterone

	dissociated hypertropia	DICC	dynamic infusion
	Dobhoff tube		cavernosometry and
DHTF	Dobhoff tube		cavernosography
	feeding	DICE	dexamethasone,
DI	(Beck) Depression		ifosfamide, cisplatin,
	Inventory		and etopside, with
	date of injury		mesna
	Debrix Index	DICLOX	dicloxacillin
	detrusor instability	DICP	demyelinated
	diabetes insipidus		inflammatory chronic
	diagnostic imaging		polyneuropathy
	dorsal interossei	DICT	dose-intensive
	drug interactions		chemotherapy
D&I	debridement and irrigation	DID	death(s) from intercurrent
	dry and intact		disease
DIA	drug-induced		delayed ischemia deficit
	agranulocytosis		dissociative identity
	drug-induced amenorrhea		disorder
diag.	diagnosis		drug-induced disease
DIAP-	(causes of transient	di,di	dichorionic, diamniotic
PERS	incontinence)	DIE	died in emergency
	delirium/confusion,		department
	infection, (urinary),		drug-induced esophagitis
	atrophic	DIED	died in emergency
	urethritis/vaginitis,		department
	pharmaceuticals,	DIF	differentiation-inducing
	psychological,		factor
	excessive excretion	DIFF	differential blood count
	(e.g., CHF,	DIG	digoxin (this is a
	hyperglycemia)		dangerous abbreviation)
	restricted mobility, and	DIH	died in hospital
	stool impaction	DIJOA	dominantly inherited
DIAS	diastolic		juvenile optic atrophy
DIAS BP	diastolic blood pressure	DIL	daughter-in-law
Diath SW	diathermy short wave		dilute
DIAZ	diazepam		drug-induced lupus
DIB	disability insurance	DILC	dose-intensity limiting
	benefits		criterium
DIBC	drug-induced blood	DILD	diffuse infiltrative lung
	cytopenias		disease
DIBS	dead-in-bed syndrome		drug-induced liver
DIC	dacarbazine (DTIC-Dome)		disease
	diagnostic imaging	DILE	drug-induced lupus
	center		erythematosus
	differential interference	DILS	drug-induced lupus
	contrast		syndrome
	disseminated intravascular	DIM	diminish
	coagulation	D₅IMB	Ionosol MB with 5%
	drug information center		dextrose injection

DIMD	drug-induced movement disorders	DISIDA	diisopropyl iminodiacetic acid
DIMOAD	diabetes insipidus, diabetes mellitus, optic atrophy, and deafness	D₅ISOM	5% Dextrose and Isolyte M
		D₅ISOP	5% Dextrose and Isolyte P
DIMS	disorders of initiating and maintaining sleep	DISR	drug-induced skin reactions
DIND	delayed ischemic neurologic deficit	DIST	distal distilled
DIOS	distal ileal obstruction syndrome distal intestinal obstruction syndrome	DIT	diiodotyrosine drug-induced thrombocytopenia
DIP	desquamative interstitial pneumonia diphtheria toxoid vaccine diplopia distal interphalangeal drip infusion pyelogram drug-induced parkinsonism	DIU	death in utero
		DIV	double inlet ventricle
		DIVA	digital intravenous angiography
		Div ex	divergence excess
		DIVP	dilute intravenous Pitocin
		DJD	degenerative joint disease
DIPₐₙₜ	diphtheria antitoxin	DK	dark
DIPC	dynamic infusion pharmacocavemosometry		diabetic ketoacidosis diseased kidney
DIPJ	distal interphalangeal joint	DKA	diabetic ketoacidosis didn't keep appointment
DIR	directions	DKB	deep knee bends
DIRD	drug-induced renal disease	DKC	double knee to chest dyskeratosis congenita
DIS	Diagnostic Interview Schedule (questionnaire) digital imaging spectrophotometer dislocation	D-K-S	Damus-Kaye-Stansel (operation/procedure)
		dl	deciliter (100 mL)
		DL	danger list deciliter diagnostic laparoscopy direct laryngoscopy drug level
DISC	disabled infectious single cycle (virus) dynamic integrated stabilization chair	D_L	maximal diffusing capacity
		DLB	dementia with Lewy bodies direct laryngoscopy and bronchoscopy
disch.	discharge		
DISCUS	Dyskinesia Identification System Condensed User Scale	DLBCL	diffuse large B-cell lymphoma
DISH	diffuse idiopathic skeletal hyperostosis	DLBD	diffuse Lewy body disease
DISI	dorsal intercalated segmental (segment) instability	DLBL	diffuse large B-cell lymphoma
		DLC	double lumen catheter

DLCL	diffuse large cell lymphoma		dermatomyositis
DLCO sb	diffusion capacity of carbon monoxide, single breath		dextromethorphan
			diabetes mellitus
			diabetic mother
			diastolic murmur
DLD	date of last drink	DM-1	diabetes mellitus type 1
DLE	discoid lupus erythematosus	DM-2	diabetes mellitus type 2
		DMA	Director of Medical Affairs
	disseminated lupus erythematosis	DMAC	*Mycobacterium avium-intracellulare* complex
DLF	digitalis-like factor		
DLI	donor leukocyte infusions	DMAD	disease-modifying antirheumatic drug
DLIF	digoxin-like immunoreactive factors	DMAE	dimethylaminoethanol
		DMAIC	disseminated *Mycobacterium avium-intracellulare* complex
DLIS	digoxin-like immunoreactive substance		
		DMARD	disease modifying antirheumatic drug
DLMP	date of last menstrual period	DMAS	Drug Management and Authorization Section
DLNG	dl-norgestrel		
DLNMP	date of last normal menstrual period	DMAT	disaster medical assistance team
DLP	dislocation of patella	DMB	data monitoring board
	double-limb progression	DMBA	dimethylbenzanthracene
DLPD	diffuse lymphocytic poorly differentiated	DMC	dactinomycin, methotrexate, and cyclophosphamide
DLPFC	dorsolateral prefrontal cortex		diabetes management center
D5LR	dextrose 5% in lactated Ringer's injection	DMD	disciform macular degeneration
DLROW	a test used in mental status examinations (patient is asked to spell WORLD backwards)		Doctor of Dental Medicine
			drowsiness monitoring device
			Duchenne's muscular dystrophy
DLS	daily living skills	DMD w/ SRNM	disciform macular degeneration with subretinal neovascular membrane
	digitalis-like substances		
	dynamic light scattering		
DLSC	double lumen subclavian catheter	DME	diabetic macular edema
			Director of Medical Education
DLST	drug-induced lymphocyte stimulation test		durable medical equipment
DLT	dose-limiting toxicity		
	double-lung transplant		
DLU	diffused lung uptake		
DLV	delavirdine (Rescriptor)		
DM	dehydrated and malnourished	DMEM	Dulbecco's Modified Eagle Medium

DMF	decayed, missing, or filled	D₅ 1/2NS	dextrose 5% in 0.45%
	dimethylformamide		sodium chloride
	Drug Master File		injection
DMFS	decayed, missing, or filled	DNA	deoxyribonucleic acid
	surfaces		did not answer
DMH	Department of Mental		did not attend
	Health		does not apply
DMI	desipramine (Norpramin)	DNA ds	deoxyribonucleic acid
	diaphragmatic myocardial		double strand
	infarction	DNA ss	deoxyribonucleic acid
DM Isch	diaphragmatic myocardial		single strand
	ischemia	DNCB	dinitrochlorobenzene
DMKA	diabetes mellitus	DNC	did not come
	ketoacidosis	DND	died a natural death
DMO	dimethadone	DNE	diabetes nurse educator
DMOOC	diabetes mellitus out of	DNEPTE	did not exist prior to
	control		enlistment
DMP	dimethyl phthalate	DNET	dysembryoplastic
DMPA	depot-medroxypro-		neuroepithelial tumor
	gesterone acetate	DNFC	does not follow
DMPC	dimyristoylphosphatidyl		commands
	choline	DNI	do not intubate
DMPG	dimyristoylphosphatidyl	DNIC	diffuse noxious inhibitory
	glycerol		control
DMPS	dimercaptopropane-	DNIF	duties not including flying
	sulfonic acid	DNKA	did not keep appointment
D-MRI	dynamic magnetic	DNN	did not nurse
	resonance imaging	DNP	did not pay
DMS	dimethylsulfide		dinitrophenylhydrazine
DMSA	succimer		do not publish
	(dimercaptosuccinic acid)	DNR	daunorubicin
DMSO	dimethyl sulfoxide		did not respond
DMT	dimethyltryptamine		do not report
DMV	disk, macula, and vessels		do not resuscitate
	Doctor of Veterinary		dorsal nerve root
	Medicine	DNS	deviated nasal septum
DMVP	disk, macula, vessel,		Director of Nursing
	periphery		Services
DMX	diathermy, massage, and		doctor did not see
	exercise		patient
DN	denuded		do not show
	diabetic nephropathy		dysplastic nevus
	dicrotic notch		syndrome
	down	D₅ 1/4 NS	dextrose 5% in 1/4 normal
	dysplastic nevus (nevi)		saline (0.225% sodium
D & N	distance and near (vision)		chloride) injection
D5NS	dextrose 5% in 0.9%	D₅NS	5% dextrose in normal
	sodium chloride		saline (0.9% sodium
	injection		chloride) injection

DNT	did not test	DOLV	double-outlet left ventricle
DO	diet order		
	dissolved oxygen	DOM	Doctor of Oriental Medicine
	distocclusal		
	Doctor of Osteopathy		domiciliary
	doctor's order		domiciliary care
D/O	disorder	DON	Director of Nursing
✓DO	check doctor's order	DOOC	diabetes out of control
DO₂	oxygen delivery	DOP	dopamine
DOA	date of admission	DOPS	diffuse obstructive pulmonary syndrome
	dead on arrival		
	dominant optic atrophy		dihydroxyphenylserine
	driver of automobile		Director of Pharmacy Service(s)
	duration of action		
DOA-DRA	dead on arrival despite resuscitative attempts	DOR	date of release
		DORV	double-outlet right ventricle
DOB	dangle out of bed		
	date of birth	DORx	date of treatment
	Dobrava hantavirus	DOS	date of surgery
	dobutamine		doctor's order sheet
	doctor's order book	DOSA	day of surgery admission
DOC	date of conception		
	diabetes out of control	DOSAK	Central Tumor Registry operated by the German-Austrian-Swiss Association for Head and Neck Tumors
	died of other causes		
	diet of choice		
	drug of choice		
DOCA	desoxycorticosterone acetate		
		DOSS	docusate sodium (dioctyl sodium sulfosuccinate)
DOCP	desoxycorticosterone pivalate		
		DOT	date of transcription
DOD	date of death		date of transfer
	dead of disease		died on table
	Department of Defense		directly observed therapy
	drug overdose		
DODD	demand oxygen delivery device		Directory of Occupational Titles
DOE	date of examination		Doppler ophthalmic test
	disease-oriented evidence	DOTS	directly observed treatment, short course
	dyspnea on exertion		
DOES	disorders of excessive somnolence	DOV	date of visit
			distribution of ventilation
DOH	Department of Health	DOX	doxepin
DOI	date of implant (pacemaker)		doxorubicin (Adriamycin)
		doz	dozen
	date of injury	DP	dental prosthesis
DO₂I	oxygen delivery index		diastolic pressure
DOJ	Department of Justice		disability pension
DOL	days of life		discharge planning
DOL #2	second day of life		dorsalis pedis (pulse)

D

103

DPA	Department of Public Assistance	DPOA	durable power of attorney
	dipropylacetic acid	DPOAHC	durable power of attorney for health care
	dual photon absorptiometry	DPP	dorsalis pedal pulse
	durable power of attorney		duration of positive pressure
DPAP	diastolic pulmonary artery pressure	DPPC	colfosceril palmitate (dipalmitoylphosphati-dylcholine)
DPB	days postburn		
DPBS	Dulbecco's phosphate-buffered saline	DPR	Department of Professional Regulation
DPC	delayed primary closure		diagnostic procedure room
	discharge planning coordinator	DPS	disintegration per second
	distal palmar crease	DPSS	Department of Public Social Service
DPD	dihydropyrimidine dehydrogenase	DPsy	Doctor of Psychology
DPDL	diffuse poorly differentiated lymphocytic lymphoma	DPT	Demerol®, Phenergan®, and Thorazine® (this is a dangerous abbreviation)
2,3-DPG	2,3-diphosphoglyceric acid		diphtheria, pertussis, and tetanus (immunization)
DPH	Department of Public Health		Driver Performance Test
	diphenhydramine (Benadryl)	DPTPM	diphtheria, pertussis, tetanus, poliomyelitis, and measles
	Doctor of Public Health		
	phenytoin (diphenylhydantoin)	DPU	delayed pressure urticaria
DPI	dietary protein intake	DPUD	duodenal peptic ulcer disease
	Doppler perfusion index	DPVSs	dilated perivascular spaces
	dry powder inhaler		
DPIL	dextrose (percentage), protein (grams per kilogram) Intralipid® (grams per kilogram)	DPXA	dual-photon x-ray absorptiometry
		D/Q	deep quiet
		D&Q	deep and quiet
DPL	diagnostic peritoneal lavage	DQOL	diabetes quality of life
		Dr	doctor
D5PLM	dextrose 5% and Plasmalyte M® injection	DR	delivery room
			diabetic retinopathy
			diagnostic radiology
DPM	distintegrations per minute (dpm)		dining room
			diurnal rhythm
	Doctor of Podiatric Medicine		drug resistant
		DRA	distal rectal adenocarcinoma
	drops per minute		
DPN	¹¹C-diprenorphine		drug-related admissions
	diabetic peripheral neuropathy	DRAPE	drug-related adverse patient event

DRC	dose-response curve	D/S	5% dextrose and 0.9% sodium chloride (saline) injection
DRE	digital rectal examination		
	Drug Recognition Expert (for detection of impaired drivers)	D&S	diagnostic and surgical dilation and suction
DRESS	depth resolved surface coil spectroscopy	D5S	dextrose 5% in 0.9% sodium chloride (saline) injection
DREZ	dorsal root entry zone		
DRG	diagnosis-related groups	D_5-1/2S	5% dextrose in 0.45% sodium chloride (saline) injection
	dorsal root ganglia		
DRGE	drainage		
DRI	defibrillation response interval	DSA	digital subtraction angiography (angiocardiography)
	Discharge Readiness Index		
	dopamine reuptake inhibitor	DSAP	disseminated superficial actinic porokeratosis
DRM	drug-related morbidity	DSB	drug-seeking behavior
DRN	drug-related neutropenia	DSBs	double strand (DNA) breaks
DRP	drug-related problem		
DRPLA	dentatorubral-pallidolluysian atrophy	DSC	differential scanning calorimeter
			Down syndrome child
DRR	drug regimen review	DSD	digital selenium drum (radiology)
DRS	Disability Rating Scale		
	disease-related symptoms		discharge summary dictated
	Duane's retraction syndrome		dry sterile dressing
DRSG	dressing	DSDB	direct self-destructive behavior
DRSI	disease-related symptom improvement	DSF	doxorubicin, streptozocin, and fluorouracil
DRSP	drug-resistant *Streptococcus pneumoniae*	DSG	desogestrel
			dressing
		DSG	deoxyspergualin
DRT	drug-related thrombocytopenia	DSHEA	Dietary Supplement Health and Education Act of 1994
DRUB	drug screen-blood		
DRUJ	distal or radial ulnar joint	DSHR	delayed skin hypersensitivity reaction
dRVVT	diluted Russell viper venom time	DSHS	Department of Social and Health Services
DS	deep sleep	DSI	deep shock insulin
	Dextrostix®		Depression Status Inventory
	discharge summary		
	disoriented	DSIAR	double-stapled ileoanal reservoir
	distant supervision		
	double strength	DSM	disease state management
	Down syndrome		drink skim milk
	drug screen		

DSM-IV	Diagnostic and Statistical Manual of Mental Disorders, 4th edition	DSWI	deep sternal wound infection
DSMB	Data and Safety Monitoring Board		deep surgical wound infection
DSO	distal-lateral subungual onychomycosis	DT	delirium tremens
DSP	digital signal processor		dietary thermogenesis
DSPC	distearoylphosphatidyl choline		dietetic technician
			diphtheria and tetanus toxoids, adsorbed, pediatric strength
D-SPINE	dorsal spine		discharge tomorrow
DSPN	distal symmetric polyneuropathy		docetaxel (Taxotere)
DSPS	delayed sleep phase syndrome	D/T	date/time
		d/t	due to
DSRCT	desmoplastic small round cell tumor	d4T	stavudine (Zerit)
		D & T	diagnosis and treatment
DSRF	drainage subretinal fluid		dictated and typed
DSS	dengue shock syndrome	DTaP	diphtheria and tetanus toxoids with acellular pertussis vaccine
	Department of Social Services		
	Disability Status Scale	DTBC	tubocurarine (D-tubocurarine)
	discharge summary sheet	DTBE	Division of Tuberculosis Elimination
	disease-specific survival	DTC	day treatment center
	distal splenorenal shunt		diticarb (diethyldithio-carbamate)
	docusate sodium (dioctyl sodium sulfosuccinate)		tubocurarine (D-tubocurarine)
DSSLR	double, seated straight leg raise	DTD #30	dispense 30 such doses
DSSN	distal symmetric sensory neuropathy	DTF	deep transverse friction
		DTH	delayed-type hypersensitivity
DSSP	distal symmetric sensory polyneuropathy	DTI	diffusion-tensor imaging
DSST	Digit-Symbol Substitution Test	DTIC	dacarbazine (DTIC-Dome)
DST	daylight saving time	D TIME	dream time
	dexamethasone suppression test	DTM	deep tissue massage
			dermatophyte test medium
	digit substitution test	DTO	danger to others
	donor-specific (blood) transfusion		deodorized tincture of opium (warning: this is *NOT* paregoric)
DSU	day stay unit		
	day surgery unit	DTOGV	dextral-transposition of great vessels
DSUH	direct suggestion under hypnosis	DTP	differential time to positivity
DSV	digital subtraction ventriculography		

D

	diphtheria, tetanus toxoids, pertussis (antigens unspecified) vaccine	D&UE	dilation and uterine evacuation
	distal tingling on percussion (+Tinel's sign)	DUF	Doppler ultrasonic flowmeter
DTPA	pentetic acid (diethylenetriaminepen-taacetic acid)	DUI	driving under the influence
		DUID	driving under the influence of drugs
DTP$_a$	diphtheria, tetanus toxoids, acellular pertussis vaccine	DUII	driving under the influence of intoxicants
DTP$_w$	diphtheria, tetanus toxoids, whole-cell pertussis vaccine	DUIL	driving under the influence of liquor
		DUKM	dialysate urea kinetic modeling
DTR	deep tendon reflexes Dietetic Technician Registered	DUM	drug use monitoring
		DUN	dialysate urea nitrogen
DTs	delirium tremens	DUNHL	diffuse undifferentiated non-Hodgkins lymphoma
DTS	danger to self donor specific transfusion	DUO	Duotube®
3D TSE	three-dimensional turbo-spin echo (images)	DUR	drug utilization review duration
DTT	diphtheria tetanus toxoid dithiothreitol	DUS	digital ultrasound distal urethral stenosis Doppler ultrasound stethoscope
DTUS	diathermy, traction, and ultrasound	3DUS	three-dimensional ultrasound
DVG	double vein graft	DUSN	diffuse unilateral subacute neuroretinitis
DTV	due to void		
DTVP	Developmental Test of Visual Perception	DV	distance vision double vision
DTwP	diphtheria and tetanus toxoids with whole-cell pertussis vaccine	D&V	diarrhea and vomiting disks and vessels
DTX	detoxification	DVA	Department of Veterans Affairs directional vacuum-assisted (biopsy) distance visual acuity vindesine (Eldisine; desacetyl vinblastine amide sulfate)
DU	decubitus ulcer developmental unit diabetic urine diagnosis undetermined duodenal ulcer duroxide uptake		
DUB	Dubowitz (score) dysfunctional uterine bleeding	DVC	direct visualization of vocal cords
DUD	dihydrouracil dehydrogenase	D V® Cream	dienestrol vaginal cream
DUE	drug use evaluation	DVD	dissociated vertical deviation

	double vessel disease	D70W	70% dextrose (in water) injection
DVI	atrioventricular sequential pacing	5 DW	5% dextrose (in water) injection
	digital vascular imaging	DWDL	diffuse well-differentiated lymphocytic lymphoma
DVIU	direct vision internal urethrotomy	DWI	diffusion-weighted (magnetic resonance) imaging
DVPX	divalproex sodium (Depakote)		driving while intoxicated
DVM	Doctor of Veterinary Medicine		driving while impaired
DVMP	disks, vessels, and macula periphery	DWI/PI	diffusion-weighted imaging/perfusion imaging
DVPA	daunorubicin, vincristine, prednisone, and asparaginase	DWMRI	diffusion-weighted magnetic resonance imaging
DVR	Division of Vocational Rehabilitation	DWRT	delayed work recall test
	double valve replacement	DWSCL	daily-wear soft contact lens
DVSA	digital venous subtraction angiography	DWV	Dandy-Walker variant (a congenital anomaly)
DVT	deep vein thrombosis	DWW	dynamic wall walk
DVTS	deep venous thromboscintigram	Dx	diagnosis
			disease
DVVC	direct visualization of vocal cords	DXA	dual-energy x-ray absorptiometry
DW	daily weight	DXG	dioxalane guanine
	deionized water	DxLS	diagnosis responsible for length of stay
	detention warrant		
	dextrose in water	DXM	dexamethasone
	diffusion-weighted (imaging)		dextromethorphan
	distilled water	DXR	delayed xenograft rejection
	doing well	DXT	deep x-ray therapy
	double wrap	DXRT	deep x-ray therapy
D/W	dextrose in water	DXS	Dextrostix®
	discussed with	DY	dusky (infant color)
D-W	Dandy-Walker (deformity/malformation)		dysprosium
	Danis-Weber (classification for ankle fractures)	DYF	drag your feet (author's note: see you in court)
D_5W	5% dextrose (in water) injection	DYFS	Division of Youth and Family Services
D10W	10% dextrose (in water) injection	DYTRO	dynamic tone-reducing orthosis
D20W	20% dextrose (in water) injection	DZ	diazepam (valium)
			disease
D50W	50% dextrose (in water) injection		dizygotic
			dozen

DZP	diazepam
DZT	dizygotic twins
DZX	dexrazoxane (Zinecard)

E

E	East (as in the location e.g., 2E, would be second floor, East wing)
	edema
	effective
	eloper
	enema
	engorged
	eosinophil
	Escherichia
	esophoria for distance
	evaluation
	evening
	expired
	eye
	methylenedioxyme-thamphetamine (MDMA; Ecstasy)
E′	elbow
	esophoria for near
E_1	estrone
E_2	estradiol
E_3	estriol
4E	4 plus edema
E20	Enfamil 20®
E → A	say E,E,E, comes out as A,A,A upon auscultation of lung showing consolidation
EA	early amniocentesis
	elbow aspiration
	electroacoustic analysis
	enteral alimentation
	epidural anesthesia
	episodic ataxia
	esophageal atresia
E/A	ratio of peak mitral early diastolic and atrial contraction velocity
	European-American
E&A	evaluate and advise
EAA	electrothermal atomic absorption

E

	essential amino acids	EBB	electron beam boosts
EAB	elective abortion		equal breath bilaterally
	Ethical Advisory Board	EBBS	equal bilateral breath sounds
EAC	erythema annulare centrifugum	EBC	early (stage) breast cancer
	esophageal adenocarcinoma		esophageal balloon catheter
	external auditory canal	EBCT	electron-beam computed tomography
EACA	aminocaproic acid (epsilon-aminocaproic acid)	EBD	endocardial border delineation
EADL	extended activities of daily living		endoscopic balloon dilation
EADs	early after-depolarizations		evidence-based decision (making)
EAE	experimental autoimmune encephalomyelitis	EBE	equal bilateral expansion
		EBEA	Epstein-Barr (virus) early antigen
EAEC	enteroaggregative *Escherichia coli*	EBF	erythroblastosis fetalis
EAggEC	enteroaggregative *Escherichia coli*	EBL	estimated blood loss
		EBL-1	European bat lyssavirus 1
EAHF	eczema, allergy, and hay fever	EBM	evidence-based medicine
			expressed breast milk
EAL	electronic artificial larynx	EBMT	European Bone Marrow Transplant (registry group)
EAM	external auditory meatus		
EAP	Employment (Employee) Assistance Programs	EBNA	Epstein-Barr (virus) nuclear antigen
	erythrocyte acid phosphatase	EBO	evidence-based outcomes
	etoposide, doxorubicin (Adriamycin), and cisplatin (Platinol)	EBP	epidural blood patch
		EBR	external beam radiotherapy
EARLIES	early decelerations	EBRs	evidence-based recommendations
EART	extended abdominal radiation therapy	EBRT	external beam radiation therapy
EAR OX	ear oximetry	EBS	epidermolysis bullosa
EAS	external anal sphincter	EBSB	equal breath sounds bilaterally
EAST	external rotation, abduction stress test		
EAT	Eating Attitudes Test	EBT	erythromycin breath test
	ectopic atrial tachycardia	EBV	Epstein-Barr virus
EATL	enteropathy-associated T-cell lymphoma	EBVCA	Epstein-Barr viral capsid antigen
EAU	experimental autoimmune uveitis	EBVEA	Epstein-Barr virus, early antigen
EB	epidermolysis bullosa	EBVNA	Epstein-Barr virus, nuclear antigen
	Epstein-Barr (virus)		
EBA	epidermolysis bullosa acquisita	EC	ejection click

endocervical

enteric coated

Escherichia coli

etopside and carboplatin

European Community

extracellular

eye care

eyes closed

E & C education and counseling

ECA enteric coated aspirin (tablets)

Epidemiological Catchment Area

ethacrynic acid

external carotid artery

ECASA enteric coated aspirin (tablets)

ECBD exploration of common bile duct

ECBO enterocytopathogenic bovine orphan (virus)

ECC edema, clubbing, and cyanosis

embryonal cell cancer

emergency cardiac care

Emergency Communications Center

endocervical curettage

estimated creatinine clearance

external cardiac compression

extracorporeal circulation

ECCE extracapsular cataract extraction

ECD endocardial cushion defect

equivalent current dipole

ECDB encourage to cough and deep breathe

ECE extracapsular extension

ECEMG evoked compound electromyography

ECF epirubicin, cisplatin, and fluorouracil

extended care facility

extracellular fluid

ECF-A eosinophil chemotactic factors of anaphylaxis

ECG electrocardiogram

ECGE extracorporeal gas exchange

ECHINO echinocyte

ECHO echocardiogram

enterocytopathogenic human orphan (virus)

etoposide, cyclophosphamide, doxorubicin (hydroxydaunomycin), and vincristine (Oncovin)

ECHO (2D) echocardiogram (2-dimensional)

EChoG electrocochleography

ECHO/ RV echocardiography/ radionuclide ventriculography

ECI extracorporeal irradiation

ECIB extracorporeal irradiation of blood

ECIC external carotid and internal carotid

extracranial to intracranial (anastamosis)

EC/IC extracranial/intracranial

ECID European Centre for Infectious Disease

ECK1 *Escherichia coli* K1

ECL electrochemiluminescence

enterochromaffin-like

extend of cerebral lesion

extracapillary lesions

ECLA extracorporeal lung assist

ECLP extracorporeal liver perfusion

ECM erythema chronicum migrans

extracellular mass

extracellular matrix

ECM/BCM extracellular mass, body cell mass ratio

ECMO enterocytopathogenic monkey orphan (virus)

extracorporeal circulation membrane oxygenation (oxygenator)

ECN extended care nursery

ecNOS	endothelial constitutive nitric oxide synthetase		elbow disarticulation
ECochG	electrocochleography		emergency department
ECOG	Eastern Cooperative Oncology Group		emotional disorder
			epidural
ECoG	electrocochleography		erectile dysfunction
	electrocorticogram		ethynodiol diacetate
E coli	*Escherichia coli*		every day (this is a dangerous abbreviation)
ECO~tox~	*Escherichia coli* (heat-labile toxin) vaccine		extensive disease
			extensor digitorum
ECP	emergency care provider	ED₅₀	median effective dose
	emergency contraceptive pills	EDA	elbow disarticulation
		EDAM	edatrexate
	extracorporeal photochemotherapy	EDAP	Emergency Department Approved for Pediatrics
	extracorporeal photopheresis	EDAS	encephalodural arterio-synangiosis
ECPL	endocavitary pelvic lymphadenectomy	EDAT	Emergency Department Alert Team
ECPD	external counterpressure device	EDAX	energy-dispersive analysis of x-rays
ECPP	extracorporeal photophoresis	EDB	ethylene dibromide
			extensor digitorum brevis
ECR	emergency chemical restraint	EDC	effective dynamic compliance
	extensor carpi radialis		electrodesiccation and curettage
ECRB	extensor carpi radialis brevis		end diastolic counts
			estimated date of conception
ECRL	extensor carpi radialis longus		estimated date of confinement
ECS	elective cosmetic surgery		extensor digitorum communis
	electrocerebral silence	EDCF	endothelium-derived constricting factor
ECT	electroconvulsive therapy		
	emission computed tomography	EDCP	eccentric dynamic compression plates
	enhanced computed tomography	EDD	esophageal detector device
ECU	electrocautery unit		expected date of delivery
	emotional care units		
	environmental control unit	EDENT	edentulous
	extensor carpi ulnaris	EDF	elongation, derotation, and flexion
ECV	emergency center visits		
	external cephalic version	EDH	epidural hematoma
ECVE	extracellular volume expansion		extradural hematoma
		EDHF	endothelium-derived hyperpolarizing factor
ECW	extracellular water		
ED	eating disorder(s)		
	education		
	effective dose		

EDI	Eating Disorders Inventory	EDXRF	energy-dispersive x-ray fluorescence
	electrodeionization	EE	emetic episodes
EDITAR	extended-duration topical arthropod repellent		end to end
			equine encephalitis
EDL	extensor digitorum longus		erosive esophagitis
ED/LD	emotionally disturbed and learning disabled		esophageal endoscopy
			ethinyl estradiol
EDLF	endogenous digitalis-like factors		external ear
		E & E	eyes and ears
EDLS	endogenous digitalis-like substance	EEA	electroencephalic audiometry
EDM	early diastolic murmur		elemental enteral alimentation
	esophageal Doppler monitor		end-to-end anastomosis
	extensor digiti minimi		energy expended with activity
EDNO	endothelium-related nitric oxide	EEC	ectrodactyly-ectodermal dysplasia (cleft syndrome)
EDP	emergency department physician		endogenous erythroid colony
	end-diastolic pressure	EECP	enhanced external counter-pulsation
EDQ	extensor digiti quinti (tendon)	EEE	eastern equine encephalomyelitis
EDQM	European Directorate for the Quality of Medicines		edema, erythema, and exudate
EDQV	extensor digiti quinti five		external eye examination
EDR	edrophonium (Tensilon)	EEG	electroencephalogram
	extreme drug resistance	EELS	electron energy loss spectrometry
EDRF	endothelium derived relaxing factor (nitric oxide)	EEN	estimated energy needs
		EENT	eyes, ears, nose, and throat
EDS	Ehlers-Danlos syndrome	EEP	end expiratory pressure
	excessive daytime somnolence	EER	extended endocardial resection
EDSS	Expanded Disability Status Scale (Score)	EES®	erythromycin ethylsuccinate
EDT	exposure duration threshold	EET	early exercise testing
EDTA	edetic acid (ethylenedi-aminetetraacetic acid)	EEV	encircling endocardial ventriculotomy
EDTU	emergency diagnostic and treatment unit	EF	eccentric fixation
			ejection fraction
EDU	eating disorder unit		endurance factor
EDV	end-diastolic volume		erythroblastosis fetalis
	epidermal dysplastic verruciformis		extended-field (radiotherapy)
EDW	estimated dry weight		
EDX	edatrexate		

E

EFA	essential fatty acid	EGJ	esophagogastric junction
EFAD	essential fatty acid deficiency	EGL	eosinophilic granuloma of the lung
E-FAP	Emory Functional Ambulation Profile	EGS	ethylene glycol succinate
		EGSs	external guide sequences
EFBW	estimate fetal body weight	EGTA	esophageal gastric tube airway
EFD	episode free day		ethyleneglycoltetracetic acid
EFE	endocardial fibroelastosis		
	epidemic fatal encephalopathy	EH	eccentric hypertrophy
			educationally handicapped
EFF	effacement		enlarged heart
EFR	effective filtration rate		essential hypertension
EFS	event-free survival		extramedullary hematopoiesis
EFHBM	eosinophilic fibrohistiocytic lesion of bone marrow	EHB	elevate head of bed
			extensor hallucis brevis
EFM	electronic fetal monitor(ing)	EHBA	extrahepatic biliary atresia
	external fetal monitoring	EHBF	extrahepatic blood flow
EFMM	external fetal maternal monitor	EHC	enterohepatic circulation
		EHDA	etidronate sodium
EFMT	electric field mediated transfer	EHDP	etidronate disodium (Didronel)
EFN	effusion	EHE	epithelioid hemangioendothelioma
EFV	efavirenz (Sustiva)		
EFW	estimated fetal weight	EHEC	enterohemorrhagic *Escherichia coli*
EF/WM	ejection fraction/wall motion	EHF	epidemic hemorrhagic fever
e.g.	for example		extremely high frequency
EGA	esophageal gastric (tube) airway	EHH	esophageal hiatal hernia
	estimated gestational age	EHI	exertional heat illness
EGBUS	external genitalia, Bartholin, urethral, and Skene's glands	EHL	electrohydraulic lithotripsy
			extensor hallucis longus
EGC	early gastric carcinoma	EHN	ethotoin
EGCG	epigallocatechin gallate	EHO	extrahepatic obstruction
EGFR	epidermal growth factor receptor	EHPH	extrahepatic portal hypertension
EGD	esophagogastroduodeno-scopy	EHS	employee health service
			exertional heat stroke
EGDT	esophagogastric devascularization and transection	EHT	electrohydrothermosation
		EI	environmental illness
			enzyme immunoassay
EGF	epidermal growth factor		extensor indicis
EGF-R	epidermal growth factor receptor	E/I	expiratory to inspiratory (ratio)
EGG	electrogastrography	E & I	endocrine and infertility

EIA	enzyme immunoassay	EJV	external jugular vein
	exercise induced asthma	EK	Ektachem 400 (see page 358)
EIAB	extracranial-intracranial arterial bypass		erythrokinase
EIB	exercise-induced bronchospasm	EKC	epidemic keratoconjunctivitis
EIC	electrical impedance cardiography	EKG	electrocardiogram
	endometrial intraepithelial carcinoma	EKO	echoencephalogram
		EKY	electrokymogram
	epidermal inclusion cyst	EL	exercise limit
	extensive intraductal component	E-L	external lids
		ELA	Establishment License Application
EICA	extra-intracranial artery (bypass)	ELAD	extracorporeal liver-assist device
EID	electroimmunodiffusion	ELAFF	extended lateral arm free flap
	electronic infusion device		
EIDC	extreme intervertebral disk collapse	ELAM	endothelial leukocyte adhesion molecule
EIEC	enteroinvasive *Escherichia coli*	ELAMS	Electronic Laboratory Animal Monitoring System
EIL	elective induction of labor	ELB	early light breakfast
eIND	Electronic Investigational New Drug (application)		elbow
		ELBW	extremely low birth weight (less than 1000 g)
EIOA	excessive intake of alcohol		
EIP	elective interruption of pregnancy	ELC	earlobe creases
		ELCA	excimer laser coronary angioplasty
	end-inspiratory pressure		
	extensor indicis proprius	ELEC	elective
eIPV	enhanced inactivated polio vaccine	ELF	elective low forceps
			endoscopic laser foraminotomy
EIR	entomological inoculation rate		epithelial lining fluid
EIS	endoscopic injection scleropathy		etoposide, leucovorin, and fluorouracil
EITB	enzyme-linked immunoelectrotransfer blot	ELFA	enzyme-linked fluorescent immunoassay
EIV	external iliac vein	ELG	endolumenal gastroplication
EJ	ejection		endoluminal graft
	elbow jerk		
	external jugular	ELH	endolymphatic hydrops
EJB	ectopic junctional beat	ELI	endomyocardial lymphocytic infiltrates
EJN	extended jaundice of newborn		
		ELIG	eligible
EJP	excitatory junction potential	ELISA	enzyme-linked immunosorbent assay

ELITT	endometrial laser intrauterine thermal therapy	EMB	endometrial biopsy endomyocardial biopsy ethambutol (Myambutol) Explanation of Medicare Benefits
Elix	elixir		
ELLIP	ellipotocytosis		
ELM	epiluminescent microscopy	EMC	encephalomyocarditis endometrial currettage essential mixed cryoglobulinemia extraskeletal myxoid chondrosarcoma
ELND	elective lymph node dissection		
ELOP	estimated length of program		
ELOS	estimated length of stay	EMD	electromechanical dissociation
ELP	electrophoresis		
ELPS	excessive lateral pressure syndrome	EMDA	electromotive drug administration
ELS	Eaton-Lambert syndrome	EMDR	eye movement desensitization and reprocessing
ELSI	ethical, legal, and social implications		
ELSS	emergency life support system	EME	extreme medical emergency
ELT	endoscopic laser therapy euglobulin lysis time	EMEA	European Medicines Evaluation Agency
ELTR	European Liver Transplant Registry	EMF	elective midforceps electromagnetic field(s) electromagnetic flow electromotive forces endomyocardial fibrosis erythrocyte maturation factor evaporated milk formula
ELVIS™	Enzyme Linked Virus Inducible System		
EM	early memory ejection murmur electron microscope emergency medicine emmetropia eosinophilia-myalgia (syndrome) erythema migrans erythema multiforme esophageal manometry estramustine (Emcyt) extensive metabolizers external monitor		
		EMG	electromyograph emergency essential monoclonal gammopathy
		EMI	elderly and mentally infirm electromagnetic interference
		EMIC	emergency maternity and infant care
E & M	Evaluation and Management (coding system)	E-MICR	electron microscopy
		EMIT	enzyme-multiplied immunoassay technique (test)
EMA	early morning awakening endomysial antibody		
EMA-CO	etoposide, methotrexate, dactinomycin (actinomycin-D), cyclophosphamide, and vincristine (Oncovin)	EMLA®	eutectic mixture of local anesthetics (lidocaine and prilocaine in an emulsion base)
		EMLB	erythromycin lactobionate

E

EMMA	eye-movement measuring apparatus	EMV	equine morbilli virus
EMMV	extended mandatory minute ventilation		eye, motor, verbal (grading for Glasgow Coma Scale)
EMo	ear mold	EMVC	early mitral valve closure
EMP	electromolecular propulsion	EMW	electromagnetic waves
	estramustine phosphate (Emcyt)	EN	enema
			enteral nutrition
EMR	educable mentally retarded		erythema nodosum
		E/N	eggnog
	electrical muscle stimulation	E 50% N	extension 50% of normal
	electronic medical record	ENA	extractable nuclear antigen
	emergency mechanical restraint	ENB	esthesioneuroblastoma
		ENC	encourage
	empty, measure, and record	ENDO	endodontia
			endodontics
	endoscopic mucosal resection		endoscopy
			endotracheal
	eye movement recording	EndoCAB	plasma antiendotoxin core antibody
EMS	early morning specimen		
	early morning stiffness	ENF	Enfamil®
	electrical muscle stimulation	ENF c Fe	Enfamil® with iron
		ENG	electronystagmogram
	emergency medical services		engorged
		ENL	enlarged
	eosinophilia myalgia syndrome		erythema nodosum leprosum
EMSA	electrophoretic mobility shift assay	ENMG	electroneuromyography
		ENOG	electroneurography
EMSU	early morning specimen of urine	ENP	extractable nucleoprotein
		ENS	exogenous natural surfactant
EMT	emergency medical technician		
		ENT	ears, nose, throat
	epithelial-mesenchymal transformation	ENTIS	European Network of Teratology Information Services
	estramustine (Emcyt)		
EMTA	Emergency Medical Technician, Advanced	ENVD	elevated new vessels on the disk
EMTC	emergency medical trauma center	ENVE	elevated new vessels elsewhere
EMT-D	emergency medical technician-defibrillation	ENVT	environment
		EO	elbow orthosis
EMTP	Emergency Medical Technician, Paramedic		embolic occlusion
			eosinophilia
EMU	early morning urine		ethylene oxide
	electromagnetic unit		eyes open
	epilepsy monitoring unit	EOA	erosive osteoarthritis

E

117

	esophageal obturator airway	EOS	end of study
			eosinophil
	examine, opinion, and advice	EP	ectopic pregnancy
			electrophysiologic
	external oblique aponeurosis		elopement precaution
			endogenous pyrogen
EOAE	evoked otoacoustic emissions		Episcopalian
			esophageal pressure
EOB	edge of bed		etoposide and cisplatin (Platinol AQ)
	end of bed		
	explanation of benefits		evoked potentials
EOC	Emergency Operations Center	E&P	estrogen and progesterone
	enema of choice	EPA	eicosapentaenoic acid
	epithelial ovarian cancer		Environmental Protection Agency
EOD	end of day		
	end organ damage	EPAB	extracorporeal pneumoperititoneal access bubble
	every other day (this is a dangerous abbreviation)	E-Panel	electrolyte panel (See page 358)
	extent of disease		
EOE	extraosseous Ewing's sarcoma	EPAP	expiratory positive airway pressure
EOFAD	early-onset form of familial Alzheimer's disease	EPB	extensor pollicis brevis
		EPC	erosive prephloric changes
E of I	evidence of insurability		external pneumatic compression
EOG	electro-oculogram		
	Ethrane, oxygen, and gas (nitrous oxide)	EPD	electrode placement device
EOL	end of file		equilibrium peritoneal dialysis
EOM	error of measurement		
	external otitis media	EPEC	enteropathogen *Escherichia coli*
	extraocular movement		
	extraocular muscles	EPEG	etoposide (VePesid)
EOMB	explanation of Medicare benefits	EPEs	extrapyramidal effects
		EPF	Enfamil Premature Formula®
EOMI	extraocular muscles intact		
EOO	external oculomotor ophthalmoplegia	EPG	electronic pupillography
			Episodic Payment Group
EOP1	end-of-phase 1	EPI	echoplanar imaging
EOP2	end-of-phase 2		epinephrine
EOR	emergency operating room		epirubicin (Ellence)
			epitheloid cells
	end of range		exercise pressure index
EORA	elderly onset rheumatoid arthritis		exocrine pancreatic insufficiency
EORTC	European Organization for Research on the Treatment of Cancer		Expanded Program of Immunizations, (World Health Organization)

	Eysenck Personality Inventory		extrapyramidal syndrome (symptom)
EPIC	etoposide, prednisolone, ifosfamide, and cisplatin	EPSA	evoked potential signal averaging
EPID	epidural	EPSCCA	extrapulmonary small cell carcinoma
epiDX	epirubicin (4'-epidoxorubicin; Ellence)	EPSDT	early periodic screening, diagnosis, and treatment
EPIG	epigastric	EPSE	extrapyramidal side effects
EPIS	epileptic postictal sleep episiotomy	EPSP	excitatory postsynaptic potential
epith.	epithelial	EPSS	E point septal separation
EPL	effective patent life extensor pollicis longus (tendon)	EPT	electroporation therapy endpoint temperature
EPM	electronic pacemaker	EPT®	early pregnancy test
EPMR	electronic patient medical record	EPTE	existed prior to enlistment
		EPTS	existed prior to service
EPN	estimated protein needs	ER	emergency room
EPO	epoetin alfa (erythropoietin; Epogen)		end range estrogen receptors extended release
	evening primrose oil		extended external rotation
	exclusive provider organization		external resistance
		E & R	equal and reactive
EPOCH	etoposide, prednisone, vincristine (Oncovin), cyclophosphamide, doxorubicin (hydroxydaunorubicin)		examination and report
		ER+	estrogen receptor-positive
		ER−	estrogen receptor-negative
		ERA	estrogen receptor assay evoked response audiometry
EPP	erythropoietic protoporphyria	%ERAD	eradication rates
EPQ-R	Eysenck Personality Questionnaire—Revised	ERAS	Electronic Residency Application Service
EPR	electronic prescription record	ERBD	endoscopic retrograde biliary drainage
	electron paramagnetic (spin) resonance	ER by ICA	estrogen receptor immunocytochemistry assay
	electrophrenic respiration		
	emergency physical restraint	ERC	endoscopic retrograde cholangiography
	epirubicin (Ellence)	ERCP	endoscopic retrograde cholangiopancreatography
	estimated protein requirement	ERCT	emergency room computerized tomography
EPS	electrophysiologic study expressed prostatic secretions		
		ERD	early retirement with disability
	extrapulmonary shunt		

E

ERE	external rotation in extension		emergency service
			endoscopic sclerotherapy
ERF	external rotation in flexion		endoscopic
ERFC	erythrocyte rosette forming cells		sphincterotomy
			end-to-side
ERG	electroretinogram		Ewing's sarcoma
ERI	elective replacement indicator		ex-smoker
			extra strength
ERL	effective refractory length	ESA	early systolic acceleration
ERLND	elective regional lymph node dissection		end-to-side anastomosis
			ethmoid sinus adenocarcinoma
ERM	epiretinal membrane	ESADDI	estimated safe and adequate daily dietary intake
ERMS	exacerbating-remitting multiple sclerosis		
ERNA	equilibrium radionuclide angiocardiography	ESAP	evoked sensory (nerve) action potential
ERP	effective refractory period	ESAS	Edmonton System Assessment System
	emergency room physician	ESAT	extrasystolic atrial tachycardia
	endocardial resection procedure	ESBL	extended-spectrum beta-lactamases
	endoscopic retrograde pancreatography	ESC	end systolic counts
	event-related potentials	ESCC	esophageal squamous cell carcinoma
	estrogen receptor protein		
ERPF	effective renal plasma flow	ESCOP	European Scientific Cooperative on Phytotherapy
ER/PR	estrogen receptor/ progesterone receptor		
ERS	endoscopic retrograde sphincterotomy	ESCS	electrical spinal cord stimulation
	evacuation of retained secundines (afterbirth)	ESD	Emergency Services Department
			esophagus, stomach, and duodenum
ERSR	Electronic Regulatory Submission and Review	ESF	external skeletal fixation
ERT	estrogen replacement therapy	ESFT	Ewing's sarcoma family of tumors
	external radiotherapy	ESHAP	etopside, methylprednisolone (Solu-Medrol), high-dose cytarabine (ara-C), and cisplatin (Platinol AQ)
ERTD	emergency room triage documentation		
ERUS	endorectal ultrasound		
ERV	expiratory reserve volume		
e-Rx	electronic prescription	ESI	epidural steroid injection
ERYTH	erythromycin	ESI-MS	electrospray ionization-mass spectrometry
ES	electrical stimulation		
	Eleutherococcus senticosus (Siberian Ginseng)	ESIN	elastic stable intramedullary nailing
	embryonic stem (cells)		

ESL	English as a second language	embryo transfer
ESLD	end-stage liver disease	endometrial thickness
	end-stage lung disease	endothelin
ESM	ejection systolic murmur	endotoxin
	endolymphatic stromal myosis	endotracheal
		endotracheal tube
	ethosuximide (Zarontin)	enterostomal therapy (therapist)
ESN	educationally subnormal	esotropia
ESN(M)	educationally subnormal-moderate	essential thrombocythemia
		essential tremor
ESN(S)	educationally subnormal-severe	eustachian tube
		Ewing's tumor
ESO	esophagus	exchange transfusion
	esotropia	exercise treadmill
ESO/D	esotropia at distance	*et*	and
ESO/N	estropia at near	ET′	esotropia at near
ESP	endometritis, salpingitis, and peritonitis	E(T)	intermittent esotropia at infinity
	end systolic pressure	E(T′)	intermittent esotropia at near
	especially		
	extrasensory perception	ET-1	endothelin-1
ES/PNET	Ewing's sarcomas and peripheral neuroectodermal tumor	ET @ 20′	esotropia at 6 meters (infinity)
ESR	early sheath removal	ETA	endotracheal airway
	erythrocyte sedimentation rate		ethionamide
		et al	and others
ESRD	end-stage renal disease	ETBD	etiology to be determined
ESRF	end-stage renal failure	ETC	and so forth
ESS	emotional, spiritual, and social		Emergency and Trauma Center
	endoscopic sinus surgery		estimated time of conception
	Epworth Sleepiness Scale	ETCO$_2$	end tidal carbon dioxide
	essential	ETD	endoscopic transformational diskectomy
	euthyroid sick syndrome		
EST	Eastern Standard Time		eustachian tube dysfunction
	endoscopic spincterotomy		eye-tracking dysfunction
	electroshock therapy		
	electrostimulation therapy	ETDLA	esophageal-tracheal double lumen airway
	established patient		
	estimated	ETE	end-to-end
	exercise stress test	ETEC	enterotoxigenic *Escherichia coli*
	expressed sequence tag		
E-stim	electrical stimulation	ETF	eustachian tubal function
ESU	electrosurgical unit		
ESWL	extracorporeal shock wave lithotripsy	ETG	Episodic Treatment Group
ET	ejection time		

ETH	elixir terpin hydrate		European Union
	ethanol		excretory urography
	Ethrane	EUA	examine under anesthesia
ETHc̄C	elixir terpin hydrate with codeine	EUCD	emotionally unstable character disorder
ETI	ejective time index	EUD	external urinary device
	endotracheal intubation	EUG	extrauterine gestation
ETKTM	every test known to man	EUL	extra uterine life
		EUM	external urethral meatus
ETLE	extratemporal lobe epilepsy	EUP	Experimental Use Permit extrauterine pregnancy
ETO	estimated time of ovulation	EUS	endoscopic ultrasonography
	ethylene oxide		esophageal ultrasound
	etoposide (VePesid)		external urethral sphincter
	eustachian tube obstruction	EV	epidermodysplasia verruciformis
EtOH	alcohol		esophageal varices
	alcoholic		etoposide and vincristine
ETOP	elective termination of pregnancy		eversion
ETP	elective termination of pregnancy	eV	electron volt (unit of radiation energy)
		EV71	enterovirus-71
ETS	elevated toilet seat	EVA	Entry and Validation Application
	endoscopic transthoracic sympathectomy		ethylene vinyl acetate
	endotracheal suction		etoposide, vinblastine, and doxorubicin (Adriamycin)
	end-to-side		
	environmental tobacco smoke	EVAC	evacuation
	erythromycin topical solution	EVAc	ethylene-vinyl acetate copolymer
ETT	endotracheal tube	eval	evaluate
	esophageal transit time	EVG	endovascular grafting
	exercise tolerance test	EWB	emotional well-being
	exercise treadmill test (time)	EWBH	extracorporeal whole body hyperthermia
	extrathyroidal thyroxine	EXC	excision
ETT-Tl	exercise treadmill test with thallium	EVD	external ventricular (ventriculostomy) drain
ETU	emergency and trauma unit	EVE	evening
	emergency treatment unit	EXEC 22	Executive 22 chemistry profile (see page 358)
ETX	edatrexate	EVER	eversion
ETYA	eicosatetraynoic acid	EVG	endovascular grafting
EU	Ehrlich units	EVH	endoscopic (saphenous) vein harvesting
	equivalent units		
	esophageal ulcer		
	etiology unknown		

EVL	endoscopic variceal ligation		extrav	extravasation
EVS	endoscopic variceal sclerosis		ext. rot.	external rotation
			EXTUB	extubation
EW	expiratory wheeze elsewhere		EX U	excretory urogram
			EZ	Edmonston-Zagreb (vaccine)
EWB	estrogen withdrawal bleeding		EZ-HT	Edmonston-Zagreb high-titer (vaccine)
EWCL	extended-wear contact lens			
EWE	Eastern and Western encephalomyelitis vaccine			
EWHO	elbow-wrist-hand orthosis			
EWL	estimated weight loss			
EWSCLs	extended-wear soft contact lenses			
EWT	erupted wisdom teeth			
ex	examined example excision exercise			
exam.	examination			
EXECHO	exercise echocardiography			
EXEF	exercise ejection fraction			
EXGBUS	external genitalia, Bartholin (glands), urethral (glands), and Skene (glands)			
EXH VT	exhaled tidal volume			
EXL	elixir			
EXOPH	exophthalmos			
EXP	experienced expired exploration expose			
expect	expectorant			
exp. lap.	exploratory laparotomy			
EXT	extension external extract extraction extremities extremity			
Ext mon	external monitor			

E

F

F   facial
Fahrenheit
fair
false
fasting
father
feces
female
finger
firm
flow
fluoride
French
fundi
fundus

F/   full upper denture
/F   full lower denture
(F)   final
°F   degrees Fahrenheit
F=   firm and equal
F_1 offspring from the first generation
F_2 offspring from the second generation
F_3 Fluothane
14 F   14-hour fast required
F II–F XIII   factor 2 through 13
FA   fatty acid
femoral artery
fetus active
first aid
fludarabine (Fludara)
fluorescein angiogram
fluorescent antibody
folic acid
forearm
Friedreich ataxia
functional activities
FAA   febrile antigen agglutination
folic acid antagonist
FAAH   fatty acid amide hydrolase
FAAP   family assessment adjustment pass

FAA SOL   formalin, acetic, and alcohol solution
FAAN   Fellow of the American Academy of Nursing
FAAP   Fellow of the American Academy of Pediatrics
FAB   digoxin immune Fab (Digibind®)
French-American-British Cooperative group
functional arm brace
FABER   flexion, abduction, and external rotation
FABF   femoral artery blood flow
FAC   ferrite ammonium citrate
fluorouracil, doxorubicin (Adriamycin), and cyclophosphamide
fractional area change
fractional area concentration
functional aerobic capacity
FACA   Fellow of the American College of Anaesthetists
FACAG   Fellow of the American College of Angiology
FACAL   Fellow of the American College of Allergists
FACAN   Fellow of the American College of Anesthesiologists
FACAS   Fellow of the American College of Abdominal Surgeons
FACC   Fellow of the American College of Cardiology
FACCP   Fellow of the American College of Chest Physicians
FACCPC   Fellow of the American College of Clinical Pharmacology & Chemotherapy
FACD   Fellow of the American College of Dentists
FACEM   Fellow of the American College of Emergency Medicine

FACEP	Fellow of the American College of Emergency Physicians	FACT-G	....–General
		FACT-L	....–Lung
		FACT-P	....–Prostate
FACES	pain scale for assessing pain intensity	FAD	familial Alzheimer's disease
FACG	Fellow of the American College of Gastroenterology		Family Assessment Device
			fetal abdominal diameter
			fetal activity determination
FACH	forceps to after-coming head		flavin adenine dinucleotide
FACLM	Fellow of the American College of Legal Medicine	FAE	fetal alcohol effect
		FAGA	full-term appropriate for gestational age
FACN	Fellow of the American College of Nutrition	FAH	fumarylacetoacetase hydrolase
FACNP	Fellow of the American College of Neuropsychopharma-cology	FAI	Functional Assessment Inventory
		FAK	focal adhesion kinase
FACO	Fellow of the American College of Otolaryngology	FAL	femoral arterial line
		FALL	fallopian
		FALS	familial amyotrophic lateral sclerosis
FACOG	Fellow of the American College of Obstetricians & Gynecologists	FAM	family
			fluorouracil, doxorubicin (Adriamycin), and mitomycin
FACOS	Fellow of the American College of Orthopedic Surgeons		full allosteric modulators
FACP	Fellow of the American College of Physicians	FAMA	fluorescent antibody to membrane antigen
FACPRM	Fellow of the American College of Preventive Medicine	FAME	fluorouracil, doxorubicin (Adriamycin), and semustin (methyl CCNU)
FACR	Fellow of the American College of Radiology	FAMMM	familial atypical multiple mole melanoma
FACS	Fellow of the American College of Surgeons	FAM-S	fluorouracil, doxorubicin (Adriamycin), mitomycin, and streptozotocin
	fluorescent-activated cell sorter		
FACSM	Fellow of the American College of Sports Medicine	FAMTX	fluorouracil, doxorubicin (Adriamycin), and methotrexate
FACT	focused appendix computed tomography	FANA	fluorescent antinuclear antibody
FACT-An	Functional Assessment of Cancer Therapy–Anemia	FANG	fluorescent angiography
		FANSS&M	fundus anterior, normal size and shape and mobile
FACT-B	....–Breast		
FACT-F	....–Fatigue		

F

FAO	Food and Agriculture Organization	FBH	hydroxybutyric dehydrogenase
FAP	familial adenomatous polyposis	FBHH	familial benign hypocalciuric hypercalcemia
	familial amyloid polyneuropathy	FBI	flossing, brushing, and irrigation
	femoral artery pressure		full bony impaction
	fibrillating action potential	FBL	fecal blood loss
FAQ	frequently asked question(s)	FBM	felbamate (Felbatol)
F-ara-A	fludarabine phosphate (Fludara)		fetal breathing motion
			foreign body, metallic
FAS	fetal alcohol syndrome	FBRCM	fingerbreadth below right costal margin
FASC	fasciculations		
FASHP	Fellow of the American Society of Health-System Pharmacists	FBS	failed back syndrome
			fasting blood sugar
			fetal bovine serum
FASPS	familial advanced sleep-phase syndrome		foreign body sensation (eye)
FAST	fetal acoustic stimulation testing	FBU	fingers below umbilicus
		FBW	fasting blood work
	fluorescent allergosorbent technique	FC	family conference
			febrile convulsion
FAT	Fetal Activity Test		female child
	fluorescent antibody test		fever, chills
	food awareness training		financial class
FAV	facio-auricular vertebral		finger clubbing
FAZ	foveal avascular zone		finger counting
FB	fasting blood (sugar)		flexion contractor
	finger breadth		flucytosine (Ancobon)
	flexible bronchoscope		foam cuffed (tracheal or endotracheal tube)
	foreign body		
F/B	followed by		Foley catheter
	forward/backward		follows commands
	forward bending		foster care
FBC	full (complete) blood count		functional capacity
			functional class
FBCOD	foreign body, cornea, right eye	5FC	flucytosine (this is a dangerous abbreviation as it can be seen as 5FU)
FBCOS	foreign body, cornea, left eye		
		F + C	flare and cells
FBD	familial British dementia	F & C	foam and condom
	fibrocystic breast disease	FCA	Federal False Claims Act
		F. cath.	Foley catheter
	functional bowel disease	FCBD	fibrocystic breast disease
FBF	forearm blood flow	FCC	familial cerebral cavernoma
FBG	fasting blood glucose		familial colonic cancer
	foreign-body-type granulomata		family centered care

F

	femoral cerebral catheter	FCSNVD	fever, chills, sweating,
	follicular center cells		nausea, vomiting, and
	fracture compound		diarrhea
	comminuted	FCU	flexor carpi ulnaris
FCCA	Final Comprehensive		(tendon)
	Consensus Assessment	FCV	feline calicivirus
FCCC	fracture complete,	FD	familial dysautonomia
	compound, and		fetal demise
	comminuted		fetal distress
FCCL	follicular center cell		focal distance
	lymphoma		forceps delivery
FCCU	family centered care unit		free drain
FCD	feces collection device		full denture
	fibrocystic disease		fully dilated
FCDB	fibrocystic disease of the	F & D	fixed and dilated
	breast	FDA	Food and Drug
FCE	fluorouracil, cisplatin, and		Administration
	etoposide		fronto-dextra anterior
	functional capacity	FDB	first-degree burn
	evaluation		flexor digitorum brevis
FCFD	fluorescence capillary-fill	FDBL	fecal daily blood loss
	device	FDCA	Food, Drug, and Cosmetic
FCH	familial combined		Act
	hyperlipidemia	FDCs	follicular dendritic
	fibrosing cholestatic		cells
	hepatitis	FDE	fixed-drug eruption
FCHL	familial combined	FDF	flexor digitorum
	hyperlipemia		profundus (tendon)
FCL	fibular collateral ligament	FDG	feeding
F-CL	fluorouracil and calcium		fluorine-18-labeled
	leucovorin		deoxyglucose
FCM	flow cytometry		(^{18}fluorodeoxyglucose)
FCMC	family centered maternity	FDGB	fall down, go boom
	care	FDG-PET	positron emission
FCMD	Fukiyama's congenital		tomography with
	muscular dystrophy		^{18}fluorodeoxyglucose
FCMN	family centered maternity	FDGS	feedings
	nursing	FDI	food-drug interaction
F/C/N/V	fever, cough, nausea, and		Functional Disability
	vomiting		Index
FCOU	finger count, both eyes	FDIU	fetal death in utero
FCP	formocresol pulpotomu	FDL	flexor digitorum longus
FCR	flexor carpi radialis	FDLMP	first day of last menstrual
	fractional catabolic rate		period
FCRB	flexor carpi radialis brevis	FDM	fetus of diabetic mother
FCRT	fetal cardiac reactivity test		flexor digiti minimi
	focal cranial radiation	FDP	fibrin-degradation
	therapy		products
FCS	fever, chills, and sweating		fixed-dose procedure

F

	flexor digitorum profundus	FEM-POP	femoral popliteal (bypass)
FDPCA	fixed-dose patient-controlled analgesia	FEM-TIB	femoral tibial (bypass)
		FERGs	focal electroretinograms
FD-PET	fluorodopa-positron emission tomography	FEN	fluid, electrolytes, and nutrition
FDQB	flexor digiti quinti brevis	FENa	fractional extraction of sodium
FDR	first-dose reaction	FEN-PHEN	fenfluramine and phentermine
FDS	flexor digitorum superficialis	FENS	field-electrical neural stimulation
	for duration of stay	FEOM	full extraocular movements
FDT	fronto-dextra transversa (right frontotransverse)	FEP	free erythrocyte porphyrins
Fe	female		free erythrocyte protoporphorin
	iron		functional exercise program
F & E	full and equal		
FEB	febrile	FER	flexion, extension, and rotation
FEC	fluorouracil, epirubicin, and cyclophosphamide	FES	fat embolism syndrome
	fluorouracil, etoposide, and cisplatin		forced expiratory spirogram
	forced expiratory capacity		functional electrical stimulation
FECG	fetal electrocardiogram	$FeSO_4$	ferrous sulfate
FeCh	ferrochelatase	FESS	functional endonasal sinus surgery
FECP	free erythrocyte coproporphyrin		functional endoscopic sinus surgery
FECT	fibroelastic connective tissue	FET	fixed erythrocyte turnover
FED	fish eye disease	FETI	fluorescence (fluorescent) energy transfer immunoassay
FEES	fiberoptic endoscopic evaluation of swallowing	FEUO	for external use only
FEF	forced expiratory flow rate	FEV	familial exudative vitreoretinopathy
$FEF_{25\%-75\%}$	forced expiratory flow during the middle half of the forced vital capacity	FEV_1	forced expiratory volume in one second
FEF_{x-y}	forced expiratory flow between two designated volume points in the forced vital capacity	$FEV_{1\%VC}$	forced expiratory volume in one second as percent of forced vital capacity
FEHBP	Federal Employee Health Benefits Plan		
FEL	familial erythrophagocytic lymphohistiocytosis	FEVR	familial exudative vitreoretinopathy
FeLV	feline leukemia virus	FF	fat free
FEM	femoral		fecal frequency
FEM-FEM	femoral femoral (bypass)		filtration fraction

	finger-to-finger	FFTP	first full-term pregnancy
	five-minute format	FFU/1	fundus firm 1 cm below umbilicus
	flat feet		
	force fluids	FFU/2	fundus firm 2 cm below umbilicus
	formula fed		
	forward flexion	FG	fibrin glue
	foster father	FGC	full gold crown
	Fox-Fordyce (disease)	FGF	fibroblast growth factor
	fundus firm	FGM	female genital mutilation
	further flexion	FGP	fundic gland polyps
F/F	face to face	FGS	fibrogastroscopy
F&F	fixes and follows		focal glomerulosclerosis
F{rarr}F	finger to finger	FH	familial hypercholesterolemia
FF1/U	fundus firm 1 cm above umbilicus		family history
FF2/U	fundus firm 2 cm above umbilicus		favorable histology
			fetal head
FF@u	fundus firm at umbilicus		fetal heart
FFA	free fatty acid		fundal height
	fundus fluorescein angiogram	FH+	family history positive
		FH−	family history negative
FFAT	Free Floating Anxiety Test	FHA	filamentous hemagglutinin
		FHB	flexor hallucis brevis
FFB	flexible fiberoptic bronchoscopy	FHC	familial hypertrophic cardiomyopathy
FFD	fat-free diet		family health center
	focal-film distance	FHCIC	Fuchs' heterochromic iridocyclitis
FFDM	freedom from distant metastases	FHD	family history of diabetes
		FHF	fulminant hepatic failure
FFE	free-flow electrophoresis	FHH	familial hypocalciuric hypercalcemia
FFF	field-flow fractionation		
FFI	fast food intake		fetal heart heard
	fatal familial insomnia	FHI	frontal horn index
FFM	fat-free mass		Fuch's heterochromic iridocyclitis
	five finger movement		
	freedom from metastases	FHL	flexor hallucis longus
FFP	free from progression	FHM	familial hemiplegic migraine
	fresh frozen plasma		
FFPE	formalin-faxed, paraffin-embedded	FHN	family history negative
		FHNH	fetal heart not heard
FFR	freedom from relapse	FHO	family history of obesity
FFROM	full, free range of motion	FHP	family history positive
FFS	failure-free survival	FHR	fetal heart rate
	fee-for-service	FHRB	fetal heart rate baseline
	Fight For Sight	FHRV	fetal heart rate variability
	flexible fiberoptic sigmoidoscopy	FHS	fetal heart sounds
			fetal hydantoin syndrome
FFT	fast-Fourier transforms	FHT	fetal heart tone
	flicker fusion threshold		

F

FHVP	free hepatic vein pressure	FISH	fluorescent (fluorescence) *in situ* hybridization
FHX	fluorouracil, hydroxyurea, and radiotherapy	FISP	fast imaging with steady state precision
FHx	family history	FITC	fluorescein isothiocyanate conjugated
FI	fiscal intermediary		
FIA	familial intracranial aneurysms	FIV	feline immunodeficiency virus
	Family Independence Agency (formerly Department of Social Services)		*in vitro* fertilization (French)
		FIVC	forced inspiratory vital capacity
FIAC	fiacitabine	FIX	factor IX (nine)
FIAU	fialuridine	FJB	facet joint block
FIB	fibrillation	FJN	familial juvenile nephrophthisis
	fibula		
FICA	Federal Insurance Contributions Act (Social Security)	FJP	familial juvenile polyposis
		FJROM	full joint range of motion
$FiCO_2$	fraction of inspired carbon dioxide	FJS	finger joint size
		FJV	first jejunal vein
FICS	Fellow of the International College of Surgeons	FK506	tacrolimus (Prograf)
		FKA	formally known as
FID	father in delivery	FKBP	FK-506 binding protein (tacrolimus; Prograf)
	free induction decay		
FIF	forced inspiratory flow	FKD	Kinetic Family Drawing
FiF	Functional Intact Fibrinogen (test)	FKE	full knee extension
		FL	fatty liver
FIGE	field inversion gel electrophoresis		femur length
			fetal length
FIGLU	formiminoglutamic acid		fluid
FIGO	International Federation of Gynecology and Obstetrics		fluorescein
			flutamide and leuprolide acetate
FIL	father-in-law		focal laser
	Filipino		focal length
FIM	functional independence measure		follicular lymphoma
			full liquids
FIN	flexible intramedullary nail	fL	femtoliter (10^{-15} liter)
		F/L	father-in-law
FIND	follow-up intervention for normal development	FLA	free-living amebic (ameba)
FiO_2	fraction of inspired oxygen		low-friction arthroplasty
		FLAIR	fluid-attenuated inversion recovery
FIP	feline infectious peritonitis		
	flatus in progress	FLAP	fluorouracil, leucovorin, doxorubicin (Adriamycin), and cisplatin (Platinol AQ)
FIRI	fasting insulin resistance index		

F

130

	5-lipoxygenase activating protein
FLASH	fast low-angle shot
FLAVO	flavopiridol
FLB	funny looking beat
FLBS	funny looking baby syndrome (see note under FLK)
FLC	follicular large cell lymphoma
FLD	fatty liver disease
	fluid
	flutamide and leuprolide acetate depot
	full lower denture
FL Dtr	full lower denture
FLE	frontal lobe epilepsy
FLe	fluorouracil and levamisole
flexsig	flexible sigmoidoscopy
FLF	funny looking facies (see note under FLK)
FLGA	full-term, large for gestational age
FLIC	Functional Living Index–Cancer
FLIE	Functional Living Index—Emesis
FLK	funny looking kid (should never be used: unusual facial features, is a better expression)
FLM	fetal lung maturity
fl. oz.	fluid ounce
FLP	fasting lipid profile
	Functional Limitations Profile
FL REST	fluid restriction
FLS	flashing lights and/or scotoma
FLT	fluorothymidine
FLU	fluconazole (Diflucan)
	fludarabine (Fludara)
	flunisolide (Aero Bid)
	fluoxetine (Prozac)
	fluticasone propionate (Flonase)
	influenza
FLU A	influenza A virus

FLUO	Fluothane
fluoro	fluoroscopy
FLUT	flutamide (Eulexin)
FLV	Friend leukemia virus
FLW	fasting laboratory work
FLZ	flurazepam (Dalmane)
FM	face mask
	fat mass
	fetal movements
	fine motor
	floor manager
	fluorescent microscopy
	foster mother
F & M	firm and midline (uterus)
F-MACHOP	fluorouracil, methotrexate, cytarabine (ara-C), cyclophosphamide, doxorubicin (hydroxydaunorubicin), vincristine (Oncovin), and prednisone
FMC	fetal movement count
FMD	family medical doctor
	fibromuscular dysplasia
	foot-and-mouth disease
FMDV	foot-and-mouth disease virus
FME	Frühsommer-meningoenzephalitis vaccine
	full-mouth extraction
FMF	familial Mediterranean fever
	fetal movement felt
	forced midexpiratory flow
FMG	fine mesh gauze
	foreign medical graduate
FMH	family medical history
	fibromuscular hyperplasia
FmHx	family history
FML®	fluorometholone
FMN	first malignant neoplasm
	flavin mononucleotide
FMOL	femtomole (10^{-15} mole)
FMP	fasting metabolic panel
	first menstrual period
	functional maintenance program
FMPA	full-mouth periapicals

F

FMR	fetal movement record	FNMTC	familial nonmedullary thyroid carcinoma
	focused medical review		
	functional magnetic resonance (imaging)	FNP	Family Nurse Practitioner
FMRD	full-mouth restorative dentistry	FNR	false negative rate
		FNS	food and nutrition services
fMRI	functional magnetic resonance imaging		functional neuromuscular stimulation
FMS	fibromyalgia syndrome	F/NS	fever and night sweats
	fluorouracil, mitomycin, and streptozocin	FNT	finger-to-nose (test)
		FNTC	fine needle transhepatic cholangiography
	full-mouth series		
F & MS	frontal and maxillary sinuses	FO	foot orthosis
			foramen ovale
FMT	functional muscle test		foreign object
FMTC	familial medullary thyroid carcinoma		fronto-occipital
		FOB	father of baby
FMU	first morning urine		fecal occult blood
FMV	fluorouracil, semustine (methyl-CCNU), and vincristine		feet out of bed
			fiberoptic bronchoscope
			foot of bed
FMX	full-mouth x-ray	FOBT	fecal occult blood test
FMZ	flumazenil (Romazicon)	FOC	father of child
FN	facial nerve		fluid of choice
	false negative		fronto-occipital circumference
	febrile neutropenia		
	femoral neck	FOD	fixing right eye
	finger-to-nose (test)		free of disease
	flight nurse	FOEB	feet over edge of bed
F/N	fluids and nutrition	FOG	Fluothane, oxygen and gas (nitrous oxide)
F to N	finger-to-nose		
FNA	fine-needle aspiration		full-on gain
FNa	filtered sodium	FOH	family ocular history
FNAB	fine-needle aspiration biopsy	FOI	flight of ideas
		FOIA	Freedom of Information Act
FNAC	fine-needle aspiratory cytology		
		FOID	fear of impending doom
FNB	femoral nerve block	FOL	fiberoptic laryngoscopy
FNCJ	fine-needle catheter jejunostomy	FOM	floor of mouth
		FOMi	fluorouracil, Oncovin, (vincristine), and mitomycin
FND	fludarabine, mitoxantrone (Novantrone), and dexamethasone		
		FONSI	finding of no significant impact
	focal neurological deficit		
FNF	femoral-neck fracture	FOOB	fell out of bed
	finger-nose-finger (test)	FOOSH	fell on outstretched hand
FNH	focal nodular hyperplasia	FOP	fibrodysplasia ossificans progressiva
FNHL	follicular non-Hodgkin's lymphoma		

FOPS	fiberoptic proctosigmoidoscopy	FPM	full passive movements
		FPNA	first-pass nuclear angiocardiography
FORMIL	foreign military		
FOS	fiberoptic sigmoidoscopy	FPOR	follicle puncture for oocyte retrieval
	fixing left eye		
	fosphenytoin (Cerebyx)	FPU	family participation unit
	future order screen	FPZ	fluphenazine
FOSC	freestanding outpatient surgery center	FPZ-D	fluphenazine decanoate
		FQ	fluoroquinolones
FOT	form of thought	FR	fair
	frontal outflow tract		father
FOV	field of view		Father (priest)
FOVI	field of vision intact		Federal Register
FOW	fenestration of oval window		first responder
			flow rate
FP	fall precautions		fluid restriction
	false positive		fluid retention
	familial porencephaly		fractional reabsorption
	family planning		freestyle, no head or lower-extremity fixation (aquatic therapy)
	family practice		
	family practitioner		
	family presence		frequent relapses
	fibrous proliferation		Friends
	flat plate		frothy
	fluorescence polarization		full range
	fluticasone propionate	Fr	French (catheter gauge)
	food poisoning	F/R	fire/rescue
	frozen plasma	F & R	force and rhythm (pulse)
F/P	fluid/plasma (ratio)		
F-P	femoral popliteal	FRA	fall risk assessment
fpA	fibrinopeptide A		fluorescent rabies antibody
FPAL	full term, premature, abortion, living		
		FRAC	fracture
FPB	femoral-popliteal bypass	FRACTS	fractional urines
	flexor pollicis brevis	FRAG	fragment
FPC	familial polyposis coli	FRAG-X	Fragile X Syndrome
	family practice center	FRAP	family risk assessment program
FPD	feto-pelvic disproportion		
	fixed partial denture		fluorescence recovery after photobleaching
FPDL	flashlamp-pumped pulsed dye laser		
		FRC	frozen red cells
FPE	first-pass effect		functional residual capacity
FPG	fasting plasma glucose		
FPHx	family psychiatric history	FRCPC	Fellow of the Royal College of Physicians of Canada
FPIA	fluorescence-polarization immunoassay		
FPL	flexor pollicis longus (tendon)	FRCPE	Fellow of the Royal College of Physicians of Edinburgh
	final printed labeling		

F

FRCSC	Fellow of the Royal College of Surgeons of Canada	FSALT	Fletcher suite after loading tandem
FRCSE	Fellow of the Royal College of Surgeons of Edinburgh	FSB	fetal scalp blood full spine board
		FSBG	fingerstick blood glucose
		FSBM	full strength breast milk
FRCSI	Fellow of the Royal College of Surgeons of Ireland	FSBS	fingerstick blood sugar
		FSC	Fatigue Symptom Checklist
FRE	flow-related enhancement		flexible sigmoidoscopy
FRET	fluoresence resonance energy transfer		fracture, simple, and comminuted
FRF	filtration replacement fluid		fracture, simple and complete
FRG	Functional Related Groups	FSCC	fracture, simple, complete, and comminuted
FRJM	full range of joint movement	FSD	female sexual dysfunction focal-skin distance
FRN	fetal rhabdomyomatous nephroblastoma		fracture, simple and depressed
FRNT	focus-reduction neutralization test	FSE	fast spin-echo fetal scalp electrode
FROA	full range of affect	FSF	fibrin stabilizing factor
FROM	full range of motion	FSG	fasting serum glucose
FROMAJE	functioning, reasoning, orientation, memory, arithmetic, judgment, and emotion (mental status evaluation)		focal and segmental glomerulosclerosis
		FSGA	full-term, small for gestational age
		FSGN	focal segmental glomerulonephritis
FRP	follicle regulatory protein functional refractory period	FSGS	focal segmental glomerulosclerosis
		FSH	facioscapulohumeral follicle-stimulating hormone
FRSN	fluoroquinolone-resistant *Streptococcus pneumoniae*	FSHMD	facioscapulohumeral muscular dystrophy
FS	fetoscope fibromyalgia syndrome fingerstick flexible sigmoidoscopy foreskin fractional shortenings frozen section full strength functional status	FSIQ	Full-Scale Intelligence Quotient (part of Wechsler test)
		FSL	fasting serum level
		FSM	functional status measures
		F-SM/C	fungus, smear and culture
		FSME	Frühsommer-meningoencephalitis
F & S	full and soft	FSO	for screws only (prosthetic cups)
FSA	Family Services Association		
FSALO	Fletcher suite after loading ovoids	FSOP	French Society of Pediatric Oncology

FSP	fibrin split products	FTFTN	finger-to-finger-to-nose
FSR	fractionated stereotactic radiosurgery	FTG	full-thickness graft
		FTI	farnesyltransferase inhibitor
	fusiform skin revision		force-time integral
FSRT	fractionated stereotactic radiotherapy		free thyroxine index
FSS	fetal scalp sampling	F TIP	finger tip
	French steel sound (dilated to #24FSS)	FTIUP	full-term intrauterine pregnancy
	frequency-selective saturation	FTKA	failed to keep appointment
		FTLB	full-term living birth
	full-scale score	FTLD	frontotemporal lobar degeneration
FSW	feet of sea water (pressure)	FTLFC	full-term living female child
	field service worker	FTLMC	full-term living male child
FT	family therapy	FTM	fluid thioglycollate medium
	fast-twitch	FTN	finger-to-nose
	feeding tube		full-term nursery
	filling time	FTNB	full-term newborn
	finger tip	FTND	Fagerstrom Test for Nicotine Dependence
	flexor tendon		
	fluidotherapy		
	follow through		full-term normal delivery
	foot (ft)	FTNSD	full-term, normal, spontaneous delivery
	free testosterone		
	full-term	FTO	full-time occlusion (eye patch)
F_3T	trifluridine (Viroptic)		
FT_3	free triiodothyronine	FTP	failure to progress
FT_4	free thyroxine		full-term pregnancy
FT_4I	free thyroxine index	FTR	father
FTA	fluorescent titer antibody		failed to report
	fluorescent treponemal antibody		failed to respond
			for the record
FTB	fingertip blood	FTRAM	free transverse rectus abdominis myocutaneous (flap)
FTBD	full-term born dead		
FTBI	fractionated total body irradiation		
		FTSD	full-term spontaneous delivery
FTC	emtricitabine (Coviracil)		
	Federal Trade Commission	FTSG	full-thickness skin graft
		FTT	failure to thrive
	frames to come		fetal tissue transplant
	full to confrontation	Ftube	feeding tube
FTD	failure to descend	FTUPLD	full-term uncomplicated pregnancy, labor, and delivery
	frontotemporal dementia		
	full-term delivery		
FTE	failure to engraft	FTV	functional trial visit
FTEs	full-time equivalents	FTW	failure to wean
FTF	finger-to-finger	FU	fraction unbound
	free thyroxine fraction		

F

	fluorouracil
F & U	flanks and upper quadrants
F/U	follow-up
	fundus at umbilicus
F↑U	fingers above umbilicus
F↓U	fingers below umbilicus
5-FU	fluorouracil
FUB	function uterine bleeding
FUCO	fractional uptake of carbon monoxide
FUD	fear, uncertainty, and doubt
	full upper denture
FUDR®	floxuridine
FU Dtr	full upper denture
FUFA	fluorouracil and leucovorin (folinic acid)
FU/FL	full upper denture, full lower denture
FUFOL	fluorouracil and leucovorin calcium (folinic acid)
FUL	federal upper limit (price list)
FULG	fulguration
5FU/LV	fluorouracil and leucovorin
FUN	follow-up note
FUNG-C	fungus culture
FUNG-S	fungus smear
FUO	fever of undetermined origin
FUOV	follow-up office visit
FU/LP	full upper denture, partial lower denture
FUP	follow-up
FUS	fusion
FUV	follow-up visit
FV	femoral vein
FVC	false vocal cord(s)
	forced vital capacity
FVFR	filled voiding flow rate
FVH	focal vascular headache
F VIII	factor VIII (eight)
FVL	femoral vein ligation
	flow volume loop
FVR	feline viral rhinotracheitis

	forearm vascular resistance
FW	fetal weight
F/W	followed with
F waves	fibrillatory waves
	flutter waves
FVWs	flow-velocity waveforms (umbilical artery Doppler)
FWB	full weight bearing
	functional well-being
FWCA	functional work capacity assessment
FWD	fairly well developed
FWHM	full width at half maximum
FWS	fetal warfarin syndrome
FWW	front wheel walker
Fx	fractional urine
	fracture
Fx-BB	fracture both bones
Fx-dis	fracture-dislocation
F XI	Factor XI (eleven)
FXN	function
FXR	fracture
FY	fiscal year
FYC	facultative yeast carrier
FYI	for your information
FZ	flutamide and goserelin acetate (Zoladex®)
FZRC	frozen red (blood) cells

F

G

G	gallop
	gastrostomy
	gauge
	gavage feeding
	gingiva
	good
	grade
	gram (g)
	gravida
	guaiac
	guanine
G +	gram-positive
	guaiac positive
G −	gram-negative
	guaiac negative
↑g	increasing
↓g	decreasing
G1–4	grade 1–4
G-11	hexachlorophene
GA	Gamblers Anonymous
	gastric analysis
	general anesthesia
	general appearance
	gestational age
	ginger ale
	glycyrrhetinic acid
	granuloma annulare
	glucose/acetone
Ga	gallium
^{67}Ga	gallium citrate Ga 67
GABA	gamma-aminobutyric acid
GABHS	group A beta hemolytic streptococci
GAD	generalized anxiety disorder
	glutamic acid decarboxylase
GAF	geographic adjustment factors
	Global Assessment of Functioning (scale)
GAG	glycosaminoglycan
GAL	galanthamine hydrobromide
	gallon
G'ale	ginger ale
GALI-PUT	galactose-1-phosphate uridye transferase enzyme
GALT	gut-associated lymphoid tissue
GAMT	guanidinoacetate methyltransferase
GAO	General Accounting Office
GAP	GTPase activating protein
GAP-43	growth-associated protein-43
GAR	gonnococcal antibody reaction
GARFT	glycinamide ribonucleotide formyl transferase
GAS	general adaption syndrome
	ginseng-abuse syndrome
	Glasgow Assessment Schedule
	Global Assessment Scale
	group A streptococcal (*Streptococcus pyogenes*) disease vaccine
	group *A* streptococci
Gas Anal F&T	gastric analysis, free and total
Ga scan	gallium scan
Gastroc	gastrocnemius
GAT	geriatric assessment team
	group adjustment therapy
GATB	General Aptitude Test Battery
GAU	geriatric assessment unit
Gaw	airway conductance
GB	gallbladder
	Ginkgo biloba
	Guillain-Barré (syndrome)
G & B	good and bad
GBA	gingivobuccoaxial
	ganglionic-blocking agent
GBBS	group B beta hemolytic streptococcus

G

137

GBE	*Ginkgo biloba* extract	GCDFP	gross cystic disease fluid protein
GBG	gonadal-steroid binding globulin	GCI	General Cognitive Index
GBH	gamma benzene hexachloride (lindane)	GCIIS	glucose control insulin infusion system
GBIA	Guthrie bacterial inhibition assay	GCM	good central maintained
GBL	gamma butyrolactone	GCMD	generalized cardiovascular metabolic disease
GBM	glioblastoma multiforme glomerular basement membrane	GC-MS	gas chromatography-mass spectroscopy
GBMI	guilty but mentally ill	GCP	gentamicin, clindamycin, and polymyxin topical preparation
GBP	gabapentin (Neurontin) gastric bypass		good clinical practices
	gated blood pool (imaging)	GCR	gastrocolonic response glucocerebrosidase
GBPS	gated blood pool scan	GCS	Glasgow Coma Scale
GBR	gamma band response (audiology)	G-CSF	filgrastim (granulocyte colony-stimulating factor)
	good blood return	GCST	Gibson-Cooke sweat test
GBS	gallbladder series	GCT	general care and treatment
	gastric bypass surgery group B streptococcal (*Streptococcus agalactiae*) disease vaccine		germ cell tumor giant cell tumor granulosa cell tumor
	group B streptococci	GCU	gonococcal urethritis
	Guillain-Barré syndrome	GCV	ganciclovir (Cytovene) great cardiac vein
GBW	generalized body weakness	GCVF	great cardiac vein flow
GBX	gall bladder extraction (cholecystectomy)	GD	gastric distension Gaucher's disease
GC	gas chromatography gastric cancer		generalized delays gestational diabetes
	geriatric chair (Gerichair®)		good gravely disabled
	gingival curettage		Graves' disease
	gonococci (gonorrhea)	Gd	gadolinium
	good condition	G & D	growth and development
	graham crackers	GDA	gastroduodenal artery
G−C	gram-negative cocci	GDB	Guide Dogs for the Blind
G+C	gram-positive cocci	Gd-	gadolinium
GCA	ghost cell ameloblastoma	BOPTA	benzyloxypropionic tetra acetate
	giant cell arteritis	GDC	Guglielmi detachable coil
GCBP	gated cardiac blood pool	Gd-DTPA	gadopentetate (Magnevist)
GCC	guanylyl cyclase C	Gd-DTPA-	gadodiamide
GCE	general conditioning exercise	BMA	
		GD FA	grandfather

G

GDH	glutamic dehydrogenase	GEP	gastroenteropancreatic
Gd-HPD03A	gadoteridol	GEQ	generic equivalent
		GER	gastroesophageal reflux
g/dl	grams per deciliter	GERD	gastroesophageal reflux disease
GDM	gestational diabetes mellitus	GES	gastric emptying scan
GDM A-1	gestational diabetes mellitus, insulin controlled, Type I	GET	gastric emptying time graded exercise test
		GET 1/2	gastric emptying half-time
GDM A-2	gestational diabetes mellitus, diet controlled, Type II	GETA	general endotracheal anesthesia
		GEU	geriatric evaluation unit
Gd-MRI	gadolinium-enhanced magnetic resonance imaging	GF	gastric fistula gluten free grandfather
GDNF	glial-derived neurotrophic factor	GFAP	glial fibrillary acid protein
		GF-BAO	gastric fluid, basal acid output
GDP	gel diffusion precipitin		
GD MO	grandmother	GFCL	Goldmann fundus contact lens
GDR	glucose disposal rate		
GDS	Global Deterioration Scale	GFD	gluten-free diet
		GFJ	grapefruit juice
GE	gainfully employed gastric emptying gastroenteritis gastroesophageal	GFM	good fetal movement
		GFP	green fluorscent protein
		GFR	glomerular filtration rate grunting, flaring, and retractions
GEA	gastroepiploic artery		
GEC	galactose elimination capacity	GFS	glaucoma filtering surgery
		GG	gamma globulin guaifenesin (glyceryl guaiacolate)
GED	General Educational Development (Test)		
GEE	Global Evaluation of Efficacy glycine ethyl ester graft-enteric erosion	G=G	grips equal and good
		GGE	Gastrografin enema generalized glandular enlargement
GEF	graft-enteric fistula		
GEJ	gastroesophageal junction	GGO	ground-glass opacity
GEM	gemcitabine (Gemzar) gemfibrozil (Lopid) generalized erythema multiforme	GGS	glands, goiter, and stiffness group G streptococci
		GGT	gamma-glutamyl-transferase
GEMU	geriatric evaluation and management unit	GGTP	gamma-glutamyl-transpeptidase
GEN	genital	GH	general health genetic hemochromatosis gingival hyperplasia glenohumeral good health growth hormone
GEN/ENDO	general anesthesia with endotracheal intubation		
GENT	gentamicin		
GENTA/P	gentamicin-peak		
GENTA/T	gentamicin-trough		

G

GH₃	Gerovital	GIS	gas in stomach
GHAA	Group Health Association of America		gastrointestinal series
		GISA	glycopeptide intermediate-resistant *Staphylococcus aureus*
GHB	gamma hydroxybutyrate		
GHb	glycosylated hemoglobin	GIT	gastrointestinal tract
GHD	growth hormone deficiency	GITS	gastrointestinal therapeutic system
GHDA	growth hormone deficiency (syndrome) in adults		gut-derived infectious toxic shock
		GITSG	Gastrointestinal Tumor Study Group
GHI	growth hormone insufficiency	GITT	glucose insulin tolerance test
GHJ	glenohumeral joint	GIWU	gastrointestinal work-up
G-H jt	glenohumeral joint	giv	given
GHP(S)	gated heart pool (scan)	GJ	gastrojejunostomy
GHQ	General Health Questionnaire		grapefruit juice
		GJIC	gap junction intercellular
GHRF	growth hormone releasing factor	GJT	gastrojejunostomy tube
		G1K	greater than one thousand
GI	gastrointestinal	GL	gastric lavage
	granuloma inguinale		glaucoma
GIA	gastrointestinal anastomosis		greatest length
		GLA	gamolenic acid
GIB	gastric ileal bypass		gingivolinguoaxial
	gastrointestinal bleeding		glucose-lowering agents
GIC	general immunocompetence	GLC	gas-liquid chromatography
		GLD	Glanders (*Actinobacillus mallei*) vaccine
GID	gastrointestinal distress		
	gender identity disorder	GLIO	glioblastoma
GIDA	Gastrointestinal Diagnostic Area	GLN	glomerulonephritis
		GLOC	gravity induced loss of consciousness
GIFD #3	colonoscope		
GIFT	gamete intrafallopian (tube) transfer	GLP	Gambro Liendia Plate
			Good Laboratory Practice (Principles of)
GIH	gastrointestinal hemorrhage		group-living program
GIK	glucose-insulin-potassium	GLP-1	glucagon-like peptide-1
GIL	gastrointestinal (tract) lymphoma	GLR	gravity lumbar reduction
		GLU	glucose
GING	gingiva	GLU 5	five-hour glucose tolerance test
	gingivectomy		
G1K	greater than one thousand	GLUC	glucose
GIOP	glucocorticoid (steroid)-induced osteoporosis	GLYCOS Hb	glycosylated hemoglobin
GIP	gastric inhibitory peptide	GM	gastric mucosa
	giant cell interstitial pneumonia		general medicine
			genetically modified
GIPU	gastrointestinal procedure unit		

140

	geometric mean	GNA	*Galanthus nivalis* agglutinin
	gram (g)		
	grand mal	GNB	ganglioneuroblastoma
	grandmother		gram-negative bacilli
	gray matter		gram-negative bacteremia
GM +	gram-positive		
GM –	gram-negative	GNBM	gram-negative bacillary meningitis
gm %	grams per 100 milliliters		
GMC	general medical clinic	GNC	gram-negative cocci
	geometric mean concentration	GND	gram-negative diplococci
GMCD	grand mal convulsive disorder	GNID	gram-negative intracellular diplococci
GM-CSF	sargramostim (granulocyte-macrophage colony-stimulating factor; Leukine)	GNP	Geriatric Nurse Practitioner
		GNR	gram-negative rods
		GnRH	gonadotropin-releasing hormone
GME	gaseous microemboli	GNS	gram-negative sepsis
GMF	general medical floor	GnSAF	gonadotropin surge attenuating factor
GMH	germinal matrix hemorrhage		
GMLOS	geometric mean length of stay	GNT	Graduate Nurse Technician
GMOs	genetically modified organisms	GO	Graves' ophthalmopathy
			Greek Orthodox
GMP	general medical panel (see page 358)	GOAT	Galveston Orientation and Amnesia Test
	Good Manufacturing Practices	GOBI	growth monitoring, *o*ral rehydration, *b*reast feeding, and *i*mmunization
	guanosine monophosphate		
GMR	gallop, murmur or rub	GOCS	Global Obsessive-Compulsive Scale
GMS	galvanic muscle stimulation		
		GOD	glucose oxidase
	general medical services	GOG	Gynecologic Oncology Group
	general medicine and surgery		
		GOK	God only knows
	Gomori methenamine silver (stain)	GOMER	get out of my emergency room
GM&S	general medicine and surgery	GON	gonococcal ophthalmia neonatorum
			greater occipital neuritis
GMSPS	Glasgow Meningococcal Septicemia Prognostic Score	GONA	glaucomatous optic nerve atrophy
		GONIO	gonioscopy
GMTs	geometric mean antibody titers	GOO	gastric outlet obstruction
GN	glomerulonephritis	GOR	gastro-oesophageal reflux (United Kingdom)
	graduate nurse		
	gram-negative		general operating room

G

GORD	gastro-oesophageal reflux disease (United Kingdom)		glucose-6-phosphate isomerase
GOS	Glasgow Outcome Scale	GPi	globus pallidus interna
GOT	glucose oxidase test	G-PLT	giant platelets
	glutamic-oxaloacetic transaminase (aspartate aminotransferase)	GPMAL	gravida, para, multiple births, abortions, and live births
	goals of treatment	GPN	graduate practical nurse
GP	gabapentin (Neurontin)	GPO	group purchasing organization
	general practitioner		
	globus pallidus	GPS	Goodpasture's syndrome
	glucose polymers	GPT	glutamic pyruvic transaminase
	glycoprotein		
	gram-positive	GPX	glutathione peroxidase
	grandparent	GR	gastric resection
	gutta percha		growth rate
G/P	gravida/para	gr	grain (approximately 60 mg) (this is a dangerous abbreviation)
G₄P₃₁₀₄	four pregnancies (gravid), 3 went to term, one premature, no abortion (or miscarriage), and 4 living children (p = para)		
		G−R	gram-negative rods
		G+R	gram-positive rods
		GRA	granisetron (Kytril)
		gravida 6, para 4-0-2-3	6 pregnancies resulting in 4-full term deliveries with 0 premature births and 2 abortions or miscarriages and 3 living children
GPA	global program on AIDS		
G#P#A#	gravida (number of pregnancies) para (number of live births) abortion (number of abortions)		
		GRAS	generally recognized as safe
GPB	gram-positive bacilli	GRASE	Generally Recognized as Safe and Effective
GPC	giant papillary conjunctivitis	GRASS	gradient recalled acquisition in a steady state
	glycerophosphorylcholine		
	G-protein coupled	Grav.	gravid (pregnant)
	gram-positive cocci	GRC	gastric remnant cancers
GPCL	gas permeable contact lens	GRD	gastroesophageal reflux disease
GPCR	G protein-coupled receptors	GRD DTR	granddaughter
		GRD SON	grandson
GPC/TP	glycerylphosphorylcholine to total phosphate	GRE	graded resistive exercise
			gradient-recalled echo
G6PD	glucose-6-phosphate dehydrogenase		gradient refocused echo
		GR-FR	grandfather
GPGL	gamma probe guided lymphoscintigraphy	GR-MO	grandmother
GPI	general paralysis of the insane	GRN	granules
			green

G

GRO	growth-related oncogene	GSS	Gerstmann-Straüssler-Scheinker (syndrome)
GRP	group		
Gr$_1$P$_0$AB$_1$	one pregnancy, no births, and one abortion	GST	glutathione S-transferase
			gold sodium thiomalate
GRP HM	group home	GSTM	gold sodium thiomalate
GRT	gastric residence time	GSUI	genuine stress urinary incontinence
	glandular replacement therapy		
		GSW	gunshot wound
	Graduate Respiratory Therapist	GSWA	gunshot wound to abdomen
	grasp and release test	GT	gait
GRTT	Graduate Respiratory Therapist Technician		gait training
			gastrostomy
GS	gallstone		gastrotomy tube
	generalized seizure		glucose tolerance
	general surgery		great toe
	Gleason score		greater trochanter
	glucosamine sulfate		green tea
	gluteal sets		group therapy
	Gram stain	GTA	glutaraldehyde
	grip strength	GTB	gastrointestinal tract bleeding
G/S	5% dextrose (glucose) and 0.9% sodium chloride (saline) injection	GTC	generalized tonic-clonic (seizure)
G & S	gait and stance	GTCS	generalized tonic-clonic seizure
GSAP	greatest single allergen present		
GSCU	geriatric skilled care unit	GTD	gestational trophoblastic disease
GSD	glucogen storage disease	GTE	general therapeutic exercise
GSD-1	glycogen storage disease, type 1		
			Green tea extract
GSE	genital self-examination	GTF	gastrostomy tube feedings
	gluten sensitive enteropathy		glucose tolerance factor
		GTH	gonadotropic hormone
	grip strong and equal	GTN	gestational trophoblastic neoplasms
GSH	glutathione		
GSI	genuine stress incontinence		glomerulo-tubulo-nephritis
			glyceryl trinitrate (name for nitroglycerin in the United Kingdom)
GSK	GlaxoSmithKline		
GSM	grey-scale median		
GSMD	gestational sack and maternal date	GTO	Golgi tendon organ(s)
		GTP	glutamyl transpeptidase
GSP	generalized social phobia		guanosine triphosphate
	general survey panel	GTR	granulocyte turnover rate
GSPN	greater superficial petrosal neurectomy		gross total resection
			guided tissue regeneration
GSR	galvanic skin resistance (response)	GTS	Gilles de la Tourette syndrome
	gastrosalivary reflex	GTT	drops

G

GTT	gestational trophoblastic tumor
	glucose tolerance test
GTT agar	gelatin-tellurite-taurocholate agar
GTT3H	glucose tolerence test 3 hours (oral)
GTTS	drops
G-tube	gastrostomy tube
GU	genitourinary
	gonococcal urethritis
GUAR	guarantor
GUD	genital ulcer disease
GUI	genitourinary infection
GUS	genitourinary sphincter
	genitourinary system
GUSTO	Global Utilization of Streptokinase and TPA for Occluded Arteries
GV	gentian violet
GVF	Goldmann visual fields
	good visual fields
GVG	vigabatrin (gamma-vinyl GABA)
GVH	generalized visceral hypersensitivity
GVHD	graft-versus-host disease
GVL	graft-versus leukemia
GVN	gentamicin, vancomycin, and nystatin
GVS	gastric vertical stapling
G/W	dextrose (glucose) in water
G&W	glycerin and water (enema)
GWA	gunshot wound of the abdomen
GWBI	General Well-Being Index
GWD	Guinea worm disease
GWS	Gulf war syndrome
GWT	gunshot wound of the throat
GWX	guide wire exchange
GXP	graded exercise program
GXT	graded exercise test
Gy	gray (radiation unit)
GYN	gynecology
GZTS	Guilford-Zimmerman Temperament Survey

H

H	*Haemophilis*
	head
	heart
	height
	Helicobacter
	heroin
	Hispanic
	hour
	husband
	hydrogen
	hyperopia
	hypermetropia
	hyperphoria
	hypodermic
	objective angle
H′	hip
Ⓗ	hypodermic injection
H²	hiatal hernia
H₂	hydrogen
3H	high, hot, and a helluva lot
HA	headache
	hearing aid
	heart attack
	hemadsorption
	hemagglutination
	hemolytic anemia
	Hispanic American
	hospital admission
	hyaluronan
	hyaluronic acid
	hyperalimentation
	hypermetropic astigmatism
	hypothalmic amenorrhea
H/A	head-to-abdomen (ratio)
	holding area
HA-1A®	nebacumab
HAA	hepatitis-associated antigen
HAAB	hepatitis A antibody
HAART	highly active antiretroviral treatment
HABF	hepatic artery blood flow

HAc	acetic acid	HAL	hemorrhoidal artery ligation
HACA	human antichimeric antibodies		hyperalimentation
HACCP	Hazard Analysis Critical Control Point(s)	HALO	halothane (Fluothane)
			hours after light onset
HACE	hepatic artery chemoembolization	HALRI	hospital-acquired lower respiratory infections
	high-altitude cerebral edema	HAM	HTLV-1-associated myelopathy
HACEK group	*Haemophilus parainfluenzae, H. aphrophilus,* and *H. paraphrophilus, Actinobacillus actinomycetemcomitans, Cardiobacterium hominis, Eikenella corrodens,* and *Kingella kingae*		human albumin microspheres
		HAMA	human antimurine antibody
		HAM-A	Hamilton Anxiety (scale)
		HAM D	Hamilton Depression (scale)
		HAMS	hamstrings
		HAN	heroin associated nephropathy
HACS	hyperactive child syndrome	HANE	hereditary angioneurotic edema
HAD	HIV (human immunodeficiency virus)-associated dementia	HAO	hearing aid orientation
		HAP	hearing aid problem
			heredopathia atactica polyneuritiformis
	human adjuvant disease		hospital-acquired pneumonia
	hypertonic acetate dextran		
HADS	Hospital Anxiety and Depression Scale	HAPC	hospital-acquired penetration contact
HAE	hearing aid evaluation	HAPD	home-automated peritoneal dialysis
	hepatic artery embolization	HAPE	high-altitude pulmonary edema
	herb-related adverse event		
	hereditary angioedema	HAPS	hepatic arterial perfusion scintigraphy
HAEC	Hirschprung's associated enterocolitis	HAPTO	haptoglobin
HAF	hyperalimentation fluid	HAQ	Headache Assessment Questionnaire
HAFM	hospital-acquired *Plasmodium falciparum* malaria		Health Assessment Questionnaire
HAGG	hyperimmune antivariola gamma globulin	HAR	high-altitude retinopathy
			hyperacute rejection
HAH	high-altitude headache	HARH	high-altitude retinal hemorrhage
HAI	hemagglutination inhibition assay	HARP	hypoprebetalipoproteinemia, acanthocytosis, retinitis pigmentosa, and pallidale degeneration (syndrome)
	hepatic arterial infusion		
HAIC	hepatic arterial infusional chemotherapy		
HAK	hyperalimentation kit		

H

HARS	Hamilton Anxiety Rating Scale	HBcAb	hepatitis B core antibody (antigen)
HAS	Hamilton Anxiety (Rating) Scale	HBc AB	hepatitis B core antibody
	home assessment service	HBc Ag	hepatitis B core antigen
	hyperalimentation solution	HbCO	carboxyhemoglobin
HASCI	head and spinal cord injury	HB core	hepatitis B core antigen
		HbCV	*Haemophilus* b conjugate vaccine
HASCVD	hypertensive arteriosclerotic cardiovascular disease	HBD	has been drinking
			hydroxybutyrate dehydrogenase
HASHD	hypertensive arteriosclerotic heart disease	HBDH	hydroxybutyrate dehydrogenase
HAT	head, arms, and trunk	HBE	hepatitis B epsilon
	heterophile antibody titer		human bronchial epithelial (cells)
	histone acetyltransferase		hypopharyngoscopy, bronchoscopy, and esophagoscopy
	hospital arrival time		
	human African trypanosomiasis (sleeping sickness)	HBeAb	hepatitis Be antibody (antigen)
HAV	hallux abducto valgus	HBED	hydroxybenzylethylene-diamine diacetic acid
	hepatitis A vaccine		
	hepatitis A virus	HbF	fetal hemoglobin
HAZWO PER	Hazardous Waste Operations and Emergency Response	HBF	hepatic blood flow
		HBGA	had it before, got it again
HB	heart-beating (donor)	HBGM	home blood glucose monitoring
	heart block		
	heel to buttock	HBH	Health Belief Model
	hemoglobin (Hb)	HBHC	hospital based home care
	hepatitis B	HBI	Harvey-Bradshaw Index
	high calorie		hemibody irradiation
	hold breakfast	HBID	hereditary benign intraepithelial dyskeratosis
	housebound		
	hydrocodone bitartrate		
1^0HB	first degree heart block	HBIG	hepatitis B immune globulin
HB1°	first degree heart block		
HB2°	second degree heart block	Hb Kansas	mutant hemoglobin with a low affinity for oxygen
HB3°	third degree heart block	HBLV	B-lymphotropic virus human
HBAB	hepatitis B antibody		
Hb A$_{1c}$	glycosylated hemoglobin	HBM	human bone marrow
HBAC	hyperdynamic beta-adrenergic circulatory	HBNK	heparin-binding neurotrophic factor
HbAS	sickle cell trait	HBO	hyperbaric oxygen (HBO$_2$ preferred)
HBBW	hold breakfast for blood work		
		HBO$_2$	hyperbaric oxygen
HBC	hereditary breast cancer	HbO$_2$	hemoglobin, oxygenated

	hyperbaric oxygen (HBO$_2$ preferred)		hypercalcemia
HBOC	hemoglobin-based oxygen carrier		hypothermic circulatory arrest
	hereditary breast and ovarian cancer	H-CAP	altretamine (hexamethyl-melamine), cyclophosphamide, doxorubicin (Adriamycin), and cisplatin (Platinol AQ)
HBOT	hyperbaric oxygen treatment/therapy (HBO$_2$T preferred)		
HBO$_2$T	hyperbaric oxygen treatment	HCB	hexachlorobenzene
HBP	high blood pressure	HCC	hepatocellular carcinoma
HBPM	home blood pressure monitoring	HCD	herniate cervical disk
			hydrocolloid dressing
HBS	Health Behavior Scale	HCFA	Health Care Financing Administration
HbS	sickle cell hemoglobin		
HBsAg	hepatitis B surface antigen	HCFC	hydrochlorofluorocarbon
HbSC	sickle cell hemoglobin C	hCG	human chorionic gonadotropin
HBSS	Hank's balanced salt solution	HCH	hexachlorocyclohexane
HbSS	sickle cell anemia		hygroscopic condenser humidifier
HBT	hydrogen breath test	HCI	home care instructions
HBV	hepatitis B vaccine	HCL	hairy cell leukemia
	hepatitis B virus	HCl	hydrochloric acid
	honey-bee venom		hydrochloride
HBVP	high biological value protein	HCLF	high carbohydrate, low fiber (diet)
HBW	high birth weight	HCLs	hard contact lenses
H/BW	heart-to-body weight (ratio)	HCLV	hairy cell leukemia variant
HC	hairy cell	HCM	health care maintenance
	handicapped		heterogeneous cation-exchange membrane
	head circumference		hypercalcemia of malignancy
	heart catheterization		hypertrophic cardiomyopathy
	heel cords		
	Hickman catheter	HCMV	human cytomegalovirus
	home care	HCO$_3$	bicarbonate
	hot compress	HCP	handicapped
	housecall		healthcare provider
	Huntington's chorea		hearing conservation programs
	hydrocephalus		hereditary coporphyria
	hydrocortisone		hexachlorophene
4-HC	4-hydroperoxycyclo-phosphamide		home chemotherapy program
H & C	hot and cold		hospital chemistry profile
HCA	health care aide		
	heterocyclic antidepressant		

HCPCS	HCFA (Health Care Financing Administration) Common Procedural Coding System		house dust Huntington's disease
HCQ	hydroxychloroquine (Plaquenil)	HDA	high-dose arm
		HD-AC	high-dose cytarabine
		HD-ara-C	high-dose cytarabine (ara-C)
HCR	health care review		
HCS	heel-cord stretches human chorionic somatomammotropin	HDBQ	Hilton Drinking Behavior Questionnaire
		HDC	habilitative day care high-dose chemotherapy
17-HCS	17-hydroxycorticosteroids	HDC-ASCS	high-dose chemotherapy with autologous stem cell support
HCSE	horse chestnut seed extract		
HCT	head computerized (axial) tomography hematocrit	HDCC	high-dose combination chemotherapy
		HD-CPA	high-dose cyclophosphamide
	histamine challenge test human chorionic thyrotropin	HDCPT	high-dose cyclophosphamide therapy
	hydrochlorothiazide (this is a dangerous abbreviation)	HDC-SCR	high-dose chemotherapy with stem-cell rescue
		HDCT	high-dose chemotherapy
	hydrocortisone	HDCV	rabies virus vaccine, human diploid (human diploid cell vaccine)
HCTU	home cervical traction unit		
HCTZ	hydrochlorothiazide (this is a dangerous abbreviation)	HDF	hemodiafiltration
		HDG	hydrogel (dressing)
		HDH	high-density humidity
HCV	hepatitis C vaccine hepatitis C virus	HDI	high-definition image
		HDL	high-density lipoprotein
HCVD	hypertensive cardiovascular disease	HDL-C	high-density lipoprotein cholesterol
HCWs	health-care workers	HDLW	hearing distance for watch to be heard in left ear
HCY	homocysteine		
HCYS	homocysteine		
HD	haloperidol decanoate Hansen's disease	HDM	home-delivered meals house dust mite
	hearing distance heart disease	HDMEC	human dermal microvascular endothelial cells
	Heller-Dor (procedure) heloma durum	HD-MTX	high-dose methotrexate
	hemodialysis herniated disk	HD-MTX-CF	high-dose methotrexate and leucovorin (citrovorum factor)
	high dose hip disarticulation	HD-MTX/LV	high-dose methotrexate and leucovorin
	Hodgkin's disease hospital day hospital discharge	HDN	hemolytic disease of the newborn

148

	heparin dosing nomogram	HEDIS	Health Employer Data
	high-density nebulizer		and Information Set
HDNS	Hodgkin's disease,	HEENT	head, eyes, ears, nose,
	nodular sclerosis		and throat
HDP	high-density polyethylene	HEK	human embryonic kidney
	hydroxymethyline	HEL	*Helicobacter pylori*
	diphosphonate		vaccine
HDPAA	heparin-dependent		human embryonic lung
	platelet-associated	HeLa	Helen Lake (tumor cells)
	antibody	HELLP	hemolysis, elevated liver
HDPC	hand piece	Syn-	enzymes, and low
HDR	heparin dose response	drome	platelet count
	husband to delivery room	HEMA	hydroxyethylmethacrylate
HDRA	histoculture drug response	HEMI	hemiplegia
	assay	HEMOSID	hemosiderin
HDRB	high-dose rate	HEMPAS	hereditary erythrocytic
	brachytherapy		multinuclearity with
HDRS	Hamilton Depression		positive acidified serum
	Rating Scale		test
HDRW	hearing distance for watch	HEMS	helicopter emergency
	to be heard in right ear		medical services
HDS	Hamilton Depression	HEN	hemorrhages, exudates,
	(Rating) Scale		and nicking
	herniated disk syndrome		home enteral nutrition
HDSCR	health deviation self-care	He-Ne	helium-neon
	requisite	HEP	hemoglobin
HDT	habilitative day treatment		electrophoresis
HDU	hemodialysis unit		heparin
	high-dependency unit (an		hepatic
	intensive care unit)		hepatoerythropoietic
HDV	hepatitis D virus		porphyria
HDW	hearing distance (with)		hepatoma
	watch		histamine equivalent
HDYF	how do you feel		prick
HE	hard exudate		home exercise program
	health educator	HEPA	hamster egg penetration
	hepatic encephalopathy		assay
H&E	hematoxylin and eosin		high-efficiency particulate
	hemorrhage and exudate		air (filter)
	heredity and environment	hep cap	heparin cap
HEA	health	HERP	human exposure
HEAR	hospital emergency		(dose)/rodent potency
	ambulance radio		(dose)
HEAT	human erythrocyte	HES	hetastarch (hydroxyethyl
	agglutination test		starch; Hespan)
HEB	hydrophilic emollient base		hypereosinophilic
HEC	Health Education Center		syndrome
HeCOG	Hellenic Cooperative	HEs	hypertensive emergencies
	Oncology Group	HETF	home enteral tube feeding

H

HEV	hepatitis E vaccine hepatitis E virus high endothelial venule	HFMD	hand-foot-and-mouth disease (often caused by coxsackievirus A16)
Hex	altretamine (hexamethylmelamine; Hexalen)	HFO	high-frequency oscillation
		HFOV	high-frequency oscillatory ventilation
Hexa-CAF	altretamine (hexamethylmelamine), cyclophosphamide, methotrexate (amethopterin), and fluorouracil	HFP	hepatic functional panel (see page 358) Hoffa fat pad
		HFPPV	high-frequency positive pressure ventilation
		HFR	hemorrhagic fever with renal syndrome vaccine
HF	Hageman factor hard feces hay fever head of fetus heart failure high frequency Hispanic female hot flashes house formula	HFRS	hemorrhagic fever with renal syndrome
		HFS	hand-foot syndrome
		HFSH	human follicle-stimulating hormone
		HFST	hearing-for-speech test
		HFUPR	hourly fetal urine production rate
		HFV	high-frequency ventilation high-fruit/vegetable (diet)
HFA	health facility administrator hydrofluoroalkane-134a	HFX RT	hyperfractionated radiation therapy
HFAS	hereditary flat adenoma syndrome	HG	handgrasp handgrip hemoglobin
HFB	high-frequency band	Hg	mercury
HFC	hydrofluorocarbon	HGA	high-grade astrocytomas
HFCB	horizontal flow clean bench	Hgb	hemoglobin
HFCC	high-frequency chest compression	Hgb ELECT	hemoglobin electrophoresis
HFD	high-fiber diet high-forceps delivery high-frequency discharges	Hgb F	fetal hemoglobin
		Hgb S	sickle cell hemoglobin
		HGE	human granulocytic ehrlichiosis
hFH	heterozygous familial hypercholesterolemia	HGES	handgrasp equal and strong
HFHL	high-frequence hearing loss	HGF	hepatocyte growth factor
		HGG	human gamma globulin
HFI	hereditary fructose intolerance	HGH	human growth hormone
		HGI	Human Genome Initiative
HFIP	hexafluoro-isopropranolol	HGM	home glucose monitoring
HFJV	high-frequency jet ventilation	HGN	hypogastric nerve
		HGO	hepatic glucose output hip guidance orthosis
H flu	*Haemophilus influenzae*		
HFM	hand-foot-and-mouth (disease) (often caused by coxsackievirus A16)	HGP	Human Genome Project

H

HGPRT	hypoxanthine-guanine phosphoribosyl-transferase		HHNS	hyperosmolar-hyperglycemic nonketotic syndrome
HGSIL	high-grade squamous intraepithelial lesion		HHS	Health and Human Service (US Department of)
HGV	hepatitis G vaccine			
	hepatitis G virus		HHT	hereditary hemorrhagic telangiectasis
HH	hard of hearing			
	head hood		HHTC	high-humidity trach collar
	hiatal hernia		HHTM	high-humidity trach mask
	home health		HHTS	high-humidity tracheostomy shield
	homonymous hemiopia			
	household		HHV-8	human herpesvirus 8
	hypogonadotropic hypogonadism		HI	*Haemophilus influenzae*
				head injury
	hypoeninemic hypoaldosteronism			health insurance
				hearing impaired
H/H	hemoglobin/hematocrit			hemagglutination inhibition
H&H	hematocrit and hemoglobin			
				homicidal ideation
HHA	health hazard appraisal			hospital insurance
	hereditary hemolytic anemia			human insulin
			HIA	hemagglutination inhibition antibody
	home health agency			
	home health aid		HIAA	hydroxyindoleacetic acid
HH Assist	hand held assist		5-HIAA	5-hydroxyindoleacetic acid
HHC	home health care			
HHCA	home health care agency		HIAP	human intracisternal A-type particle
	hypothermic hypokalemic cardioplegic arrest		HIB	*Haemophilus influenzae* type b (vaccine)
HHD	Doctor of Holistic Health		HIB$_{cn}$	*haemophilus influenzae* type b conjugate vaccine
	home hemodialysis			
	hypertensive heart disease			
HHFM	high-humidity face mask		HIB$_{HbOC}$	*Haemophilus influenzae* type b vaccine, HbOC conjugate vaccine
HHH	hypermethionemia, hyperammonemia, and homocitrolinemia (syndrome)			
			HIB$_{PRP-D}$	*haemophilus influenzae* type b vaccine, PRP-D conjugate vaccine
HHM	high-humidity mask			
	humoral hypercalcemia of malignancy		HIB$_{PRP-OMP}$	*haemophilus influenzae* type b vaccine, PRP-OMP conjugate vaccine
HHN	hand held nebulizer			
HHNC	hyperosmolar hyperglycemic nonketotic coma		HIB$_{PRP-T}$	*haemophilus influenzae* type b vaccine, PRP-T conjugate vaccine
HHNK	hyperglycemic hyperosmolar nonketotic (coma)		HIB$_{ps}$	*haemophilus influenzae* type b polysaccharide vaccine

H

HIC	Human Investigation Committee	HIPAA	Health Insurance Portability and Accountability Act of 1996
hi-cal	high caloric		
HID	headache, insomnia, and depression	HIPC	hormone-independent prostate cancer
	herniated intervertebral disk	HIPPS	Health Insurance Prospective Payment System
HIDA	hepato-iminodiacetic acid (lidofenin)	hi-pro	high-protein
HiDAC	high-dose cytarabine (ara-C)	HIR	head injury routine
HIDS	hyperimmunoglobulinemia D syndrome	HIS	Hanover Intensive Score
			Health Intention Scale
HIE	hyperimmunoglobulinemia E		high-intermittent suction
			histidine
	hypoxic-ischemic encephalopathy		Home Incapacity Scale
			hospital (healthcare) information system
HIF	*Haemophilus influenzae*	HISMS	How I See Myself Scale
	higher integrative functions	HISTO	histoplasmin skin test
			histoplasmosis
HIFU	high-intensity focused ultrasonography	HIT	heparin induced thrombocytopenia
HIHA	high impulsiveness, high anxiety		histamine inhalation test
			home infusion therapy
HIHARS	hyperventilation-induced high-amplitude rhythmic slowing	HITS	high-intensity transient signals
HII	hepatic-iron index	HITTS	heparin-induced thrombotic thrombocytopenia syndrome
HIIC	heated intraoperative intraperitoneal chemotherapy		
		HIU	head injury unit
HIL	hypoxic-ischemic lesion	HIV	human immunodeficiency virus
HILA	high impulsiveness, low anxiety		human immunodeficiency virus vaccine
HILP	hyperthermic isolated limb perfusion	HIV-1	human immunodeficiency virus type 1
HIM	health information management	HIV-2	human immunodeficiency virus type 2
HIN	*haemophilus influenzae* nontypable strain(s) vaccine	HIVAT	home intravenous antibiotic therapy
		HIVD	herniated intervertebral disk
HINI	hypoxic-ischemic neuronal injury	HIV-D	human immunodeficiency virus-related dementia
HIO	health insuring organization	hi-vit	high-vitamin
	hepatic iron overload	HIVMP	high-dose intravenous methylprednisolone
HIP	health insurance plan		

152

HJB	Howell-Jolly bodies	HLT	heart-lung transplantation (transplant)
HJR	hepatojugular reflux		
HK	hand-to-knee	HLV	herpes-like virus
	heel-to-knee		hypoplastic left ventricle
	hexokinase	HM	hand motion
HKAFO	hip-knee-ankle-foot orthosis		head movement
			heart murmur
HKAO	hip-knee-ankle orthosis		heavily muscled
HKMN	Hickman (catheter)		heloma molle
HKO	hip-knee orthosis		Hispanic male
HKS	heel-knee-shin (test)		Holter monitor
HKT	heterotopic kidney transplant		human milk
			human semisynthetic insulin
HL	hairline		humidity mask
	half-life	HMA	hemorrhages and microaneurysms
	hallux limitus		
	haloperidol	HMB	beta-hydroxy-beta methylbutyrate (a leucine metabolite)
	harelip		
	hearing level		
	hearing loss		homatropine methylbromide
	heavy lifting		
	hemilaryngectomy	HMBA	hexamethylene bisacetamide
	heparin lock		
	hepatic lipase	HMD	hyaline membrane disease
	Hickman line	HMDP	hydroxymethyline diphosphonate
H&L	heart and lung		
HLA	human leukocyte antigen	HME	heat and moisture exchanger
	human lymphocyte antigen		
			heat, massage, and exercise
HLA nega-tive	heart, lungs, and abdomen negative		home medical equipment
			human monocytic ehrlichiosis
HLB	head, limbs, and body		
HLD	haloperidol decanoate	HMETSC	heavy metal screen
	herniated lumbar disk	HMF	human milk fortifier
HLDP	hypoglossia-limb deficiency phenotype	HMG	human menopausal gonadotropin
HLGR	high-level gentamicin resistance	HMG CoA	hydroxymethyl glutaryl coenzyme A
HLH	hemophagocytic lymphohistiocytosis	HMI	healed myocardial infarction
	human luteinizing hormone		history of medical illness
HLHS	hypoplastic left-heart syndrome	HMIS	hospital medical information system
HLK	heart, liver, and kidneys	HMK	homemaking
HLM	hemosiderin-laden macrophages	HM & LP	hand motion and light perception
HLP	hyperlipoproteinemia		
hLS	human lung surfactant		

H

HMM	altretamine (hexamethyl-melamine)	HNKDC	hyperosomolar nonketotic diabetic coma
HMO	Health Maintenance Organization	HNKDS	hyperosmolar nonketotic diabetic state
HMP	health maintenance plan	HNLN	hospitalization no longer necessary
	hexose monophosphate		
	hot moist packs	HNN	hybrid neural network
HMPAO	hexylmethylpropylene aminoxine	HNP	herniated nucleus pulposus
HMR	histocytic medullary reticulosis	HNPCC	heredity nonpolyposis colorectal cancer
	Hoechst Marion Roussel	HNPP	hereditary neuropathy with liability to pressure palsies
^{1}H-MRS	proton magnetic resonance spectroscopy	HNRNA	heterogeneous nuclear ribonucleic acid
HMS	hyperactive malarial splenomegaly	HNS	0.45% sodium chloride injection (half normal saline)
	hypodermic morphine sulfate (this is a dangerous abbreviation)		head and neck surgery
			head, neck, and shaft
HMS®	medrysone	HNSCC	squamous cell carcinoma of the head and neck
hMSCs	human mesenchymal stem cells		
HMSN I	hereditary motor and sensory neuropathy type I	HNSN	home, no services needed
		HNT	hantaan (hantavirus) vaccine
HMSR	high medical-social risk	HNV	has not voided
HMSS	hyperactive malarial splenomegaly syndrome	HNWG	has not worn glasses
		HO	hand orthosis
HMWK	high-molecular weight kininogen		Hemotology-Oncology
			heterotropic ossification
HMX	heat massage exercise		hip orthosis
HN	head and neck		house officer
	head nurse	H/O	history of
	high nitrogen	H_2O	water
	home nursing	H_2O_2	hydrogen peroxide
H&N	head and neck	HOA	hip osteoarthritis
HN2	mechlorethamine HCl	HOB	head of bed
HNC	head and neck cancer	HOB UPSOB	head of bed up for shortness of breath
	human neutrophil collagenase		
		HOC	Health Officer Certificate
	hyperosmolar nonketotic coma	HOCM	high-osmolality contrast media
HNCa	head and neck cancer		
HNCCG	Head and Neck Cancer Cooperative Group		hypertrophic obstructive cardiomyopathy
		HOG	halothane, oxygen, and gas (nitrous oxide)
HNE	human neutrophil elastase		
HNI	hospitalization not indicated	HOH	hard of hearing
		HOI	hospital onset of infection

H

HOM	high-osmolar contrast media	HPD	high-protein diet
			home peritoneal dialysis
HONK	hyperosmolar nonketotic (coma)	HpD	hematoporphyrin derivative
HOP	hourly output	HP&D	hemoprofile and
HOPI	history of present illness		differential
HORF	high-output renal failure	HPE	hemorrhage, papilledema, exudate
HORS	Hemiballism/Hemichorea Outcome Rating Score		history and physical examination
HOSP	hospital	HPET	*Helicobacter pylori*
	hospitalization		eradication therapy
HOTV	letter symbols used in pediatric visual acuity testing	HPF	high-power field
		HPFH	hereditary persistence of fetal hemoglobin
HOVT	letter symbols used in pediatric visual acuity testing	HPG	human pituitary gonadotropin
		HPI	history of present illness
HP	hard palate	HPIP	history, physical, impression, and plan
	Harvard pump		
	Helicobacter pylori	HPL	human placenta lactogen
	hemipelvectomy		hyperplexia
	hemiplegia	HPLC	high-performance (pressure) liquid chromatography
	high-protein (supplement)		
	hot packs		
	house physician	HPM	hemiplegic migraine
	hydrogen peroxide	HPMC	high-performance membrane chromatography
	hydrophilic petrolatum		
Hp	*Helicobacter pylori*		
H&P	history and physical		hydroxypropyl methylcellulose
HPA	hybridization protection assay		
		HPN	home parenteral nutrition
	hypothalamic-pituitary-adrenal (axis)		
		HPNI	hemodialysis prognostic nutrition index
HPAE-PAD	high-pH anion exchange chromatography coupled with pulsed amperometric detection		
		HPNS	high pressure nervous syndrome
		HPO	hydrophilic ointment
HPAT	home parenteral antibiotic therapy		hypertrophic pulmonary osteoarthropathy
HPB	Health Protection Branch (the Canadian equivalent of the U.S. Food and Drug Administration)	HPOA	hypertrophic pulmonary osteoarthropathy
		2HPP	2-hour postprandial (blood sugar)
		2HPPBS	2-hour postprandial blood sugar
HPC	hereditary prostate cancer history of present condition (complaint)	HPPM	hyperplastic persistent pupillary membrane
HPCE	high-performance capillary electrophoresis	hPRL	prolactin, human

H

HPS	hantavirus pulmonary syndrome	HRCT	high-resolution computed tomography
	hepatopulmonary syndrome	HRD	human retroviral disease
	hypertrophic pyloric stenosis	HRE	high-resolution electrocardiography
HpSA	*Helicobacter pylori* stool antigen	HRF	Harris return flow health-related facility histamine releasing factor
HPT	heparin protamine titration histamine provocation test		hypertensive renal failure
	home pregnancy test hyperparathyroidism	HRIF	histamine inhibitory releasing factor
HPTD	highly permeable transparent dressing	HRL	head rotated left
		HRLA	human reovirus-like agent
hPTH	human parathyroid hormone I$_{34}$ (teriparatide)	HRLM	high-resolution light microscopy
		hRLX-2	synthetic human relaxin
HPTM	home prothrombin time monitoring	HRMPC	hormone-refractory metastatic prostate cancer
HPTX	hemopneumothorax		
HPV	human papilloma virus human papilloma virus vaccine	HRNB	Halstead-Reitan Neuropsychological Battery
	human parvovirus	HRP	high-risk pregnancy horseradish peroxidase
H pylori	*Helicobacter pylori*		
HPZ	high pressure zone	HRP-2	histidine-rich protein-2
HQC	hydroquinone cream	HRPC	hormone-refractory prostate cancer
HQL	health-related quality of life		
		HRQL	health-related quality of life
HR	hallux rigidus		
	Harrington rod	HRQOL	health-related quality of life
	hazard ratio		
	heart rate	HRR	head rotated right
	hemorrhagic retinopathy	HRRC	Human Research Review Committee
	hospital record		
	hour	HRS	Haw River syndrome
Hr 0	zero hour (when treatment starts)		hepatorenal syndrome Hodgkin-Reed-Sternberg (cells)
Hr -2	minus two hours (two hours prior to treatment)	HRSD	Hamilton Rating Scale for Depression
H & R	hysterectomy and radiation	HRST	heat, reddening, swelling, or tenderness
HRA	high-right atrium histamine releasing activity	HRT	heart rate heparin response test high-risk transfer
H2RA	histamine$_2$-receptor antagonist		hormone replacement therapy
HRC	Human Rights Committee	HRV	heart rate variability

	heterogeneous resistance to vancomycin	HSE	herpes simplex encephalitis
HS	bedtime (must specify if a dose is to be given one time [HS × 1 dose today] or nightly [HS nightly])		human skin equivalent hypertonic saline-epinephrine
	half strength	HSES	hemorrhagic shock and encephalopathy
	hamstrings	HSG	herpes simplex genitalis
	hamstring sets		hysterosalpingogram
	Hartman's solution (lactated Ringer's)	HSGYV	heat, steam, gum, yawn, and Valsalva's maneuver (for otitis media)
	heart size		
	heart sounds		
	heavy smoker	H-SIL	high-grade squamous intraepithelial lesions
	heel spur	HSK	herpes simplex keratitis
	heel stick	HSL	herpes simplex labialis
	hereditary spherocytosis		hormone sensitive lipase
	herpes simplex		
	hidradenitis suppurativa	HSM	hepatosplenomegaly
	high school		holosystolic murmur
	hippocampal sclerosis	HSN	Hansen-Street nail
	Hurlers syndrome		heart sounds normal
H → S	heel-to-shin		hereditary sensory neuropathy
H&S	hearing and speech		
	hemorrhage and shock	HSP	heat shock protein
	hysterectomy and sterilization		Henoch-Schönlein purpura hereditary spastic paraplegia
HSA	Health Services Administration (Administrator)		hysterosalpingography
		HSPC	hydrogenated soy phosphatidyl choline
	Health Systems Agency		
	human serum albumin	HSPE	high-strength pancreatic enzymes
	hypersomnia-sleep apnea	HSQ	Health Status Questionnaire
HSAN	hereditary sensory and autonomic neuropathy (types I–IV)	HSR	heated serum reagin hypersensitivity reaction hypofractionated stereotactic radiotherapy
HSB	husband		
HSBS	evening blood sugar		
HSBG	heel stick blood gas		
HSC	hematopoietic stem cell	HSS	half-strength saline (0.45% Sodium Chloride)
HSCL	Hopkins Symptom Check List		
HSD	Honestly Significant Difference (test) (Turkey)	HSSE	high soap suds enema
		HS-tk	herpes simplex thymidine kinase
	hypoactive sexual desire (disorder)	HSV	herpes simplex virus highly selective vagotomy

157

HSV-1	herpes simplex virus type 1	HTM	*Haemophilus* test medium
	herpes simplex virus type 1 vaccine		high threshold mechanoceptors
HSV₂	herpes simplex virus type 2 vaccine	HTML	hypertext markup language
		HTN	hypertension
HSV₁₂	herpes simplex virus types 1, 2 vaccine	HTO	high tibial osteotomy
		HTP	House-Tree-Person-test
HSV-2	herpes simplex virus type 2	5-HTP	serotonin (5-hydroxytryptophan)
HSVE	herpes simplex virus encephalitis	HTR	hard tissue replacement
HT	hammertoe	hTRT	human telomerase reverse transcriptase
	hearing test		
	heart	HTS	head traumatic syndrome
	heart transplant		heel-to-shin (test)
	height		Hematest® stools
	high temperature		high-throughput screening
	hormonotherapy	HTSCA	human tumor stem cell assay
	Hubbard tank		
	hypermetropia	H-TSH	human thyroid-stimulating hormone
	hyperopia		
	hypertension	HTT	hand thrust test
	hyperthermia	HTV	herpes-type virus
	hyperthyroid	HTVD	hypertensive vascular disease
H/T	heel and toe (walking)		
H&T	hospitalization and treatment	HTX	hemothorax
		HTx	heart transplant
H(T)	intermittent hypertropia	HU	head unit
5-HT₁	serotonin (5-hydroxytryptamine)		hydroxyurea
			hypertensive urgencies
HTA	hypertension (French)	Hu	Hounsfield units
ht. aer.	heated aerosol	HUAEC	human umbilical endothelial cells
HTAT	human tetanus antitoxin		
HTB	hot tub bath	HUCB	human umbilical cord blood
HTC	heated tracheostomy collar		
		HUH	Humana Hospital
	hypertensive crisis	HUI	Health Utilities Index
hTERT	human telomerase reverse transcriptase	HUIFM	human leukocyte interferon meloy
HTF	house tube feeding	HUK	human urinary kallikrein
HTGL	hepatic triglyceride lipase	HUM	heat, ultrasound, and massage
HTK	heel-to-knee (test)		
HTL	hearing threshold level	HUM 70/30	human insulin, regular 30 units/mL with human insulin isophane suspension 70 units/mL (Humulin® 70/30 insulin)
	honey-thick liquid (diet consistency)		
	human T-cell leukemia		
	human thymic leukemia		
HTLV III	human T-cell lymphotrophic virus type III	HUMARA	human androgen receptor assay

H

HUM L	human insulin zinc suspension (Humulin® L Insulin)	HVPG	hepatic venous pressure gradient
HUM N	human insulin isophane suspension (Humulin® N Insulin)	HYPT	hyperventilation provocation test
		HVS	hyperventilation syndrome
HUM R	human insulin, regular (Humulin® R Insulin)	HVS-TK	herpes simplex virus thymidine kinase
HUR	hydroxyurea	HW	heparin well
HUS	head ultrasound		homework
	hemolytic uremic syndrome		housewife
	husband	HWB	hot water bottle
husb	husband	HWFE	housewife
HUT	head-upright tilt (test)	HWG	has worn glasses
	hyperplasia of usual type	HWH	halfway house
HUVEC	human umbilical vein endothelial cells	HWP	hot wet pack
		HWPG	has worn prescription glasses
HV	hallux valgus	Hx	history
	Hantavirus		hospitalization
	has voided	HXM	altretamine (hexamethylmelamine)
	Hemovac®		
	hepatic vein	Hx & Px	history and physical (examination)
	herpesvirus		
	home visit	Hy	hypermetropia
H&V	hemigastrectomy and vagotomy	HYDRO	hydronephrosis
			hydrotherapy
HVA	homovanillic acid	HYG	hygiene
HVD	hypertensive vascular disease	HYPER	above
			higher than
HVDO	hypovitaminosis D osteopathy	Hyper Al	hyperalimentation
		Hyper K	hyperkalemia
HVE	high-voltage electrophoresis	HYPER T & A	hypertrophic tonsils and adenoids
HVES	high-voltage electrical stimulation	HYPO	below
			hypodermic injection
			lower than
HVF	Humphrey visual field	Hypo K	hypokalemia
HVGS	high-voltage galvanic stimulation	hypopit	hypopituitarism
		HYs	healthy years of life
HVI	hollow viscus injury	Hyst	hysterectomy
HVL	half-value layer	Hz	Hertz
	hippocampal volume loss	HZ	herpes zoster
HVOD	hepatic veno-occlusive disease	HZD	herpes zoster dermatitis
		HZO	herpes zoster ophthalmicus
HVOO	hepatic venous outflow obstruction	HZV	herpes zoster virus
HVPC	high-voltage pulsed current		

H

I

I	impression
	incisal
	incontinent
	independent
	initial
	inspiration
	intact (bag of waters)
	intermediate
	iris
	one
I_2	iodine
I^{131}	radioactive iodine
I-3+7	idarubicin and cytarabine
IA	ideational apraxia
	incidental appendectomy
	incurred accidentally
	intra-amniotic
	intra-arterial
I & A	irrigation and aspiration
IAA	ileoanal anastomosis
	insulin autoantibodies
	interrupted aortic arch
IAB	incomplete abortion
	induced abortion
	intermittent androgen blockade
IABC	intra-aortic balloon counterpulsation
IABCP	intra-aortic balloon counterpulsation
IABP	intra-aortic balloon pump
	intra-arterial blood pressure
IAC	internal auditory canal
	intra-arterial chemotherapy
	isolated adrenal cell
IAC-CPR	interposed abdominal compressions—cardiopulmonary resuscitation
IACG	intermittent angle-closure glaucoma

IACNS	isolated angiitis of central nervous system
IACP	intra-aortic counterpulsation
IAD	implantable atrial defibrillator
	intermittent androgen deprivation
	intractable atopic dermatitis
IADHS	inappropriate antidiuretic hormone syndrome
IADL	Instrumental Activities of Daily Living
IA DSA	intra-arterial digital subtraction arteriography
IAET	International Association for Enterostomal Therapy (Standards of Care Dermal Wounds: Pressure Ulcers)—see WOCN
IAGT	indirect antiglobulin test
IAHA	immune adherence hemagglutination
IAHC	intra-arterial hepatic chemotherapy
IAHD	idiopathic acquired hemolytic disease
IAI	intra-abdominal infection
	intra-amniotic infection
IALD	instrumental activities of daily living
IAM	internal auditory meatus
IAN	intern's admission note
IAO	immediately after onset
IAP	independent adjudicating panel
	intermittent acute porphyria
	intra-abdominal pressure
	intracarotid amobarbital procedure
IARC	International Agency for Research on Cancer
IART	intra-atrial reentrant tachycardia

IAS	idiopathic ankylosing spondylitis	IBPS	Insall-Burstein posterior stabilizer
	intermittent androgen suppression	IBR	immediate breast reconstruction
	internal anal sphincter		infectious bovine rhinotracheitis
IASD	interatrial septal defect		
IAT	immunoaugmentive therapy	IBRS	Inpatient Behavior Rating Scale
	indirect antiglobulin test	IBS	irritable bowel syndrome
	intracarotid amobarbital test	IBT	ink blot test (Rorschach test)
	intraoperative autologous transfusion		interblinking time
			immune-based therapy
IATT	intra-arterial thrombolytic therapy	IBTR	intrabreast-tumor recurrence
IAV	intermittent assist ventilation	IBU	ibuprofen
		IBW	ideal body weight
IB	ileal bypass	IC	between meals
	insulin receptor binding test		iliac crest
			immune complex
	isolation bed		immunocompromised
IB1A	interferon beta-1a (Avonex)		incipient cataract (grade 1+ to 4+)
IBAM	idiopathic bile acid malabsorption		incomplete
			indirect calorimetry
IBBB	intra-blood-brain barrier		indirect Coombs (test)
IBBBB	incomplete bilateral bundle branch block		individual counseling
			informed consent
IBC	invasive bladder cancer		inspiratory capacity
	iron binding capacity		intensive care
IBD	infectious bursal disease		intercostal
			intercourse
	inflammatory bowel disease		intermediate care
			intermittent catheterization
IBDQ	Inflammatory Bowel Disease Questionnaire		intermittent claudication
			interstitial changes
IBG	iliac bone graft		interstitial cystitis
IBI	intermittent bladder irrigation		intracerebral
			intracranial
ibid	at the same place		intraincisional
IBILI	indirect bilirubin		irritable colon
IBM	ideal body mass	I/C	imipenem-cilastatin (Primaxin®)
	inclusion body myositis		
IBMI	initial body mass index	ICA	ileocolic anastomosis
IBMTR	International Bone Marrow Transplant Registry		intermediate care area
			internal carotid artery
			intracranial abscess
IBNR	incurred but not reported		intracranial aneurysm
IBOW	intact bag of waters		islet-cell antibody

I

ICa	calcium, ionized
ICAAC	Interscience Conference on Antimicrobial Agents and Chemotherapy
ICAM	intracellular adhesion molecule
ICAM-1	intercellular adhesion molecule-1
ICAO	internal carotid artery occlusion
ICAS	intermediate coronary artery syndrome
ICAT	infant cardiac arrest tray
ICB	intracranial bleeding
ICBG	iliac crest bone graft
ICBT	intercostobronchial trunk
ICC	immunocytochemistry
	Indian childhood cirrhosis
	intracluster correlation coefficient
	intraclass correlation coefficient
	islet cell carcinoma
ICCD	intensified charge-coupled device
ICCE	intracapsular cataract extraction
ICCU	intensive coronary care unit
	intermediate coronary care unit
ICD	implantable cardioverter defibrillator
	indigocarmine dye
	informed consent document
	instantaneous cardiac death
	isocitrate dehydrogenase
	irritant contact dermatitis
ICDA	International Classification of Disease, Adapted
ICDB	incomplete database
ICDC	implantable cardioverter defibrillator catheter

ICD 9 CM	International Statistical Classification of Diseases, 9th Revision, Clinical Modification
ICD-10-PCS	International Statistical Classification of Diseases, Tenth Revision, Procedure Coding Classification System
ICDO	International Classification of Diseases for Oncology
ICE	ice, compression, and elevation
	ifosfamide, carboplatin, and etoposide
	individual career exploration
	interleukin-1 alpha converting enzyme
	interleukin-1 beta converting enzyme
	intracardiac echocardiography
+ ice	add ice
ICES	ice, compression, elevation, and support
ICF	intermediate care facility
	intracellular fluid
ICG	indocyanine green
ICGA	indocyanine green angiography
ICH	immunocompromised host
	International Council on Harmonization (of Technical Requirements for Registration of Pharmaceuticals for Human Use)
	intracerebral hemorrhage
	intracranial hemorrhage
ICIT	intensified conventional insulin therapy
ICL	intracorneal lens
	isocitrate lyase
ICLE	intracapsular lens extraction

I

ICM	intercostal margin	ICTX	intermittent cervical
	intercostal muscle		traction
ICN	infection control nurse	ICU	intensive care unit
	intensive care nursery		intermediate care unit
ICN2	neonatal intensive care	ICV	intracerebroventricular
	unit level II	ICVH	ischemic cerebrovascular
ICP	inductively coupled		headache
	plasma	ICW	in connection with
	intercostal position (for		intercellular water
	chest lead)	ID	identification
	intracranial pressure		identify
ICP-MS	inductively-coupled		idiotype
	plasma—mass		ifosfamide, mesna
	spectrometer		uroprotection, and
ICP-OES	inductively-coupled		doxorubicin
	plasma—optical		immunodiffusion
	emission spectrometry		induction delivery
ICPP	intubated continuous		infectious disease
	positive pressure		(physician or
ICR	intercostal retractions		department)
	intrastromal corneal		initial diagnosis
	ring		initial dose
ICRC	International Committee		internal derangement
	of the Red Cross		intradermal
ICRF-159	razoxane	*id*	the same
ICS	ileocecal sphincter	I & D	incision and drainage
	inhaled corticosteroid(s)	IDA	idarubicin (Idamycin)
	intercostal space		iron deficiency
ICSC	idiopathic central serous		anemia
	choroidopathy	IDAM	infant of drug abusing
ICSH	interstitial cell-stimulating		mother
	hormone	IDB	incomplete database
ICSI	intracytoplasmic sperm	IDC	idiopathic dilated
	injection		cardiomyopathy
ICSR	Individual Case Safety		invasive ductal cancer
	Reports	IDCF	immunodiffusion
	intercostal space		complement fixation
	retractions	IDCM	idiopathic dilated
ICT	icterus		cardiomyopathy
	indirect Coombs' test	IDD	insulin-dependent
	inflammation of		diabetes
	connective tissue		iodine-deficiency
	intensive conventional		disorders
	therapy	IDDM	insulin-dependent diabetes
	intermittent cervical		mellitus
	traction	IDDS	implantable drug delivery
	intracranial tumor		system
	intracutaneous test	IDE	Investigational Device
	islet cell transplant		Exemption

163

IDEA	Individuals with Disabilities Education Act		international unit (European abbreviation)
IDET	intradiskal electrothermal therapy	I & E	ingress and egress (tubes) internal and external
IDFC	immature dead female child	*i.e.*	that is
IDH	isocitric dehydrogenase	IEC	independent ethics committee inpatient exercise center intradiskal electrothermal coagulation
IDI	Interpersonal Dependency Inventory intrathecal drug infusion		
IDK	internal derangement of knee	IEF	isoelectric focusing
IDL	intermediate-density lipoprotein	IEI	idiopathic environmental intolerance
IDM	infant of a diabetic mother	IEL	intestinal-intraepithelial lymphocyte
IDMC	immature dead male child	IEM	immune electron microscopy inborn errors of metabolism
IDNA	iron-deficient, not anemic		
IDP	initiate discharge planning inosine diphosphate	iEMG	integrated electromyography
IDPN	intradialytic parenteral nutrition	IEP	immunoelectrophoresis Individualized Education Plan
IDR	idarubicin idiosyncratic drug reaction intradermal reaction	IEPA	immunoelectrophoresis analysis
IDS	infectious disease service integrated delivery system	I:E ratio	inspiratory to expiratory time ratio
IDT	intensive diabetes treatment interdisciplinary team intradermal test	IES	Impact of Event Scale
		IET	infantile estropia
		IF	idiopathic flushing ifosfamide (Ifex) immunofluorescence injury factor interferon interfrontal intermaxillary fixation internal fixation intrinsic factor involved field (radiotherapy)
IDTP	immunodiffusion tube precipitin		
IDU	idoxuridine infectious disease unit injecting drug user		
IDV	indinavir (Crixivan) intermittent demand ventilation		
IDVC	indwelling venous catheter	IFA	immunofluorescent assay indirect fluorescent antibody
IE	ifosfamide, and etoposide with mesna immunoelectrophoresis induced emesis infective endocarditis inner ear	IFAT	immunofluorescence antibody test (technique)
		IFC	interferential current

I

IFE	immunofixation electrophoresis			infusion hepatic arteriography
	in-flight emergency	IHC		idiopathic hypercalciuria
IFL	indolent follicular lymphoma			immobilization hypercalcemia
IFM	internal fetal monitoring			immunohistochemistry
IFN	interferon			inner hair cell
IFNB	interferon beta-1 b (Betaseron®)			(in cochlea)
IFO	ifosfamide (Ifex)	IHD		intraheptic duct (ule)
	in front of			ischemic heart disease
IFOS	ifosfamide (Ifex)	IHDN		integrated health delivery network
IFP	inflammatory fibroid polyps	IHH		idiopathic hypogonadotrophic hypogonadism
IFSAC	Inventory of Functional Status After Childbirth	IHO		idiopathic hypertrophic osteoarthropathy
IFSE	internal fetal scalp electrode	IHP		idiopathic hypoparathyroidism
IgA	immunoglobulin A			inferior hypogastric plexus
IGCS	inpatient geriatric consultation services	IHPH		intrahepatic portal hypertension
IgD	immunoglobulin D			
IGDE	idiopathic gait disorders of the elderly	IHPS		infantile hypertrophic pyloric stenosis
IGDM	infant of gestational diabetic mother	IHR		inguinal hernia repair intrinsic heart rate
IgE	immunoglobulin E	IHS		Indian Health Service
IGF-I	insulin-like growth factor I			integrated healthcare system
IGFA	indocyanine-green fundus angiography			International Headache Society (criteria)
IgG	immunoglobulin G			Iodiopathic Headache Score
IGIM	immune globulin intramuscular	IHs		iris hamartomas
IGIV	immune globulin intravenous	IHSA		iodinated human serum albumin
IgM	immunoglobulin M	IHSS		idiopathic hypertrophic subaortic stenosis
IGP	interstitial glycoprotein			
IGR	intrauterine growth retardation	IHT		insulin hypoglycemia test
IGT	impaired glucose tolerance	IHU		inpatient hospice unit
		IHW		inner heel wedge
IGTN	ingrown toenail	II		internal iliac (artery)
IH	indirect hemagglutination	IIA		internal iliac artery
	infectious hepatitis	IICP		increased intracranial pressure
	inguinal hernia			
	in-house	IICU		infant intensive care unit
IHA	immune hemolytic anemia	IIEF		International Index of Erectile Function
	indirect hemagglutination			

I

IIF	indirect immunofluorescence		indentation load deflection
IIH	idiopathic infantile hypercalcemia		intermediate density lipoproteins
IIH	iodine-induced hyperthyroidism		interstitial lung disease ischemic leg disease
IIHT	iodide-induced hyperthyroidism	ILE	infantile lobar emphysema
		ILF	indicated low forceps
IIM	idiopathic inflammatory myopathies	ILFC	immature living female child
IINB	iliohypogastric ilioinguinal nerve block	ILHP	ipsilateral hemidiaphragmatic paresis
IIP	idiopathic interstitial pneumonitis	ILI	influenza-like illness
		ILM	internal limiting membrane
IIPF	idiopathic interstitial pulmonary fibrosis	ILMC	immature living male child
IJ	ileojejunal internal jugular	ILMI	inferolateral myocardial infarct
I&J	insight and judgment	ILP	interstitial laser photocoagulation
IJC	internal jugular catheter		
IJD	inflammatory joint disease		isolated limb perfusion
IJO	idiopathic juvenile osteoporosis	ILQTS	idiopathic long QT (interval) syndrome
IJP	internal jugular pressure	ILVEN	inflammatory linear verrucous epidermal nevus
IJR	idiojunctional rhythm		
IJT	idiojunctional tachycardia		
IJV	internal jugular vein	IM	ice massage
IK	immobilized knee interstitial keratitis		infectious mononucleosis intermetatarsal
IL	immature lungs interleukin (1, 2, etc.) intralesional Intralipid®		internal medicine intramedullary intramuscular
IL-2	aldesleukin (Proleukin; interleukin-2)	IMA	inferior mesenteric artery internal mammary artery
IL-11	oprelvekin (Neumega; interleukin-11)	IMAC	ifosfamide, mesna uroprotection, doxorubicin (Adriamycin), and cisplatin
ILA	inferior lateral angle insulin-like activity		
ILB	incidental Lewy body		immobilized metal affinity chromatography
ILBBB	incomplete left bundle branch block		
ILBW	infant, low birth weight (less than 2,500 g)	IMAE	internal maxillary artery embolization
ILC	interstitial laser coagulation	IMAG	internal mammary artery graft
	invasive lobular cancer	IMARD	immunomodulating antirheumatic drugs
ILD	immature lung disease		

IMB	intermenstrual bleeding	important
IMBP	immobilized mismatch binding protein	impression
		improved
IMC	intermittent catheterization	inosine monophoshate
	intramedullary catheter	IMPX impaction
IMCI	Integrated Management of Childhood Illness	IMR infant mortality rate
		IMRA immunoradiometric assay
IMCU	intermediate care unit	
IME	important medical event	IMS immunosuppressants
	independent medical examination (evaluation)	incurred in military service
		IMT inspiratory muscle training
IMF	idiopathic myelofibrosis	
	ifosfamide, mesna uroprotection, methotrexate, and fluorouracil	intimal medial thickness
		IMU intermediate medicine unit
	immobilization mandibular fracture	IMV inferior mesenteric vein
	inframammary fold	intermittent mandatory ventilation
	intermaxillary fixation	
IMG	internal medicine group	intermittent mechanical ventilation
IMGU	insulin-mediated glucose uptake	IMVP-16 ifosfamide, mesna uroprotection, methotrexate, and etoposide
IMH	idiopathic myocardial hypertrophy	
IMH test	indirect microhemagglutination test	IN insulin
		intranasal
IMI	imipramine	In inches
	impending myocardial infarction	indium
		INAD in no apparent distress
	inferior myocardial infarction	Investigational New Animal Drug
	intramuscular injection	INB intercostal nerve blockade
^{131}I-MIBG	iodine^{131}-metaiodobenzyl-guanidine (iobenguane ^{131}I)	INC incisal
		incision
		incomplete
		incontinent
IMIG	intramuscular immunoglobulin	increase
		inside-the-needle catheter
IMLC	incomplete mitral leaflet closure	INCC Institut National du Cancer du Canada
IMM	immune modulating nutrition (immunonutrition)	Inc Spir incentive spirometer
		IND indinavir (Crixivan)
		induced
	immunizations	Investigational New Drug (application)
IMN	internal mammary (lymph) node	
		INDA Investigational New Drug Application
IMP	impacted	

167

INDIGO	interstitial laser ablation of the prostate	INR	international normalized ratio (for anticoagulant monitoring)
INDM	infant of nondiabetic mother	INS	idiopathic nephrotic syndrome
INDO	indomethacin		inspection
^{111}In-DTPA	indium pentetate		insurance
INE	infantile necrotizing encephalomyelopathy	INST	instrumental delivery
		INT	intermittent needle therapy
INEX	inexperienced		internal
INF	infant		
	infarction	Int mon	internal monitor
	infected	INTERP	interpretation
	infection	Int Med	internal medicine
	inferior	intol	intolerance
	influenza virus vaccine, not otherwise specified	int-rot	internal rotation
		int trx	intermittent traction
	information	intub	intubation
	infused	inver	inversion
	infusion	INVOS	in vivo optical spectroscopy
	intravenous nutritional fluid	IO	inferior oblique
INF$_a$	influenza virus, attenuated live vaccine		initial opening
			intestinal obstruction
INFC	infected		intraocular pressure
	infection		intra-Ommaya
INFs	influenza virus vaccine, split virus		intraoperative
		I&O	intake and output
INF$_w$	influenza virus vaccine, whole virus	IOA	intact on admission
		IOC	intern on call
ING	inguinal		intraoperative cholangiogram
✓ing	checking	IOCG	intraoperative cholangiogram
INH	isoniazid		
INI	intranuclear inclusion	IOD	interorbital distance
inj	injection	IODM	infant of diabetic mother
	injury		
INK	injury not known	IOF	intraocular fluid
INN	International Nonproprietary Name	IOFB	intraocular foreign body
		IOFNA	intraoperative fine needle aspiration
INO	inhaled nitrous oxide		
	internuclear ophthalmoplegia	IOH	idiopathic orthostatic hypotension
INOP	internodal ophthalmoplegia	IOI	intraosseous infusion
		IOL	intraocular lens
iNOS	inducible nitric oxide synthase	IOLI	intraocular lens implantation
inpt	inpatient	IOM	Institute of Medicine
INQ	inferior nasal quadrant	ION	ischemic optic neuropathy

IONIS	indirect optic nerve injury syndrome	IPCD	idiopathic paroxysmal cerebral dysrhythmia
IONTO	iontophoresis		infantile polycystic disease
IOOA	inferior oblique overaction	IPCK	infantile polycystic kidney (disease)
IOP	intraocular pressure		
IOR	ideas of reference	IPCT	intraperitoneal chemotherapy
	immature oocyte retrieval		
	inferior oblique recession	IPD	idiopathic Parkinson's disease
IO-RB	intraocular retinoblastoma		immediate pigment darkening
IORT	intraoperative radiation therapy		inflammatory pelvic disease
IOS	intraoperative sonography		intermittent peritoneal dialysis
IOT	intraocular tension		
IOTEE	intraoperative transesophageal echocardiography		interpupillary distance
		IPF	idiopathic pulmonary fibrosis
IOUS	intraocular ultrasound		interstitial pulmonary fibrosis
IOV	initial office visit		
IP	ice pack	IPFD	intrapartum fetal distress
	incubation period	IPG	impedance plethysmography
	individualized plan		
	Infrapatellar		individually polymerized grass
	inpatient		
	in plaster	IPH	idiopathic pulmonary hemosiderosis
	interphalangeal		
	interstitial pneumonia		interphalangeal
	intestinal permeability		intraparenchymal hemorrhage
	intraperitoneal		
	invasive procedures		intraperitoneal hemorrhage
I/P	iris/pupil		
IP3	inositol triphosphate	IPHEP	independent progressive home exercise program
IPA	independent practice association		
		IPHP	intraperitoneal hyperthermic chemotherapy
	interpleural analgesia		
	invasive pulmonary aspergillosis	IPI	International Prognostic Index
	isopropyl alcohol		
IPAA	ileo-pouch anal anastamosis	IPJ	interphalangeal joint
		IPK	intractable plantar keratosis
IPAP	inspiratory positive airway pressure		
		IPM	intrauterine pressure monitor
IPB	infrapopliteal bypass		
IPC	indirect pulp cavity		interventional pain management
	intermittent pneumatic compression (boots)		
		IPMI	inferoposterior myocardial infarct
	intraperitoneal chemotherapy		

IPN	infantile periarteritis nodosa	IPVC	interpolated premature ventricular contraction
	intern's progress note	IPW	interphalangeal width
	interstitial pneumonia	IQ	intelligence quotient
IPOF	immediate postoperative fitting	IQR	interquartile range
IPOM	intraperitoneal onlay mesh	IR	immediate-release (tablets)
IPOP	immediate postoperative prosthesis		inferior rectus
IPP	inflatable penile prosthesis		infrared
	intrapleural pressure		insulin resistance
	isolated pelvic perfusion		internal reduction
IPPA	inspection, palpation, percussion, and auscultation		internal resistance
			internal rotation
		I&R	insertion and removal
		IRA	infarct-related artery
IPPB	intermittent positive-pressure breathing	IRA-EEA	ileorectal anastomoses with end-to-end anastomosis
IP-PDT	intraperitoneal photodynamic therapy	IRAP	interleukin-1 receptor antagonist protein
IPPF	immediate postoperative prosthetic fitting	IRB	Institutional Review Board
IPPI	interruption of pregnancy for psychiatric indication	IRBBB	incomplete right bundle branch block
IPPV	intermittent positive pressure ventilation	IRBC	immature red blood cell
			irradiated red blood cells
IPS	infundibular pulmonic stenosis	IRBP	interphotoreceptor retinoid-binding protein
	initial prognostic score		
	intermittent photic stimulation	IRC	indirect radionuclide cystography
IPSCs	islet-producing stem cells		infrared coagulation
IPSF	immediate postsurgical fitting		Institutional Review Committee (Board)
IPSID	immunoproliferative small intestinal disease	IRCU	intensive respiratory care unit
IPSP	inhibitory postsynaptic potential	IRD	immune renal disease(s)
		IRDM	insulin-resistant diabetes mellitus
IPSS	inferior petrosal sinus sampling	IRDS	idiopathic respiratory distress syndrome
I-PSS	International Prostate Symptom Score		infant respiratory distress syndrome
I PSY	intermediate psychiatry		
IPT	intermittent pelvic traction	IRE	internal rotation in extension
iPTH	parathyroid hormone by radioimmunoassay	IRED	infrared emission detection
IPTX	intermittent pelvic traction		
IPV	inactivated poliovirus vaccine	IRF	internal rotation in flexion

IRH	intraretinal hemorrhage		Incest Survivors Anonymous
IRI	immunoreactive insulin		intrinsic sympathomimetic activity
IRIV	immunopotentiating reconstituted influenza virosomes	ISADH	inappropriate secretion of antidiuretic hormone
IRM	magnetic resonance imaging (French)	ISB	incentive spirometry breathing
IRMA	immediate response mobile analysis (blood analysis system)	ISBP	interscalen brachial plexus
		ISC	indwelling subclavian catheter
	immunoradiometric assay		infant servo-control
	intraretinal microvascular abnormalities		infant skin control
IRMS	isotope-ratio mass spectrometry		intermittent self-catheterization
IROS	ipsilateral routing of signals		intermittent straight catheterization
			isolette servo-control
IRR	infrared radiation	ISCM	intramedullary spinal cord metastases
	intrarenal reflux		
	irregular rate and rhythm	I/SCN	urinary iodine/thiocyanate ratio
IRRC	Institutional Research Review Committee	ISCOM	immunostimulating complex
irreg	irregular		
IRR HYDRO	irreversible hydrocolloid	ISCs	irreversible sickle cells
		ISCU	infant special care unit
IRS	Information and Referral Society	ISD	inhibited sexual desire
			initial sleep disturbance
	insulin-resistance syndrome		intrinsic (urethral) sphincter deficiency
IRSB	intravenous regional sympathetic block		isosorbide dinitrate
IRSG	Intergroup Rhabdomyosarcoma Study Group	ISDN	isosorbide dinitrate
		ISE	ion-sensitive electrode
		ISEL	in situ end labeling
IRT	immunoreactive trypsin	ISF	interstitial fluid
IRV	inspiratory reserve volume	ISG	immune serum globulin (immune globulin)
	inverse ratio ventilation	ISH	isolated systolic hypertension
IS	incentive spirometer		
	induced sputum	ISHH	in situ hybridization histochemistry
	in situ		
	intercostal space	ISHLT	International Society for Heart and Lung Transplantation
	inventory of systems		
	ipecac syrup		
I-S	Ionescu-Shiley (prosthetic heart valve)	ISHT	isolated systolic hypertension
I & S	intact and symmetrical	ISI	International Sensitivity Index
I/S	instruct/supervise		
ISA	ileosigmoid anastomosis	ISK	isokinetic

ISMA	infantile spinal muscular atrophy		inhalation therapy
			inspiratory time
ISMN	isosorbide mononitrate		intensive therapy
ISMO®	isosorbide mononitrate		intermittent traction
ISMP	Institute for Safe Medication Practices		interpreted
			intertrochanteric
ISNA	iron-sufficient, not anemic		intertuberous
ISO	isodose		intrathecal (dangerous abbreviation)
	isolette		
	isoproterenol		intratracheal (dangerous, could be interupted as intrathecal)
ISOE	isoetharine		
ISOF	isoflurane (Florane)		
ISOK	isokinetic		intratumoral
ISOM	isometric	ITA	individual treatment assessment
ISOs	isoenzymes		
ISP	inferior spermatic plexus		inferior temporal artery
	interspace		itasetron
ISQ	as before; continue on (*in status quo*)	ITAG	internal thoracic artery graft
ISR	injection site reaction	ITAL	intrathoracic artificial lung
	integrated secretory response	ITB	iliotibial band
			intrathecal baclofen
ISS	idiopathic short stature	ITBC	intraluminal typical bronchial carcinoid
	Individual Self-Rating Scale		
		ITBS	iliotibial band syndrome
	Injury Severity Score		Iowa Tests of Basic Skills
	irritable stomach syndrome	ITC	Incontinence Treatment Center
	Integrated Summary of Safety		in-the-canal (hearing aid)
			isothermal titration calorimetry
IS10S	10% invert sugar in 0.9% sodium chloride (saline) injection	ITCP	idiopathic thrombocytopenic purpura
ISSP	Infant Support Services Program	ITCU	intensive thoracic cardiovascular unit
IST	injection sclerotherapy	ITE	insufficient therapeutic effect
	insulin sensitivity test		
	insulin shock therapy		in-the-ear (hearing aid)
ISU	intermediate surgical unit	ITF	inpatient treatment facility
ISW	interstitial water	ITFF	intertrochanteric femoral fracture
IS10W	10% invert sugar injection (in water)		
		ITGV	intrathoracic gas volume
ISWI	incisional surgical wound infection	ITMTX	intrathecal methotrexate
		ITN	irinotecan (Camptosar)
IT	incentive therapy	ITOC	intratracheal oxygen catheter
	individual therapy		
	inferior-temporal	ITOP	intentional termination of pregnancy
	information technology		
	Inhalation Therapist		

ITOU	intensive therapy observation unit	IUPC	intrauterine pressure catheter
ITP	idiopathic thrombocytopenic purpura	IUPD	intrauterine pregnancy delivered
	interim treatment plan	IUP,TBCS	intrauterine pregnancy, term birth, cesarean section
ITPA	Illinois Test of Psycholinguistic Ability	IUP,TBLC	intrauterine pregnancy, term birth, living child
ITQ	inferior temporal quadrant	IUR	intrauterine retardation
ITR	isotretinoin (Accutane)	IUT	intrauterine transfusion
ITRA	itraconazole (Sporanox)	IUTD	immunizations up to date
ITS	internal transcribed spacer	IV	four
	isometric trunk stabilization		interview
			intravenous (i.v.)
ITSCU	infant-toddler special care unit		intravertebral
			invasive
ITT	identical twins (raised) together		inversion
	insulin tolerance test		symbol for class 4 controlled substances
	intention-to-treat (analysis)	IVA	Intervir-A
ITU	infant-toddler unit	IVAD	implantable venous access device
	intensive therapy unit		implantable vascular access device
	intensive treatment unit		
ITVAD	indwelling transcutaneous vascular access device	IVBAT	intravascular bronchoalveolar tumor
ITX	immunotoxin(s)	IVC	inferior vena cava
ITZ	itraconazole (Sporanox)		inspiratory vital capacity
IU	international unit (this is a dangerous abbreviation as it is read as intravenous)		intravenous chemotherapy
			intravenous cholangiogram
			intraventricular catheter
IUC	intrauterine catheter		intraventricular conduction
IUCD	intrauterine contraceptive device	IVCD	intraventricular conduction defect (delay)
IUD	intrauterine death		
	intrauterine device	IVCP	inferior vena cava pressure
IUDR	idoxuridine (Herplex)	IVCV	inferior venacavography
IUFB	intrauterine foreign body	IVD	intervertebral disk
IUFD	intrauterine fetal death (demise)		intravenous drip
		IVDA	intravenous drug abuse
	intrauterine fetal distress	IVDSA	intravenous digital subtraction angiography
IUFT	intrauterine fetal transfusion		
IUGR	intrauterine growth retardation (restriction)	IVDU	intravenous drug user
IUI	intrauterine insemination	IVET	*in vivo* expression technology
IUP	intrauterine pregnancy		

I

IVF	intervertebral foramina		intravenous rider (this is a
	intravenous fluid(s)		dangerous abbreviation
	in vitro fertilization		as it has been read as
IVFA	intravenous fluorescein		IVP-intravenous push)
	angiography		isovolumic relaxation
IVFE	intravenous fat		(time)
	emulsion	IVRA	intravenous regional
IVF-ET	*in vitro* fertilization-		anesthesia
	embryo transfer	IVRAP	intravenous retrograde
IVFT	intravenous fetal		access port
	transfusion	IVRG	intravenous retrograde
IVGG	intravenous gamma	IV-RNV	intravenous radionuclide
	globulin		venography
IVGTT	intravenous glucose	IVRO	intraoral vertical ramus
	tolerance test		osteotomy
IVH	intravenous	IVRT	isovolumic relation time
	hyperalimentation	IVS	intraventricular septum
	intraventricular		irritable voiding
	hemorrhage		syndrome
IVIG	intravenous	IVSD	intraventricular septal
	immunoglobulin		defect
IVJC	intervertebral joint	IVSE	interventricular septal
	complex		excursion
IVL	intravenous lock	IVSO	intraoral vertical
IVLBW	infant of very low birth		segmental osteotomy
	weight (less than	IVSS	intravenous Soluset®
	1,500 g)	IVT	intravenous transfusion
IVMP	intravenously	IVTTT	intravenous tolbutamide
	administered		tolerance test
	methylprednisolone	IVU	intravenous urography
IVNC	isolated ventricular		(urogram)
	noncompaction	IVUC	intravenous ultrasound
IVO	intraoral vertical		catheter
	osteotomy	IVUS	intravascular ultrasound
IVOX	intravascular oxygenator	IW	inspiratory wheeze
	(oxygenation)	IWD	individual with a
IVP	intravenous push (this is		disability
	a dangerous meaning	IWI	inferior wall infarction
	as it is read as	IWL	insensible water loss
	intravenous	IWMI	inferior wall myocardial
	pyelogram)		infarct
	intravenous pyelogram	IWML	idiopathic white matter
IVPB	intravenous piggyback		lesion
IVPF	isovolume pressure flow	IWT	ice-water test
IVPU	intravenous push		impacted wisdom teeth
IVR	idioventricular rhythm		
	interactive voice-response		
	(system)		
	intravenous retrograde		

I

J

J	Jaeger measure of near vision with 20/20 about equal to J1
	jejunostomy
	Jewish
	joint
	joule
	juice
J 1-16	Jaeger near acuity notation (1 to 16 scale)
JA	joint aspiration
Jack	jacknife position
JAFAR	Juvenile Arthritis Functional Assessment Report
JAMA	*Journal of the American Medical Association*
JAMG	juvenile autoimmune myasthenia gravis
JAN	Japanese Accepted Name
JAR	junior assistant resident
JARAN	junior assistant resident admission note
JBE	Japanese B encephalitis
JBS	Johanson Blizzard syndrome
JC	junior clinicians (medical students)
JCA	juvenile chronic arthritis
JCAHO	Joint Commission on Accreditation of Healthcare Organizations
JCOG	Japanese Clinical Oncology Group
JCQ	Job Content Questionnaire
JD	jaundice
JDG	jugulodigastric
JDM	juvenile diabetes mellitus
JDMS	juvenile dermatomyositis
JE	Japanese encephalitis
JEB	junctional escape beat

JEJ	jejunum
JEN	Japanese encephalitis vaccine
JER	junctional escape rhythm
JET	jejunal extension tube junctional ectopic tachycardia
JEV	Japanese encephalitis virus
JF	joint fluid
JFS	Jewish Family Service
JGCT	juvenile granulosa cell tumor
JHR	Jarisch-Herxheimer reaction
JI	jejunoileal
JIB	jejunoileal bypass
JIS	juvenile idiopathic scoliosis
JJ	jaw jerk
J & J	Johnson & Johnson Health Care Systems, Inc.
JLP	juvenile laryngeal papillomatosis
JM-9	iproplatin
JME	juvenile myoclonic epilepsy
JMS	junior medical student
JNA	juvenile nasopharyngeal angiofibroma
JNB	jaundice of newborn
JNCL	juvenile-onset neuronal ceroid lipofuscinosis
JND	just noticeable difference
JNT	joint
JNVD	jugular neck vein distention
JODM	juvenile-onset diabetes mellitus
JOMAC	judgment, orientation, memory, abstraction, and calculation
JOMACI	judgment, orientation, memory, abstraction, and calculation intact
JP	Jackson-Pratt (drain) Jobst pump joint protection

J

JPB	junctional premature beats		
JP BS	Jackson-Pratt to bulb suction		
JPC	junctional premature contraction		

K

K	cornea
	kelvin
JPS	joint position sense		ketamine (Super K)
JR	junctional rhythm		kilodalton
JRA	juvenile rheumatoid arthritis		Kosher
			potassium
JRAN	junior resident admission note		thousand
Jr BF	junior baby food		vitamin K
JRC	joint replacement center	K′	knee
JSF	Japanese spotted fever	K^+	potassium
JT	jejunostomy tube	K_1	phytonadione
	joint	K_2	menatetrenone
	junctional tachycardia	K_3	menadione
JTF	jejunostomy tube feeding	K_4	menadiol sodium diphosphate
JTJ	jaw-to-jaw (position)		
JTP	joint projection	17K	17-ketosteroids
JTPS	juvenile tropical pancreatitis syndrome	510(k)	Medical Device Premarket Notification
J-Tube	jejunostomy tube	KA	kainic acid
JUV	juvenile		keratoacanthoma
JV	jugular vein		ketoacidosis
JVC	jugular venous catheter	Ka	first order absorption constant in hr.$^{-1}$
JVD	jugular venous distention		
JVP	jugular venous pressure	KAB	knowledge, attitude, and behavior
	jugular venous pulsation		
	jugular venous pulse	K-ABC	Kaufman Assessment Battery for Children
JVPT	jugular venous pulse tracing	KABINS	knowledge, attitude, behavior, and improvement in nutritional status
JW	Jehovah's Witness		
Jx	joint		
JXG	juvenile xanthogranuloma		
		KACT	kaolin-activated clotting time
		KAFO	knee-ankle-foot orthosis
		KAO	knee-ankle orthosis
		KAS	Katz Adjustment Scale
		KASH	knowledge, abilities, skills, and habits
		kat	katal
		K-A units	King-Armstrong units
		KB	ketone bodies
			kilobase
			knee-bearing
		KBD	Kashin-Beck disease
		KC	kangaroo care

J

	keratoconjunctivitis
	keratoconus
	knees-to-chest
	Korean conflict
kcal	kilocalorie
KCCT	kaolin cephalin clotting time
KChIPs	potassium channel-interacting proteins
kCi	kilocurie
KCl	potassium chloride
KCS	keratoconjunctivitis sicca
KCZ	ketoconazole (Nizoral)
KD	Kawasaki's disease
	Keto Diastix®
	ketogenic diet
	kidney donors
	knee disarticulation
	knowledge deficit
Kd	kilodalton
KDA	known drug allergies
KDC®	brand name of infant warmer
KDU	Kidney Dialysis Unit
KE	first order elimination rate constant in hr.$^{-1}$
KED	Kendrick extrication device
k_{el}	elimination rate constant
KET	ketoconazole (Nizoral)
	ketones
KETO	ketoconazole (Nizoral)
17 Keto	17 ketosteroids
keV	kilo-electron volts
KEVD	Krupin eye valve with disk
KF	kidney function
KFA	kinetic fibrinogen assay
KFAB	kidney-fixing antibodies
KFAO	knee-foot-ankle orthosis
KFD	Kyasanur Forrest disease
KFR	Kayser-Fleischer ring
KFS	Klippel-Feil syndrome
kg	kilogram
K-G	Kimray-Greenfield (filter)
KGF	keratinocyte growth factor
KGC	Keflin, gentamicin, and carbenicillin
17-KGS	17-ketogenic steroids
KGy	kiloGray
KHF	Korean hemorrhagic fever
K24H	potassium, urine 24 hour
kHz	kilohertz
KI	karyopyknotic index
	knee immobilizer
	potassium iodide
KID	keratitis, ichthyosis, and deafness (syndrome)
	kidney
kilo	kilogram
	thousand
KIN	kinetic
KISS	saturated solution of potassium iodide
KIT	Kahn Intelligence Test
KIU	kallikrein inhibitor units
KJ	kilojoule
	knee jerk
KJR	knee jerk reflex
KK	knee kick
	knock-knee
KLB	klebsiella vaccine
KL-BET	Kleihauer-Betke
Kleb	*Klebsiella*
KLH	keyhole limpet hemocyanin
K-Lor®	potassium chloride tablets
KLS	kidneys, liver, and spleen
KM	kanamycin
KMG	kangaroo-mother care
$KMnO_4$	potassium permanganate
KMO	Kaiser-Meyer-Olkin (measure of statistical sampling adequacy)
KMV	killed measles vaccine
KN	knee
KNO	keep needle open
KNSA	Kron Nutritive Sucking Apparatus
KO	keep open
	knee orthosis
	knocked out
KOH	potassium hydroxide
KOR	keep open rate
KP	hot pack
	keratoprecipitate
	kinetic perimetry

K

KPE	Kelman phacoemulsification	KWB	Keith, Wagener, Barker
		KWIC	keywork in context
KPM	kilopounds per minute	K-wire	Kirschner wire
KPS	Karnofsky performance status (scores) (scale)		
Kr	krypton		
K-rod	Küntscher rod		
KS	Kawasaki syndrome		
	Kaposi's sarcoma		
	kidney stone		
	Klinefelter's syndrome		
17-KS	17-ketogenic steroids		
	17-ketosteroids		
KSA	knowledge, skills, and abilities		
KSE	knee sling exercises		
KSHV	Kaposi's sarcoma-associated herpesvirus		
KS/OI	Kaposi's sarcoma and opportunistic infections		
KSP	Karolinska Scales of Personality		
KSR	potassium chloride sustained release (tablets)		
KSS	Kearns-Sayre syndrome		
KSW	knife stab wound		
KT	kidney transplant		
	kinesiotherapy		
	known to		
KTC	knee-to-chest		
KTP	potassium-titanyl-phosphate (laser)		
KTU	kidney transplant unit		
	known to us		
KTZ	ketoconazole (Nizoral)		
KUB	kidney(s), ureter(s), and bladder		
	kidney ultrasound biopsy		
KUS	kidney(s), ureter(s), and spleen		
KV	kilovolt		
KVO	keep vein open		
KVP	kilovolt peak		
KW	Keith-Wagener (ophthalmoscopic finding, graded I-IV)		
	Kimmelstiel-Wilson		

K

L

L	fifty	LABBB	left anterior bundle branch block
	left	LABC	locally advanced breast cancer
	lente insulin	LAC	laceration
	levorotatory		*lactobacillus acidophilus* vaccine
	lingual		left antecubital
	Listeria		left atrial catheter
	liter		locally advanced cancer
	liver		long arm cast
	lumbar	LAc	Licensed Acupuncturist
	lung	LACC	locally advanced cervical carcinoma
l	levorotatory	LACI	lacunar circulation infarct
L'	lumbar	LACT-ART	lactate arterial
Ⓛ	left		
L₁...L₅	lumbar nerve 1 through 5	LAD	left anterior descending
	lumbar vertebra 1 through 5		left axis deviation
			leukocyte adhesion deficiency
L1-2	lumbar spine, between first and second vertebrae (the disk space)	LADA	left anterior descending (coronary) artery
		LADCA	left anterior descending coronary artery
LA	language age	LADD	left anterior descending diagonal
	latex agglutination	LAD-MIN	left axis deviation minimal
	Latin American		
	left arm	LADPG	laparoscopically assisted distal partial gastrectomy
	left atrial		
	left atrium		
	leukoaraiosis (a radiologic finding)	LAE	left atrial enlargement
			long above elbow
	light adaptation	LAEC	locally advanced esophageal cancer
	linguoaxial		
	linoleic acid	LAF	laminar air flow
	local anesthesia		Latin-American female
	long acting		low animal fat
	lupus anticoagulant		lymphocyte-activating factor
L + A	light and accommodation		
		LAFB	left anterior fascicular block
	living and active		
LAA	left atrium and its appendage	LAFF	lateral arm free flap
		LAFM	locally acquired *Plasmodium falciparum* malaria
LAAM	levomethadyl acetate (L-alpha acetylmeth-adol, Orlaam)		
		LAFR	laminar airflow room
LAB	laboratory	LAG	lymphangiogram
	left abdomen		

LAH	left anterior hemiblock		long-acting release
	left atrial hypertrophy		low anterior resection
LAHB	left anterior hemiblock	LARM	left arm
LAIT	latex agglutination inhibition test	LARS	laparoscopic antireflux surgery
LAK	lymphokine-activated killer	LARSI	lumbar anterior-root stimulator implants
LAL	left axillary line	LAS	laxative abuse syndrome
	limulus amebocyte lysate		left arm, sitting
LALLS	low-angle laser light scattering		leucine acetylsalicylate
			long arm splint
LALT	larynx-associated lymphoid tissue		low-amplitude signal
			lymphadenopathy syndrome
	low air loss therapy (mattress)		lymphangioscintigraphy
LAM	laminectomy		lysine acetylsalicylate
	laminogram	LASA	Linear Analogue Self-Assessment (scales)
	Latin-American male		
	lymphangioleiomyomatosis		lipid-associated sialic acid
lam✓	laminectomy check	LASER	light amplification by stimulated emission of radiation
LAMB	mucocutaneous lentigines, atrial myxoma, and blue nevus (syndrome)		
		LASIK	laser *in situ* keratomileusis
L-AMB	liposomal amphotericin B	L-ASP	asparaginase (Elspar)
LAMMA	laser microprobe mass analysis	LAST	left anterior small thoracotomy
LANC	long arm navicular cast	LAT	lateral
LAN	lymphadenopathy		latex agglutination test
LAO	left anterior oblique		left anterior thigh
LAP	laparoscopy	LATCH	literature attached to chart
	laparotomy	lat.men.	lateral meniscectomy
	left abdominal pain	LATS	long-acting thyroid stimulator
	left atrial pressure		
	leucine amino peptidase	LAUP	laser-assisted uvula-palatoplasty
	leukocyte alkaline phosphatase	LAV	lymphadenopathy associated virus
	lower abdominal pain		
LAPA	locally advanced pancreatic adenocarcinoma	LAVA	laser-assisted vasal anastomosis
		LAVH	laparoscopically assisted vaginal hysterectomy
LAP-APPY	laparoscopic appendectomy		
		LAW	left atrial wall
LAP CHOLE	laparoscopic cholecystectomy	LAWER	life-terminating acts without the explicit request
LAPMS	long arm posterior molded splint		
		LAX	laxative
LAPW	left atrial posterior wall	LB	large bowel
LAQ	long arc quad		lateral bend
LAR	left arm, reclining		left breast

	left buttock		low birth weight (less
	live births		than 2,500 g)
	low back	LBWI	low birth weight
	lung biopsy		infant
	lymphoid body	LC	Laënnec's cirrhosis
	pound		laparoscopic
L&B	left and below		cholecystectomy
LB3	colonoscope		left circumflex
LBA	laser balloon angioplasty		leisure counseling
LBB	left breast biopsy		level of consciousness
	long back board		living children
LBBB	left bundle branch block		low calorie
LBBx	left breast biopsy		lung cancer
LBCD	left border of cardiac	L & C	lids and conjunctivae
	dullness	3LC	triple-lumen catheter
L/B/Cr	electrolytes, blood urea	LCA	Leber's congenital
	nitrogen, and serum		amaurosis
	creatinine (see page		left circumflex artery
	358)		left coronary artery
LBD	large bile duct		light contact assist
	left border dullness	LCAD	long-chain acyl-coenzyme
	Lewy body dementia		A dehydrogenase
	low back disability	LCAH	life-care at home
LBE	long below elbow	LCAL	large-cell anaplastic
LBG	Landry-Guillain-Barré		lymphoma
	(syndrome)	LCAT	lecithin cholesterol
LBH	length, breadth, and		acyltransferase
	height	LCB	left costal border
LBM	last bowel movement	LCCA	left circumflex coronary
	lean body mass		artery
	loose bowel movement		left common carotid
LBMI	last body mass index		artery
LBNA	lysis bladder neck		leukocytoclastic angiitis
	adhesions	LCCS	low cervical cesarean
LBNP	lower body negative		section
	pressure	LCD	coal tar solution (*liquor*
LBO	large bowel obstruction		*carbonis detergens*)
LBP	low back pain		localized collagen
	low blood pressure		dystrophy
LBQC	large base quad cane		low-calcium diet
LBS	low back syndrome	LCDC	Laboratory Centre for
	pounds		Disease Control
LBT	low back tenderness		(Canada)
	low back trouble	LCDCP	low-contact dynamic
LBV	left brachial vein		compression plate
	low biological value	LCDE	laparoscopic common
LBVO	left brachial vein		duct exploration
	occlusion	LCE	laparoscopic
LBW	lean body weight		cholecystectomy

L

	left carotid endarterectomy	LCT	low continuous wall suction
LCF	left circumflex		long-chain triglyceride
LCFA	long-chain fatty acid		low cervical transverse
LCFM	left circumflex marginal		lymphocytotoxicity
LCGU	local cerebral glucose utilization	LCTA	lungs clear to auscultation
		LCTCS	low cervical transverse cesarean section
LCH	Langerhans' cell histiocytosis	LCTD	low-calcium test diet
		LCV	leucovorin
	local city hospital		leukocytoclastic vasculitis
LCIS	lobular cancer *in situ*		low cervical vertical
LCL	lateral collateral ligament	LCX	left circumflex coronary artery
LCLC	large cell lung carcinoma		
LCM	laser-capture microdissection	LD	lactic dehydrogenase (formerly LDH)
	left costal margin		last dose
	lower costal margin		latissimus dorsi
	lymphocytic choriomeningitis		learning disability
			learning disorder
LCMI	left ventricular mass index		left deltoid
LC-MS-MS	liquid chromatography coupled to tandem mass spectrometry		Legionnaire's disease
			lethal dose
			levodopa
LCN	lidocaine		Licensed Dietician
LCNB	large-core needle biopsy		liver disease
LCO	low cardiac output		living donor
LCP	long, closed, posterior (cervix)		loading dose
			long dwell
LCPD	Legg-Calvé-Perthes disease		low density
			low dosage
LCPUFAs	long-chain polyunsaturated fatty acids		Lyme disease
		L&D	labor and deliver
		L/D	labor and delivery
LCR	cerebrospinal fluid (French)		light to dark (ratio)
		LD-1	lactic dehydrogenase 1
	late cortical response	LD-5	lactic dehydrogenase 5
	late cutaneous reaction	LD$_{50}$	median lethal dose
	ligase chain reaction	LDA	low density areas
LCRS	Living Conditions Rating Scale		low-dose arm
		LDB	Legionnaires disease bacterium
LCS	low constant suction		
	low continuous suction	LDCOC	low-dose combination oral contraceptive
LCSG	left cardiac sympathetic ganglionectomy		
		LDD	laser disk decompression
	lost child support group		Lee and Desu's D (test)
LCSS	Lung Cancer Symptom Score		light-dark discrimination
		LDDS	local dentist
LCSW	Licensed Clinical Social Worker	LDEA	left deviation of electrical axis

LDF	laser Doppler flowmetry	LEAP	Lower Extremity Amputation Prevention (program)
LDH	lactic dehydrogenase		
LDIH	left direct inguinal hernia		
LDIR	low-dose of ionizing radiation	LEB	lumbar epidural block
		LEC	lens epithelial cell
LDI-TOF-MS	laser desorption/ionization time-of-flight-mass spectrometer	LECBD	laparoscopic exploration of the common bile duct
LDL	low-density lipoprotein	LED	liposomal encapsulated doxorubicin (Doxil)
LDL-C	low-density lipoprotein cholesterol		lowest effective dose
			lupus erythematosus disseminatus
LDLT	living donor liver transplantation		
LDM	lorazepam, dexamethasone, and metoclopramide	LEEP	loop electrosurgical excision procedure
		LEF	lower extremity fracture
LDMRT	low-dose mediastinal radiation therapy	LEH	liposome-encapsulated hemoglobin
LDNF	lung-derived neurotrophic factor	LEHPZ	lower esophageal high pressure zone
l-dopa	levodopa	LEJ	ligation of the esophagogastric junction
LD-PCR	limiting dilution polymerase chain reaction		
		LEL	low-energy laser
LDR	labor, delivery, and recovery	LEM	lateral eye movements
			light electron microscope
	length-to-diameter ratio	LEMS	Lambert-Eaton myasthenic syndrome
	long-duration response		
LDR/P	labor, delivery, recovery, and postpartum	LEP	leptospirosis
			liposome-encapsulated paclitaxel
LDT	left dorsotransverse		
LD-T	lactic dehydrogenase total		lower esophageal pressure
LDUB	long double upright brace	LEP 2	leptospirosis 2
LDUH	low-dose unfractionated heparin	LE prep	lupus erythematosus preparation
LDV	laser Doppler velocimetry	L-ERX	leukoerythroblastic reaction
LE	left ear	LES	local excitatory state
	left eye		lower esophageal sphincter
	lens extraction		
	live embryo		lumbar epidural steroids
	lower extremities		lupus erythematosus systemic
	lupus erythematosus		
LEA	lower extremity amputation	LESEP	lower extremity somatosensory evoked potential
	lumbar epidural anesthesia		
		LESG	Late Effects Study Group
LEAD	lower extremity arterial disease	LESI	lumbar epidural steroid injection

L

LESP	lower esophageal sphincter pressure		low flap transverse
LET	left esotropia	LFU	limit flocculation unit
	leukocyte esterase test		lost to follow-up
	lidocaine, epinephrine and tetracaine gel	LG	large
			laryngectomy
	linear energy transfer		left gluteal
LEU	leucine		linguogingival
LEV	levamisole (Ergamisol)		lymphography
	levator muscle	L-G	Lich-Gregoire (ureteroneocystostomy)
LEVA	levamisole (Ergamisol)		
LF	laparoscopic fundoplications	LGA	large for gestational age
			left gastric artery
	Lassa fever	LGG	low-grade gliomas
	left foot	L-GG	*Lactobacillus rhamnosus* strain GG
	living female		
	low fat	LGI	lower gastrointestinal (series)
	low forceps		
	low frequency	LGIOS	low-grade intraosseous-type osteosarcoma
LFA	left femoral artery		
	left forearm	LGL	large granular lymphocyte
	left fronto-anterior		low-grade lymphoma(s)
	leukocyte function-associated antigen		Lown-Ganong-Levine (syndrome)
	low friction arthroplasty	LGLS	Lown-Ganong-Levine syndrome
	lymphocyte function-associated antigen	LGM	left gluteus medius (maximus)
LFA-1	leukocyte function-associated antigen-1	LGN	lateral geniculate leaflet
			lobular glomerulonephritis
LFB	low-frequency band	LG-NHL	low-grade non-Hodgkin's lymphoma
LFC	living female child		
	low-fat and cholesterol	LGS	Lennox-Gastaut syndrome
LFCS	low flap cesarean section		low Gomco suction
LFD	lactose-free diet	LGSIL	low-grade squamous intraepithelial lesion
	low-fat diet		
	low-fiber diet	LGV	lymphogranuloma venerum
	low forceps delivery		
	lunate fossa depression	LH	learning handicap
LFGNR	lactose fermenting gram-negative rod		left hand
			left hemisphere
LFL	left frontolateral		left hyperphoria
LFM	lateral force microscopy		luteinizing hormone
LFP	left frontoposterior	LHA	left hepatic artery
LFS	leukemia-free survival	LHC	left heart catheterization
	Li-Fraumeni syndrome	LHD	left-hand dominant
	liver function series	LHF	left heart failure
LFT	latex flocculation test	LHG	left hand grip
	left fronto-transverse	LHH	left homonymous hemianopsia
	liver function tests		

LHI	Labor Health Institute	LIG	ligament
LHL	left hemisphere lesions		lymphocyte immune
	left hepatic lobe		globulin
LHON	Leber's hereditary optic	LIGHTS	phototherapy lights
	neuropathy	LIH	laparoscopic inguinal
LHP	left hemiparesis		herniorrhaphy
LHR	leukocyte histamine		left inguinal hernia
	release	LIHA	low impulsiveness, high
LHRH	luteinizing hormone-		anxiety
	releasing hormone	LIJ	left internal jugular
LHRH-A	luteinizing hormone-	LILA	low impulsiveness, low
	releasing hormone		anxiety
	analogue	LIM	limited toxicology
LHRT	leukocyte histamine		screening
	release test	LIMA	left internal mammary
LHS	left hand side		artery (graft)
	long-handled sponge	LIMS	laboratory information
LHSH	long-handled shoe horn		management system(s)
LHT	left hypertropia	LINDI	lithium-induced
LI	lactose intolerance		nephrogenic diabetes
	lamellar ichthyosis		insipidus
	large intestine	LING	lingual
	laser iridotomy	LIO	laser-indirect
	learning impaired		ophthalmoscope
	linguoincisal		left inferior oblique
	liver involvement		(muscle)
Li	lithium	LIOU	laparoscopic
LIA	laser interference acuity		intraoperative
	left iliac artery		ultrasound
LIB	left in bottle	LIP	lithium-induced
LIC	left iliac crest		polydipsia
	left internal carotid		lymphocytic interstitial
	leisure interest class		pneumonia
LICA	left internal carotid artery	LIPV	left inferior pulmonary
LICD	lower intestinal Crohn's		vein
	disease	LIQ	liquid
LICM	left intercostal margin		liquor
Li$_2$CO$_3$	lithium carbonate		lower inner quadrant
LICS	left intercostal space	LIR	left iliac region
Lido	lidocaine		left inferior rectus
LIF	left iliac fossa	LIS	left intercostal space
	left index finger		locked-in syndrome
	leukemia-inhibiting factor		low intermittent
	liver (migration)		suction
	inhibitory factor		lung injury score
LIFE	laser-induced fluorescence	LISS	low ionic strength
	emission		saline
	lung imaging fluorescence	LISW	Licensed Independent
	endoscopy		Social Worker

L

LIT	literature
	liver injury test
LITA	left internal thoracic artery
LITH	lithotomy
LITHO	lithotripsy
LITT	laser-induced thermotherapy
LIV	left innominate vein
L-IVP	limited intravenous pyelogram
LIVB	live birth
LIVC	left inferior vena cava
LIVPRO	liver profile (see page 358)
LIWS	low intermittent wall suction
LJ	left jugular
LJL	lateral joint line
LJM	limited joint mobility
LK	lamellar keratoplasty
	left kidney
LKA	Lazare-Klerman-Armour (Personality Inventory)
LKM-3	liver-kidney microsomal antibodies type 3
LKS	Landau-Kleffner syndrome
	liver, kidneys, spleen
LKSB	liver, kidneys, spleen, and bladder
LKSNP	liver, kidneys, and spleen not palpable
LL	large lymphocyte
	left lateral
	left leg
	left lower
	left lung
	lid lag
	long leg (brace or cast)
	lower lid
	lower lip
	lower lobe
	lumbar laminectomy
	lumbar length
	lymphocytic leukemia
	lymphoblastic lymphoma
L&L	lids and lashes
LL2	limb lead two

LLA	lids, lashes, and adnexa
	limulus lysate assay
LLAT	left lateral
LLB	last living breath
	left lateral bending
	left lateral border
	long leg brace
LLC	laparoscopic laser cholecystectomy
	Lewis lung carcinoma
	long leg cast
LLBCD	left lower border of cardiac dullness
LLD	left lateral decubitus
	left length discrepancy
	leg length differential
LLE	left lower extremity
	little league elbow
LLETZ	large-loop excision of the transformation zone
LLFG	long leg fiberglas (cast)
LLG	left lateral gaze
LL-GXT	low-level graded exercise test
LLL	left lower lid
	left lower lobe (lung)
LLLE	lower lid left eye
LLLNR	left lower lobe, no rales
LLLT	low-level laser therapy
LLO	Legionella-like organism
LLOD	lower lid, right eye
	lower limit of detection
LLOS	lower lid, left eye
LLP	long leg plaster
LLPS	low-load prolonged stress
LLQ	left lower quadrant (abdomen)
LLR	left lateral rectus
LLRE	lower lid, right eye
LLS	lazy leukocyte syndrome
LLSB	left lower sternal border
LLT	left lateral thigh
	lowest level term
LLWC	long leg walking cast
LLX	left lower extremity
LM	left main
	light microscopy
	linguomesial
	living male

	lung metastases		light moving touch
L/M	liters per minute	LMW	low molecular weight
LMA	laryngeal mask airway	LMWD	low molecular weight
	left mentoanterior		dextran
	liver membrane	LMWH	low molecular weight
	autoantibody		heparins
LMB	Laurence-Moon-Biedl	LN	latent nystagmus
	syndrome		left nostril (nare)
	left main bronchus		lymph nodes
LMC	living male child	LN$_2$	liquid nitrogen
LMCA	left main coronary artery	LNA	alpha-linolenic acid
	left middle cerebral artery	LNB	lymph node biopsy
LMCAT	left middle cerebral artery	LNCs	lymph node cells
	thrombosis	LND	light-near dissociation
LMCL	left midclavicular line		lonidamine
LMD	local medical doctor		lymph node dissection
	low molecular weight	LNE	lymph node enlargement
	dextran		lymph node excision
LME	left mediolateral	LNF	laparoscopic Nissen
	episiotomy		fundoplication
LMEE	left middle ear	LNG	levonorgestrel
	exploration	LNM	lymph node metastases
LMF	left middle finger	LNMC	lymph node mononuclear
	melphalan (L-PAM),		cells
	methotrexate, and	LNMP	last normal menstrual
	fluorouracil		period
LMFT	Licensed Marriage and	LNNB	Luria-Nebraska
	Family Therapist		Neuropsychological
L/min	liters per minute		Battery
LML	left medial lateral	LNS	lymph node sampling
	left middle lobe	LNT	late neurological toxicity
LMLE	left mediolateral	LO	lateral oblique (x-ray
	episiotomy		view)
LMM	lentigo maligna melanoma		linguo-occlusal
LMN	lower motor neuron		lumbar orthosis
LMNL	lower motor neuron lesion	5-LO	5-lipoxygenase
LMP	last menstrual period	LOA	late-onset
	left mentoposterior		agammaglobulinemia
	low malignant potential		leave of absence
LMR	left medial rectus		left occiput anterior
LMRM	left modified radical		looseness of associations
	mastectomy		lysis of adhesions
LMS	lateral medullary	LOAD	late-onset Alzheimer's
	syndrome		disease
	leiomyosarcomas	LOAEL	lowest observed adverse
LMT	left main trunk		effect level
	left mentotransverse	LOB	loss of balance
	Licensed Massage	LOC	laxative of choice
	Therapist		level of care

L

	level of comfort		lower outer quadrant
	level of concern	LOR	loss of resistance
	level of consciousness	LORS-I	Level of Rehabilitation
	local		Scale-I
	loss of consciousness	LOS	length of stay
LOCF	last observation carried		loss of sight
	forward	LOT	left occiput transverse
LOCM	low-osmolality contrast		Licensed Occupational
	media		Therapist
LOD	limit of detection	LOV	loss of vision
	line of duty	LOVA	loss of visual acuity
LOE	left otitis externa	LOZ	lozenge
LOF	leaking of fluids	LP	light perception
	leave on floor		linguopulpal
LOFD	low outlet forceps		lipid panel (see page
	delivery		358)
LOG	Logmar chart		lipoprotein
LOH	loss of heterozygosity		low protein
LOHF	late-onset hepatic failure		lumbar puncture
LOHP	oxaliplatin	L/P	lactate-pyruvate
LOIH	left oblique inguinal		ratio
	hernia	LP5	Life-Pak 5
LOI	level of injury	LPA	left pulmonary artery
	Leyton Obsessional	Lp(a)	lipoprotein (a)
	Inventory	LPA%	left pulmonary artery
	loss of imprinting		oxygen saturation
LOINC	Logical Observation	L-PAM	melphalan (Alkeran)
	Identifier Names and	LPC	laser photocoagulation
	Codes		Licensed Professional
LOL	laughing out loud		Counselor
	left occipitolateral	LPCC	Licensed Professional
	little old lady		Certified Counselor
LOM	left otitis media	LPC-L	lymphoplasmacytoid
	limitation of motion		lymphoma
	little old man	LPc̄P	light perception with
	loss of motion		projection
	low-osmolar (contrast)	LPD	leiomyomatosis
	media		peritonealis
LOMSA	left otitis media,		disseminata
	suppurative, acute		low potassium dextran
LOMSC	left otitis media,		low protein diet
	suppurative, chronic		luteal phase defect
LoNa	low sodium		luteal phase deficiency
LOO	length of operation		lymphoproliferative
LOP	laparoscopic orchiopexy		disease
	leave on pass	LPDA	left posterior descending
	left occiput posterior		artery
	level of pain	LPEP	left pre-ejection period
LOQ	limit(s) of quantitation	LPF	liver plasma flow

	low-power field	LQTS	long QT (interval) syndrome
	lymphocytosis-promoting factor	LR	labor room
LPFB	left posterior fascicular block		lactated Ringer's (injection)
LPH	left posterior hemiblock		laser resection
LPHB	left posterior hemiblock		lateral rectus
LPI	laser peripheral iridectomy		left-right
			light reflex
	leukotriene pathway inhibitor		likelihood ratios
		L&R	left and right
LPICA	left posterior internal carotid artery	L → R	left to right
		LR1A	labor room 1A
LPIH	left-posterior-inferior hemiblock	LRA	left radial artery
			left renal artery
LPL	laparoscopic pelvic lymphadenectomy	LRC	lower rib cage
		LRCP	Licentiate of the Royal College of Physicians
	left posterolateral		
	lipoprotein lipase	LRCS	Licentiate of the Royal College of Surgeons
LPLC	low-pressure liquid chromatography		
		LRD	limb reduction defects
LPLND	laparoscopic pelvic lymph node dissection		living-related donor
			living renal donor
LPM	latent primary malignancy	LRDT	living-related donor transplant
	liters per minute		
LPN	Licensed Practical Nurse	LRE	localization-related epilepsy
LPO	left posterior oblique		
	light perception only	LREH	low renin essential hypertension
LPPC	leukocyte-poor packed cells		
		LRF	left rectus femoris
LPPH	late postpartum hemorrhage		left ring finger
			local-regional failure
LPR	leprosy (Hansen's disease) vaccine	L&R gtt	Levophed and Regitine drip (infusion)
LPS	last Pap smear	LRHT	living-related hepatic transplantation
	lipopolysaccharide		
LP SHUNT	lumboperitoneal shunt	LRI	lower respiratory infection
LP͞sP	light perception without projection	LRLT	living-related liver transplantation
LPT	leptospirosis (Leptospira-*Leptospires* sp.) vaccine	LRM	left radical mastectomy
			local regional metastases
	Licensed Physical Therapist	LRMP	last regular menstrual period
LPTN	Licensed Psychiatric Technical Nurse	LRND	left radical neck dissection
LPV	left portal vein	LRO	long range objective
	left pulmonary vein	Lrot	left rotation

L

LRP	laparoscopic radical prostatectomy lung-resistance protein	LSC	last sexual contact late systolic click least significant change left subclavian (artery) (vein)
LRQ	lower right quadrant		
LROU	lateral rectus, both eyes		
LRR	light reflection rheography		lichen simplex chronicus
LRRT	locoregional radiotherapy	LSCA	left scapuloanterior
LRS	lactated Ringer's solution	LSCC	laryngeal squamous cell carcinoma
LRT	living renal transplant local radiation therapy lower respiratory tract		
		LSCCB	limited-state small-cell cancer of the bladder
LRTD	living relative transplant donor	LSCM	laser-scanning confocal microscopy
LRTI	ligament reconstruction with tendon interposition lower respiratory tract infection	LSCP	left scapuloposterior
		LSCS	lower segment cesarean section
		LSD	least significant difference low-salt diet lysergide
LRV	left renal vein log reduction value		
		LSE	local side effects
LRZ	lorazepam (Ativan)	LSed	level of sedation
LS	left side legally separated Leigh's syndrome liver scan liver-spleen low salt lumbosacral lung sounds	LSF	low-saturated fat
		LSFA	low-saturated fatty acid (diet)
		LSH	laparoscopic supracervical hysterectomy leishmaniasis vaccine
		LSI	levonorgestrel subdermal implant
L/S	lecithin-sphingomyelin ratio	L-SIL	low-grade squamous intraepithelial lesions
L&S	ligation and stripping liver and spleen	LSK	liver, spleen, and kidneys
L5-S1	lumbar fifth vertebra to sacral first vertebra (where the lumbar and sacral spines join)	LSKM	liver-spleen-kidney-megalgia
		LSL	left sacrolateral left short leg (brace)
		LSLF	low sodium, low fat (diet)
LSA	left sacrum anterior lipid-bound sialic acid lymphosarcoma	LSM	laser scanning microscope late systolic murmur least squares mean limited sampling model liver, spleen masses
LSB	left scapular border left sternal border local standby lumbar spinal block lumbar sympathetic block		
		LSMFT	liposclerosing myxofibrous tumor
		LSMT	life-sustaining medical treatment
LS BPS	laparoscopic bilateral partial salpingectomy	LSO	left salpingo-oophorectomy

	left superior oblique	LTB	laparoscopic tubal
	lumbosacral orthosis		banding
LSP	left sacrum posterior		laryngotracheobronchitis
	liver-specific (membrane)	LTB$_4$	leukotriene B$_4$
	lipoprotein	LTC	left to count
L–Spar	Elspar (asparaginase)		long-term care
L-SPINE	lumbar spine		long thick closed
LSQ	Life Situation	LTC$_4$	leukotriene C$_4$
	Questionnaire	LTC-101	long-term care form-101
LSR	left superior rectus	LTCBDE	laparoscopic transcystic
L/S ratio	lecithin/sphingomyelin		common bile duct
	ratio		exploration
LSS	limb sparing surgery	LTCCS	low transverse cervical
	liver-spleen scan		cesarean section
	lumbar spinal stenosis	LTCF	long-term care facility
LSSS	Liverpool Seizure	LTC-IC	long-term culture-
	Severity Scale		initiating cells
LST	left sacrum transverse	LTCS	low transverse cesarean
LSTC	laparoscopic tubal		section
	coagulation	LTD	largest tumor dimension
LSTL	laparoscopic tubal ligation		leg transfer device
L's & T's	lines and tubes	LTD$_4$	leukotriene D$_4$
LSU	life support unit	LTE	less than effective
LSV	left subclavian vein	LTE$_4$	leukotriene E$_4$
LSVC	left superior vena cava	LTED	long-term estrogen
LSW	left-side weakness		deprivation
	Licensed Social Worker	LTFU	long-term follow-up
LT	laboratory technician	LTG	lamotrigine (Lamictal)
	left		long-term goal
	left thigh		low-tension glaucoma
	left triceps	LTGA	left transposition of great
	leukotrienes		artery
	Levin tube	LTH	luteotropic hormone
	light	LTK	laser thermal keratoplasty
	light touch	LTL	laparoscopic tubal
	low transverse		ligation
	lumbar traction	LTM	long-term memory
	lung transplantation		long-term monitoring
	lunotriquetral	LTOT	long-term oxygen therapy
	lymphotoxin	LTP	laser trabeculoplasty
L&T	lettuce and tomato		long-term plan
LT4	levothyroxine		long-term potentiation
LTA	laryngotracheal applicator	LTR	long terminal repeats
	laryngeal tracheal		lower trunk rotation
	anesthesia	LTRA	leukotriene receptor
	lateral thoracic arteries		antagonist
	local tracheal anesthesia	LTS	laparoscopic tubal
LTAC	long-term acute care		sterilization
LTAS	left transatrial septal		long-term survivors

L

191

LTT	lactose tolerance test			left ventricle
	lymphocyte transformation test			leucovorin
				live virus
LTUI	low transverse uterine incision	LVA	left ventricular aneurysm
		LVC	laser vision correction
LTV	long-term variability			low viscosity cement
	Luche tumor virus			low vision clinic
LTV+	long-term variability–average to moderate	LVAD	left ventricular assist device
		LV Angio	left ventricular angiogram
LTV 0	long-term variability–absent	L-VAM	leuprolide acetate, vinblastine, doxorubicin (Adriamycin), and mitomycin
LTVC	long-term venous catheter		
LTZ	letrozole (Femara)		
LU	left upper		
	left ureteral	LVAS	left ventricular assist system
	living unit	LVAT	left ventricular activation time
	Lutheran		
L & U	lower and upper	LVBP	left ventricle bypass pump
LUA	left upper arm	LVD	left ventricular dimension
LUD	left uterine displacement			left ventricular dysfunction
LUE	left upper extremity	LVDd	left ventricular end-diastolic diameter
Lues I	primary syphilis		
Lues II	secondary syphilis	LVDP	left ventricular diastolic pressure
Lues III	tertiary syphilis		
LUL	left upper lid	LVDs	left ventricular systolic diameter
	left upper lobe (lung)		
LUNA	laparoscopic uterosacral nerve ablation	LVDT	linear variable differential transformer
LUOB	left upper outer buttock	LVDV	left ventricular diastolic volume
LUOQ	left upper outer quadrant		
LUQ	left upper quadrant	LVE	left ventricular enlargement
LURD	living-unrelated donor		
LUS	laparoscopic ultrasonography	LVEDP	left ventricular end diastolic pressure
	lower uterine segment	LVEDV	left ventricular end-diastolic volume
LUSB	left upper scapular border		
	left upper sternal border	LVEF	left ventricular ejection fraction
LUST	lower uterine segment transverse	LVEP	left ventricular end pressure
LUT	lower urinary tract		
LUTD	lower urinary tract dysfunction	LVESD	left ventricular end-systolic dimension
LUTS	lower urinary tract symptoms	LVESVI	left ventricular end-systolic volume index
LUTT	lower urinary tract tumor	LVET	left ventricular ejection time
LUW	lungworm vaccine		
LUX	left upper extremity	LVF	left ventricular failure
LV	leave			left visual field

L

LVFP	left ventricular filling pressure	LVT	levetiracetam (Keppra)
LVFU	leucovorin and fluorouracil	LVV	left ventricular volume
			live varicella vaccine
LVG	left ventrogluteal	LVW	left ventricular wall
LVH	left ventricular hypertrophy	LVWI	left ventricular work index
LVID	left ventricular internal diameter	LVWMA	left ventricular wall motion abnormality
LVIDd	left ventricle internal diameter at end-diastole	LVWMI	left ventricular wall motion index
LVIDs	left ventricle internal dimension systole	LVWT	left ventricular wall thickness
LVL	large volume leukapheresis	LW	lacerating wound
			living will
	left vastus lateralis	L & W	Lee and White (coagulation)
LVM	left ventricular mass		
LVMI	left ventricular mass index		living and well
LVMM	left ventricular muscle mass	LWAQ	Living with Asthma Questionnaire
LVN	Licensed Visiting Nurse	LWCT	Lee-White clotting time
		LWBS	left without being seen
	Licensed Vocational Nurse	LWC	leave without consent
		LWCT	left without completing treatment
LVO	left ventricular overactivity	LWOP	leave without pay
LVOT	left ventricular outflow tract	LWOT	left without treatment
		LWP	large whirlpool
LVOTO	left ventricular outflow tract obstruction	LX	larynx local irradiation
			lower extremity
LVP	large volume parenteral	LXC	laxative of choice
	left ventricular pressure	LXT	left exotropia
LVPW	left ventricular posterior wall	LYCD	live yeast cell derivative
		LYEL	lost years of expected life
LVR	leucovorin	LYG	lymphomatoid granulomatosis
LVRS	lung-volume reduction surgery	LYM	Lyme disease vaccine
			lymphocytes
LVRT	liver volume replaced by tumor	lymphs	lymphocytes
		LYS	large yellow soft (stools)
LVS	left ventricular strain		lysine
LVS EMI	left ventricular subendocardial myocardial ischemia	lytes	electrolytes (Na, K, Cl, etc.)
			electrolyte panel (see page 358)
LVSP	left ventricular systolic pressure	LZ	landing zone
LVSW	left ventricular stroke work	LZP	lorazepam (Ativan)
LVSWI	left ventricular stroke work index		

L

M

M	male
	manual
	marital
	married
	masked (audiology)
	mass
	medial
	memory
	mesial
	meta
	meter (m)
	mild
	million
	minimum
	molar
	Monday
	monocytes
	mother
	mouth
	murmur
	muscle
	Mycobacterium
	Mycoplasma
	myopia
	myopic
	thousand
Ⓜ	murmur
M_1	first mitral sound
M1	left mastoid
	tropicamide 1% ophthalmic solution (Mydriacyl)
M1 to M7	categories of acute nonlymphoblastic leukemia
M_2	second mitral sound
m^2	square meters (body surface)
M2	right mastoid
M-2	vincristine, carmustine, cyclophosphamide, melphalan, and prednisone
M_3	third mitral sound

M-3	medical student 3rd year
3M	mitomycin, mitoxantrone, and methotrexate
M-3+7	mitoxantrone and cytarabine
M-4	medical student 4th year
MA	machine
	Master of Arts
	mean arterial (blood pressure)
	medical assistance
	medical authorization
	megestrol acetate
	menstrual age
	mental age
	Mexican-American
	microalbuminuria
	metabolic acidosis
	microaneurysms
	Miller-Abbott (tube)
	milliamps
	monoclonal antibodies
	motorcycle accident
M/A	mood and/or affect
MA-1	Bennett volume ventilator
MAA	macroaggregates of albumin
	Marketing Authorization Application (European Union)
MAB	maximum androgen blockade
Mab	monoclonal antibody
MABP	mean arterial blood pressure
MAC	macrocytic erythrocytes
	macrophage
	macula
	maximal allowable concentration
	medial arterial calcification
	membrane attack complex
	Mental Adjustment to Cancer (scale)
	methotrexate, dactinomycin (Actinomycin D), and cyclophosphamide

	mid-arm circumference	MAEW	moves all extremities
	minimum alveolar		well
	concentration	MAF	malignant ascites fluid
	monitored anesthesia care		metabolic activity factor
	multi-access catheter		Mexican-American female
	Mycobacterium avium	MAFAs	movement-associated fetal
	complex		(heart rate)
MACC	methotrexate,		accelerations
	doxorubicin,	MAFO	molded ankle/foot orthosis
	(Adriamycin)	MAFP	maternal alpha-fetoprotein
	cyclophosphamide, and	MAG	medication administration
	lomustine (Cee Nu)		guideline (record)
MACCC	Master Arts, Certified	mag cit	magnesium citrate
	Clinical Competence	MAGP	meatal advancement
MACE	Malon antegrade		glandulophaleoplasty
	continence enema	mag sulf	magnesium sulfate
MACOP-B	methotrexate,	MAHA	macroangiopathic
	doxorubicin,		hemolytic anemia
	(Adriamycin)	MAI	maximal aggregation
	cyclophosphamide,		index
	vincristine (Oncovin),		minor acute illness
	prednisone, and		*Mycobacterium avium-*
	bleomycin with		*intracellulare*
	leucovorin rescue	MAID	mesna, doxorubicin
MACRO	macrocytes		(Adriamycin),
MACS	magnetic activated cell		ifosfamide, and
	sorting		dacarbazine
MACs	malignancy-associated	MAL	malaria vaccine
	changes		malignant
MACTAR	McMaster-Toronto		midaxillary line
	Arthritis Patient	MALDI	matrix-assisted laser
	Reference (Disability		desorption ionization
	Questionnaire)	MALDI-	matrix-assisted laser
MAD	major affective disorder	TOFMS	desorption ionization–
	mind altering drugs		time-of-flight mass
	moderate atopic dermatitis		spectrometry
MADD	Mothers Against Drunk	MALG	Minnesota
	Driving		antilymphoblast
MADL	mobility activities of daily		globulin
	living	malig	malignant
MADRS	Montgomery-Åsburg	MALT	mucosa-associated
	Depression Rating		lymphoid tissue
	Scale	MALToma	lymphoma of mucosa-
MAE	medical air evacuation		associated lymphoid
	moves all extremities		tissue
MAES	moves all extremities	MAM	mammogram
	slowly		Mexican-American male
MAEEW	moves all extremities		monitored administration
	equally well		of medication

MAMC	mid-arm muscle circumference	MARE	manual active-resistive exercise
Mammo	mammography	MARSA	methicillin-aminoglycoside-resistant *Staphylococcus aureus*
MAMP	milliampere		
m-AMSA	amsacrine		
MAMTT	minimal active muscle tendon tension	MAS	macrophage activation syndrome
MAN	malignancy associated neutropenia		meconium aspiration syndrome
Mand	mandibular		Memory Assessment Scale
MANE	Morrow Assessment of Nausea and Emesis		minimum-access surgery
MANOVA	multivariate analysis of variance		mobile arm support
MAO	maximum acid output	MASA	mutant allele-specific amplification
MAO-A	monoamine oxidase type A	MASDA^{SM}	Multiple-Allele-Specific Diagnostic Assay
MAO-B	monoamine oxidase type B	MASER	microwave amplification (application) by stimulated emission of radiation
MAOI	monoamine oxidase inhibitor		
MAOP	Mid-Atlantic Oncology Program		
MAP	magnesium, ammonium, and phosphate (Struvite stones)	MASH POT	mashed potatoes
	mean airway pressure	MAST	mastectomy
	mean arterial pressure		medical antishock trousers
	Medical Assistance Program		Michigan Alcoholism Screening Test
	megaloblastic anemia of pregnancy		military antishock trousers
	Miller Assessment for Preschoolers (test for developmental delays)	MAT	manual arts therapy
			maternal
			maternity
	mitogen-activated protein		mature
	mitomycin, doxorubicin (Adriamycin), and cisplatin (Platinol)		medication administration team
			Miller-Abbott tube
			multifocal atrial tachycardia
	morning after pill (oral contraceptives)	MATHS	muscle pain, allergy, tachycardia and tiredness, and headache syndrome
	muscle-action potential		
MAPI	Millon Adolescent Personality Inventory	MAU	microalbuminuria
		MAVR	mitral and aortic valve replacement
MAPS	Make a Picture Story		
MAR	marital	max	maxillary
	medication administration record		maximal
		MAX A	maximum assistance (assist)
	mineral apposition rates		

MAXCONT	maximum contrast method	MBI	methylene blue installation
MAxL	midaxillary line		
MAYO	mayonnaise	MBL	mannose-binding lectin
MB	buccal margin		menstrual blood loss
	mandible	MBM	mother's breast milk
	Mallory body	MBNW	multiple-breath nitrogen washout
	Medical Board		
	medulloblastoma	MBO	mesiobuccal occulsion
	mesiobuccal	MBOT	mucinous borderline ovarian tumors
	methylene blue		
	myocardial bands	MBP	malignant brachial plexopathy
M/B	mother/baby		
MBA	Master of Business Administration		mannan-binding protein
			mannose-binding protein
M-BACOD	methotrexate (high-dose), bleomycin, doxorubicin (Adriamycin), cyclophosphamide, vincristine (Oncovin), and dexamethasone with leucovorin rescue		medullary bone pain
			mesiobuccopulpal
			myelin basic protein
		MBq	megabecquerels
		MBS	modified barium swallow
		MBT	maternal blood type
			multiple blunt trauma
MBC	male breast cancer	MC	male child
	maximum bladder capacity		medium-chain (triglycerides)
	maximum breathing capacity		metacarpal
			metatarso - cuneiform
	metastatic breast cancer		mini-laparotomy cholecystectomy
	methotrexate, bleomycin, and cisplatin		
			mitoxantrone and cytarabine
	minimal bactericidal concentration		
			mitral commissurotomy
MB-CK	a creatinine kinase isoenzyme		mixed cellularity
			molluscum contagiosum
MBD	metabolic bone disease		monocomponent highly purified pork insulin
	methylene blue dye		
MBEST	modulus blipped echo-planar		*Moraxella catarrhalis*
			mouth care
	single-pulse technique		myocarditis
MBD	minimal brain damage	m + c	morphine and cocaine
	minimal brain dysfunction	MCA	Medicines Control Agency (United Kingdom)
MBE	may be elevated		
	medium below elbow		megestrol, cyclophosphamide, and doxorubicin (Adriamycin)
MBF	meat base formula		
	myocardial blood flow		
MBFC	medial brachial fascial compartment		metacarpal amputation
			micrometastases clonogenic assay
MBHI	Millon Behavioral Health Inventory		

	middle cerebral aneurysm		muscle contraction
	middle cerebral artery		headache
	monoclonal antibodies	MCHC	mean corpuscular
	motorcycle accident		hemoglobin
	multichannel analyzer		concentration
	multiple congenital	MCI	mild cognitive impairment
	anomalies	mCi	millicurie
2-MCA	2-methyl citric acid	MCID	minimum clinically
MCAD	medium-chain acyl-CoA		important difference(s)
	dehydrogenase	mckat	microkatal (1 millionth
MCAF	monocyte chemoattractant		$[10^{-6}]$ of a katal)
	and activity factor	MCL	mantle cell lymphoma
MCAO	middle cerebral artery		maximum comfort level
	occlusion		medial collateral ligament
MCAT	Medical College		midclavicular line
	Admission Test		midcostal line
MCB	Medicines Control Board		modified chest lead
	(United Kingdom's		most comfortable level
	equivalent to the	mcL	microliter (1/1,000 of an
	United States Food and		mL)
	Drug Administration)	MCLL	most comfortable
	midcycle bleeding		listening level
	middle chamber bubbling	MCLNS	mucocutaneous lymph
McB pt	McBurney's point		node syndrome
MCC	microcrystalline cellulose	MCMI	Millon Clinical Multiaxial
	midstream clean-catch		Inventory
MCCU	mobile coronary care unit	mcmol	micromoles (one millionth
MCD	malformation of cortical		$[10^{-6}]$ of a mole)
	development	MCN	minimal change
	mean cell diameter		nephropathy
	minimal-change disease	MCNS	minimal change nephrotic
	multicystic dysplasia		syndrome
MCDK	multicystic dysplasia of	MCO	managed care organization
	the kidney		mupirocin calcium
MCDT	mast cell degranulation		ointment (Bactroban
	test		Nasal)
MCE	major coronary event	MCP	mean carotid pressure
MCF	multicentric foci		metacarpophalangeal joint
MCFA	medium-chain fatty		metoclopramide (Reglan)
	acid		monocyte chemotactic
mcg	microgram (μg)		protein
MCG	magnetocardiogram	MCR	Medicare
	magnetocardiography		metabolic clearance rate
MCGN	minimal-change		myocardial
	glomerular nephritis		revascularization
MCH	mean corpuscular	MC=R	moderately constricted
	hemoglobin		and equally reactive
	microfibrillar collagen	MCRC	metastatic colorectal
	hemostat		cancer

MCS	microculture and sensitivity	MDA	malondialdehyde
	moderate constant suction		manual dilation of the anus
	multiple chemical sensitivity		Medical Devises Agency (United Kingdom)
	myocardial contractile state		methylenedioxyamphet-amine
MCSA	minimal cross-sectional area		micrometastases detection assay
M-CSF	macrophage colony-stimulating factor		motor discriminative acuity
MC-SR	moderately constricted and slightly reactive	MDAC	multiple-dose activated charcoal
MCT	manual cervical traction	MDACC	MD Anderson Cancer Center
	mean circulation time	MDA LDL	malondialdehydeconju-gated low-density lipoprotein
	medium chain triglyceride		
	medullary carcinoma of the thyroid	MDC	Major Diagnostic Category
	microwave coagulation therapy		medial dorsal cutaneous (nerve)
MCTC	metrizamide computed tomography cisternogram	MDCM	mildly dilated congestive cardiomyopathy
MCTD	mixed connective tissue disease	MDD	major depressive disorder
			manic-depressive disorder
MCU	micturating cystourethrogram	MDE	major depressive episode
		MDF	myocardial depressant factor
MCV	mean corpuscular volume		
MCVRI	minimal coronary vascular resistance index	MDGF	macrophage-derived growth factor
MCYLS	marginal cost per year of life saved	MDI	manic-depressive illness
			metered-dose inhaler
MD	macula degeneration		methylenedioxyindenes
	maintenance dialysis		multiple daily injection
	maintenance dose		multiple dosage insulin
	major depression	MDIA	Mental Development Index, Adjusted
	mammary dysplasia		
	manic depression	MDII	multiple daily insulin injection
	medical doctor		
	mediodorsal	MDIS	metered-dose inhaler-spacer (device)
	Menière's disease		
	mental deficiency	MDM	mid-diastolic murmur
	mesiodistal		minor determinant mix (of penicillin)
	movement disorder		
	multiple dose	MDMA	methylenedioxy-methamphetamine (ecstasy)
	muscular dystrophy		
	myocardial damage		
MD-50®	diatrizoate sodium injection 50%	MDNT	midnight

MDO	mentally disordered offender		multiple dose vial
		MDY	month, date, and year
MDOT	modified directly observed therapy	ME	macular edema
			manic episode
MDP	methylene diphosphonate		medical events
MDPH	Michigan Department of Public Health		medical evidence
			medical examiner
MDPI	maximum daily permissible intake		mestranol
			Methodist
MDR	Medical Device Reporting (regulation)		middle ear
			myalgic encephalomyelitis
	minimum daily requirement	M/E	metabloic/endocrine
	multidrug resistance		myeloid-erythroid (ratio)
MD=R	moderately dilated and equally reactive	M&E	Mecholyl and Eserine
			mucositis and enteritis
MDR-1	multidrug resistance gene	MEA	microwave endometrial ablation
MDRE	multiple-drug-resistant enterococci		measles virus vaccine
MDREF	multidrug resistant enteric fever	MEA-I	multiple endocrine adenomatosis type I
MDRTB	multidrug-resistant tuberculosis	MEB	Medical Evaluation Board
MDS	maternal deprivation syndrome		methylene blue
		MEC	meconium
	Minimum Data Set		middle ear canal(s)
	myelodysplastic syndromes	MeCCNU	semustine
MD-SR	moderately dilated and slightly reactive	MECG	maternal electrocardiogram
MDSU	medical day stay unit	MeCP	semustine (methyl CCNU) cyclophosphamide, and prednisone
MDT	maggot debridement therapy		
	Mechanical Diagnostic Therapist	MED	medial
	motion detection threshold		median erythrocyte diameter
	multidisciplinary team		medical
	multidrug therapy		medication
MDTM	multidisciplinary team meeting		medicine
MDTP	multidisciplinary treatment plan		medium
			medulloblastoma
MDU	maintenance dialysis unit		minimal erythema dose
	microvascular Doppler ultrasonography		minimum effective dose
		MEDAC	multiple endocrine deficiency Addison's disease (autoimmune) candidiasis
MDUO	myocardial disease of unknown origin		
MDV	Marek's disease virus	MEDCO	Medcosonolator

MEDDRA	Medical Dictionary for Drug Regulatory Affairs		meningococcal (*Neisseria meningitidis*) (serogroups unspecified) vaccine
MEDEX	medication administration record	MEN (II)	multiple endocrine neoplasia (type II)
MED-LARS	Medical Literature Analysis and Retrieval System	MEN$_{cn-AC}$	meningococcal (*Neisseria meningitidis*) serogroups A, C conjugate vaccine
MEDLINE	National Library of Medicine medical database	MEN$_{cn-B}$	meningococcal (*Neisseria meningitidis*) serogroup B conjugate vaccine
MED NEC	medically necessary	MEN$_{ps}$	meningococcal (*Neisseria meningitidis*) polysaccharide vaccine, not otherwise specified
MEDS	medications		
MEE	maintenance energy expenditure		
	measured energy expenditure	MEN$_{ps-ACYW}$	meningococcal (*Neisseria meningitidis*) serogroups A, C, Y, W-135 polysaccharide vaccine
	middle ear effusion		
MEF	maximum expired flow rate	MEN$_{ps-B}$	meningococcal (*Neisseria meningitidis*) serogroup B polysaccharide vaccine
	middle ear fluid		
MEFR	mid expiratory flow rate		
MEFV	maximum expiratory flow-volume	MENS	microcurrent electrical neuromuscular stimulation
MEG	magnetoencephalogram		
	magnetoencephalography		mini-electrical nerve stimulator
Meg-CSF	megakaryocytic colony-stimulating factor		
MEGX	monoethylglycinexylidide	MEO	malignant external otitis
MeHg	methylmercury	MeOH	methyl alcohol
MEI	medical economic index	MEOS	microsomal ethanol oxidizing system
MEIA	microparticle enzyme immunoassay	MEP	maximal expiratory pressure
MEKC	micellar electrokinetic chromatography		meperidine
MEL	melatonin		motor-evoked potential
MELAS	myopathy, encephalopathy, lactic acidosis, and stroke-like episodes (syndrome)		multimodality evoked potential
		mEq	milliequivalent
MEL B	melarsoprol (Arsobal)	mEq/24 H	milleequivalents per 24 hours
MEM	memory		
	monocular estimate method (near retinoscopy)	mEq/L	milliequivalents per liter
		MER	medical evidence of record
MEN	meningeal		methanol-extracted residue (of phenol-treated BCG)
	meninges		
	meningitis		

M/E ratio	myeloid/erythroid ratio		myocardial fibrosis
MERRF	myoclonic epilepsy and ragged red fibers	M/F	male-female ratio
		M & F	male and female
MES	mesial		mother and father
MeSH	Medical Subject Headings of the National Library of Medicine	MFA	malaise, fatigue, and anorexia
MESS	Mangled Extremity Severe Score	MFAT	multifocal atrial tachycardia
MET	medical emergency treatment	MFB	metallic foreign body multiple-frequency bioimpedance
	metabolic	MFC	medial femoral condyle
	metamyelocytes	MFCU	Medicaid Fraud Control Unit
	metastasis		
	metronidazole	MFD	Memory for Designs
META	metamyelocytes		midforceps delivery
METH	methicillin		milk-free diet
MetHb	methemoglobin		multiple fractions per day
	methemoglobinemia	MFEM	maximal forced expiratory maneuver
methyl CCNU	semustine	MFFT	Matching Familiar Figures Test
methyl G	mitroguazone dihydrochloride (Zyrkamine)	MFH	malignant fibrous histiocytoma
		MFI	mean fluorescent intensity
methyl GAG	mitroguazone dihydrochloride (Zyrkamine)	MFM	multifidus muscle
		MFNS	mometasone furoate nasal spray (Nasonex)
METS	metabolic equivalents (multiples of resting oxygen uptake)	MFPS	myofascial pain syndrome
		MFR	mid-forceps rotation
	metastases		myofascial release
METT	maximum exercise tolerance test	MFS	Miller-Fisher syndrome mitral first sound
MEV	million electron volts		monofixation syndrome
MEWDS	multifocal evanescent white dot syndrome	MFT	muscle function test
		MFVNS	middle fossa vestibular nerve section
MEX	Mexican	MFVPT	Motor Free Visual Perception Test
MF	Malassezia folliculitis *Malassezia furfur*	MFVR	minimal forearm vascular resistance
	masculinity/femininity	MG	Marcus Gunn
	meat free		Michaelis-Gutmann (bodies)
	mesial facial		milligram (mg)
	methotrexate and fluorouracil		myasthenia gravis
	midcavity forceps	mg	milligram
	midforceps	Mg	magnesium
	mother and father	mG	milligauss
	mycosis fungoides		
	myelofibrosis		

μg	microgram (1/1000 of a milligram) (mcg)	*mgtt*	minidrop (60 minidrops = 1 mL)
M&G	myringotomy and grommets	MGUS	monoclonal gammopathy of undetermined significance
mg%	milligrams per 100 milliliters	MGW	multiple gunshot wound
MGBG	mitoguazone (Zyrkamine)	MGW enema	magnesium sulfate, glycerin, and water enema
MGCT	malignant glandular cell tumor	M-GXT	multistage graded exercise test
MGD	meibomian gland dysfunction	mGy	milligray (radiation unit)
MGDF	megakaryocyte growth and development factor	MH	macular hemorrhage malignant hyperthermia marital history
mg/dl	milligrams per 100 milliliters		medical history menstrual history
MGF	macrophage growth factor		mental health moist heat
	mast cell growth factor maternal grandfather	MHA	Mental Health Assistant methotrexate, hydrocortisone, and cytarabine (ara-C)
MGG	May-Grünwald-Giemsa (stain)		microangiopathic hemolytic anemia
MGGM	maternal great grandmother		microhemagglutination
MGHL	middle glenohumeral ligament	MHA-TP	microhemagglutination-*Treponema pallidum*
mg/kg	milligram per kilogram	MHB	maximum hospital benefits
mg/kg/d	milligram per kilogram per day	MHb	methemoglobin
mg/kg/hr	milligram per kilogram per hour	MHBSS	modified Hank's balanced salt solution
MGM	maternal grandmother milligram (mg is correct)	MHC	major histocompatibility complex
MGMA	Medical Group Management Association		mental health center (clinic)
MGN	membranous glomerulonephritis		mental health counselor
MgO	magnesium oxide	M/hct	microhematocrit
MG/OL	molecular genetics/oncology laboratory	mHg	millimeters of mercury
		MHH	mental health hold
MGP	Marcus Gunn pupil medical group practice	MHI	Mental Health Index (information)
MGR	murmurs, gallops, or rubs	MHIP	mental health inpatient
MGS	malignant glandular schwannoma	MH/MR	mental health and mental retardation
MgSO₄	magnesium sulfate (Epsom salt)	MHN	massive hepatic necrosis
MGT	management	MHO	medical house officer

MHRI	Mental Health Research Institute	MICN	mobile intensive care nurse
MHS	major histocompatibility system	MICR	methacholine inhalation challenge response
	malignant hyperthermia susceptible	MICRO	microcytes
	multihospital system	MICS	minimally invasive cardiac surgery
MHT	mental health team	MICU	medical intensive care unit
	Mental Health Technician		mobile intensive care unit
MHTAP	microhemagglutination assay for antibody to *Treponema pallidum*	MID	mesioincisodistal
			microvillus inclusion disease
MHV	middle hepatic vein		minimal ineffective dose
MHW	medial heel wedge		multi-infarct dementia
	mental health worker	MIDCAB	minimally invasive direct coronary artery bypass
MHX	methohexital sodium	MID EPIS	midline episiotomy
MHx	medical history	Mid I	middle insomnia
MHxR	medical history review	MIE	maximim inspiratory effort
MHz	megahertz		meconium ileus equivalent (cystic fibrosis)
MI	membrane intact		
	mental illness		
	mental institution		medical improvement expected
	mesial incisal		
	mitral insufficiency	MIEI	medication-induced esophageal injury
	myocardial infarction		
MIA	medically indigent adult	MIF	Merthiolate, iodine, and formalin
	missing in action		
MIBI	technetium Tc99m sestamibi (a myocardial perfusion agent; Cardiolite)		mifepristone (RU 486; Mifeprex)
			migration inhibitory factor
		MIFR	midinspiratory flow rate
MIBG	iobenguane sulfate I 123 (meta-iodobenzyl guanidine I 123)	MIF 50% VC	midinspiratory flow at 50% of vital capacity
		MIG	measles immune globulin
MIBK	methylisobutylketone	MIGET	multiple inert gas elimination technique
MIC	maternal and infant care		
	methacholine inhalation challenge	MIH	medication-induced headache
	medical intensive care		migraine with interparoxysmal headache
	microscope		
	microcytic erythrocytes		
	minimum inhibitory concentration		myointimal hyperplasia
MICA	mentally ill chemical abuser	MIL	military
MICE	mesna, ifosfamide, carboplatin, and etoposide		mesial incisal lingual (surface)

	mother-in-law	MIRS	Medical Improvement Review Standard
MIMCU	medical intermediate care unit	MIS	management information systems
MIN	mammary intraepithelial neoplasia		minimally invasive surgery
	melanocytic intraepidermal neoplasia		mitral insufficiency
			moderate intermittent suction
	mineral	MISC	miscarriage
	minimum		miscellaneous
	minor	M Isch	myocardial ischemia
	minute (min)	MISH	multiple *in situ* hybridization
MIN A	minimal assistance (assist)	MISO	misonidazole
MIME	mitoguazone, ifosfamide, methotrexate, and etoposide with mesna	MISS	minimally invasive spine surgery
			Modified Injury Severity Score (scale)
MINE	Medical Information Network of Europe	MIT	meconium in trachea
	mesna, ifosfamide, mitoxantrone (Novantrone), and etoposide		miracidia immobilization test
			multiple injection therapy (of insulin)
	medical improvement not expected	MITO-C	mitomycin (Mutamycin)
MINI	Mini International Neuropsychiatric Interview	MITOX	mitoxantrone (Novantrone)
		MIU	million international units
MIO	minimum identifiable odor	mIU	milli-international unit (one-thousandth of an International unit)
	monocular indirect ophthalmoscopy	MIVA	mivacurium (Mivacron)
MIP	macrophage inflammatory protein	MIW	mental inquest warrant
		mix mon	mixed monitor
	maximum inspiratory pressure	MJ	marijuana
			megajoule
	maximum-intensity projection	MJD	Machado-Joseph Disease
	mean intrathoracic pressure	MJL	medial joint line
		MJS	medial joint space
	mean intravascular pressure	MJT	Mead Johnson tube
		μkat	microkatal (micro-moles/sec)
	medical improvement possible	MKAB	may keep at bedside
	metacarpointerphalangeal	MKB	married, keeping baby
MIRD	medical internal radiation dose	MK-CSF	megakaryocyte colony-stimulating factor
MIRP	myocardial infarction rehabilitation program	MKI	mitotic-karyorrhectic index

MKM	microgram per kilogram per minute		mucocutaneous lymph node syndrome (Kawasaki syndrome)
ML	malignant lymphoma		
	mediolateral	MLO	mesiolinguo-occlusal
	middle lobe	MLP	mento-laeva posterior
	midline		mesiolinguopulpal
mL	milliliter		midlevel provider
M/L	monocyte to lymphocyte (ratio)	MLPN	Medical Licensed Practical Nurse
	mother-in-law	MLPP	maximum loose-packed position
MLA	medical laboratory assay		
	mento-laeva anterior	MLR	middle latency response
MLAC	minimum local analgesic concentration		mixed lymphocyte reaction
MLAP	mean left atrial pressure		multiple logistic regression
MLBW	moderately low birth weight	MLS	mediastinal B-cell lymphoma with sclerosis
MLC	metastatic liver cancer		
	minimal lethal concentration	MLT	melatonin
			mento-laeva transversa
	mixed lymphocyte culture	MLU	mean length of utterance
	multilevel care	MLV	monitored live voice
	multilumen catheter	MLWHF	Minnesota Living with Heart Failure (questionnaire)
	myelomonocytic leukemia, chronic		
MLD	manual lymph drainage	MM	major medical (insurance)
	masking level difference		malignant melanoma
	melioidosis (*Pseudomonas pseudomallei*) vaccine		malignant mesothelioma
			Marshall-Marchetti
			medial malleolus
	metachromatic leukodystrophy		member months
			meningococcic meningitis
	microlumbar diskectomy		mercaptopurine and methotrexate
	microsurgical lumbar diskectomy		methadone maintenance
			micrometastases
	minimal lethal dose		millimeter (mm)
MLDT	Manual Lymph Drainage Therapist		mist mask
MLE	maximum likelihood estimation		morbidity and mortality
			motor meal
	midline (medial) episiotomy		mucous membrane
			multiple myeloma
MLF	median longitudinal fasciculus		muscle movement
			myelomeningocele
MLN	manifest latent nystagmus	mM.	millimole (mmol)
		mm	millimeter
	melanoma vaccine		
MLNS	minimal lesions nephrotic syndrome	M&M	milk and molasses
			morbidity and mortality

MMA	methylmalonic acid		Minnesota Multiphasic
	methylmethacrylate		Personality Inventory
MMC	mitomycin (mitomycin C)	MMPI-D	Minnesota Multiphasic
MMD	malignant metastatic		Personality Inventory-
	disease		Depression Scale
	mucus membranes dry	6-MMPR	6-methylmercaptopurine
	myotonic muscular		riboside
	dystrophy	MMR	measles, mumps, and
MMECT	multiple monitor		rubella
	electroconvulsive		midline malignant
	therapy		reticulosis
MMEFR	maximal mid-expiratory		mismatch repair
	flow rate	MMRISK	a skin cancer mnemonic;
MMF	mean maximum flow		**m**oles that are atypical,
	mycophenolate mofetil		**m**oles that are many in
	(CellCept)		number,
MMFR	maximal mid-expiratory		**r**ed hair or freckles,
	flow rate		**i**nability to tan,
MMG	mechanomyography		**s**unburn,
mm Hg	millimeters of mercury		**k**indred
MMI	maximal medical	MMS	Mini-Mental State
	improvement		(examination)
MMK	Marshall-Marchetti-Krantz		Mohs' micrographic
	(cystourethropexy)		surgery
MMM	mitoxantrone,	MMSE	Mini-Mental State
	methotrexate, and		Examination
	mitomycin	MMT	malignant mesenchymal
	mucous membrane		tumors
	moist		manual muscle test
	myelofibrosis with		methadone maintenance
	myeloid metaplasia		treatment
mMMSE	modified version of the		Mini Mental Test
	mini mental status		mixed müllerian tumors
	examination	MMTP	Methadone Maintenance
MMMT	metastatic mixed		Treatment Program
	müllerian tumor	MMTV	malignant mesothelioma
MMN	multifocal motor		of the tunica vaginalis
	neuropathy		monomorphic ventricular
MMOA	maxillary mandibular		tachycardia
	odontectomy		mouse mammary tumor
	alveolectomy		virus
mmol	millimole	MMV	mandatory minute
μmol	micromole		volume
MMP	matrix metalloproteinase	MMWR	*Morbidity and Mortality*
	multiple medical		*Weekly Report*
	problems	MN	midnight
MMP-8	metalloproteinase-8		mononuclear
MMPI	matrix metalloproteinase	Mn	manganese
	inhibitor	M&N	morning and night

	Mydriacyl and Neo-Synephrine	MOAHI	mixed obstructive apnea and hypopnea index
MNC	monomicrobial necrotizing cellulitis	MOB	medical office building
	mononuclear leukocytes		mobility
MNCV	motor nerve conduction velocity		mobilization
MND	modified neck dissection	MOB-PT	mitomycin, vincristine (Oncovin), bleomycin, and cisplatin (Platinol AQ)
	motor neuron disease		
MNF	myelinated nerve fibers		
MNG	multinodular goiter	MOC	medial olivocochlear
MNM	mononeuritis multiplex		Medical Officer on Call
MNMCB	motor neuropathy with multifocal conduction block		metronidazole, omeprazole, and clarithromycin
			mother of child
MNNB	Monas-Nitz Neuropsychological Battery	MOCI	Maudsley Obsessive-Compulsive Inventory
		MOD	maturity onset diabetes
MNPRT	mixed neutron and photon radiotherapy		medical officer of the day
			mesio-occlusodistal
MNR	marrow neutrophil reserve		moderate
			mode of death
MNSc	Master of Nursing Science		moment of death
			multiorgan dysfunction
MnSOD	manganese superoxide dismutase	MOD A	moderate assistance (assist)
Mn SSEPS	median nerve somatosensory evoked potentials	MODM	mature-onset diabetes mellitus
		MODS	multiple organ dysfunction syndrome
MNTB	medial nucleus of the trapezoid body	MODY	maturity onset diabetes of youth
MNX	meniscectomy	MOE	movement of extremities
MNZ	metronidazole	MOF	mesial occlusal facial
MO	medial oblique (x-ray view)		methotrexate, vincristine (Oncovin), and fluorouracil
	menhaden oil		methoxyflurane (Penthrane)
	mesio-occlusal		multiple organ failure
	mineral oil	MOFS	multiple-organ failure syndrome
	month (mo)		
	months old	MOH	Ministry of Health
	morbidly obese	MOI	mechanism of injury
Mo	molybdenum	MoICU	mobile intensive care unit
MOA	mechanism of action	MOJAC	mood orientation, judgement, affect, and content
	metronidazole, omeprazole, and amoxicillin		
MoAb	monoclonal antibody	MOM	milk of magnesia

	mother	MP	malignant pyoderma
	mucoid otitis media		melphalan and prednisone
MoM	multiples of the median		menstrual period
MOMP	major outer membrane		mercaptopurine
	protein		metacarpal phalangeal
MON	maximum observation		joint
	nursery		moist park
	monitor		monitor pattern
MONO	infectious mononucleosis		monophasic
	monocyte		motor potential
	monospot		mouthpiece
mono, di	monochorionic,		myocardial perfusion
	diamniotic	M & P	Millipore and phase
mono,	monochorionic,	4 MP	methylpyrazole
mono	monoamniotic		(fomepizole; Antizol)
MOP	medical outpatient	6-MP	mercaptopurine
8 MOP	methoxsalen	MPA	main pulmonary artery
MOPP	mechlorethamine,		Medical Products Agency
	vincristine (Oncovin),		(Sweden)
	procarbazine, and		medroxyprogesterone
	prednisone		acetate
MOPV	monovalent oral	MPa	megapascal
	poliovirus vaccine	MPAC	Memorial Pain
MOR	morphine		Assessment Card
MOS	Medical Outcome Study	MPAP	mean pulmonary artery
	mirror optical system		pressure
	months	MPAQ	McGill Pain Assessment
mOsm	milliosmol		Questionnaire
MOSF	multiple organ system	MPB	male pattern baldness
	failure		mephobarbital
MOS sf-20	Medical Outcomes Study,	MPBFV	mean pulmonary-blood-
	short form 20 items		flow velocity
MOS sf-36	Medical Outcomes Study,	MPBNS	modified Peyronie bladder
	short form, 36 items		neck suspension
mOsmol	milliosmole	MPC	meperidine, promethazine,
MOT	motility examination		and chlorpromazine
MOTS	mucosal oral therapeutic		mucopurulent cervicitis
	system	MPCN	microscopically positive
MOTT	mycobacteria other than		and culturally negative
	tubercle	M-PCR	multiplex polymerase
MOU	medical oncology unit		chain reaction
	memorandum of	MPCU	medical progressive care
	understanding		unit
MOUS	multiple occurrences of	MPD	maximum permissable
	unexplained symptoms		dose
MOV	minimum obstructive		methylphenidate
	volume		(Ritalin)
	multiple oral vitamin		moisture permeable
MOW	Meals on Wheels		dressing

	multiple personality disorder	MPP	massive periretinal proliferation
	myeloproliferative disorder		maximum pressure picture
	myofascial pain dysfunction (syndrome)	MPP	multiple presentation phenotype
MPE	malignant pleural effusion	MPQ	McGill Pain Questionnaire
	mean prediction error		
	multiphoton excitation	MPPT	methylprednisolone pulse therapy
MPEC	multipolar electrocoagulation	MPR	massive periretinal retraction
MPEG	methoxypolyethylene glycol	MPS	mean particle size
MPF	methylparaben free		mononuclear phagocyte system
m-PFL	methotrexate, cisplatin (Platinol), fluorouracil, and leucovorin		mucopolysaccharidosis
			multiphasic screening
MPGN	membranoproliferative glomerulonephritis	MPS-1	mucopolysaccharidosis I
		MPSS	massively parallel signature sequencing
MPH	massive pulmonary hemorrhage		methylprednisolone sodium succinate
	Master of Public Health		
	methylphenidate (Ritalin)	MPT	multiple parameter telemetry
	miles per hour		
MPI	master patient index	MPTRD	motor, pain, touch, and reflex deficit
	Maudsley Personality Inventory	MPU	maternal pediatric unit
	myocardial perfusion imaging	MPV	mean platelet volume
		MQ	memory quotient
MPIF-1	myeloid progenitor inhibitory factor-1	MR	Maddox rod
			magnetic resonance
MPJ	metacarpophalangeal joint		manifest refraction
MPK	milligram per kilogram		may repeat
MPL	maximum permissable level		measles-rubella
			medial rectus
	mesiopulpolingual		medical record
MPL®	monophosphoryl lipid A		mental retardation
MPLC	medium pressure liquid chromatography		milliroentgen
			mitral regurgitation
MPM	malignant pleural mesothelioma		moderate resistance
		M&R	measure and record
	Mortality Prediction Model	MR × 1	may repeat times one (once)
MPN	monthly progress note	MRA	magnetic resonance angiography
	most probable number		
	multiple primary neoplasms		main renal artery
MPO	male pattern obesity		medical record administrator
	myeloperoxidase		medical research associate
MPOA	medial preoptic area		midright atrium

	multivariate regression analysis	MRHD	maximum recommended human dose
mrad	millirad	MRHT	modified rhyme hearing test
MRAN	medical resident admitting note	MRI	magnetic resonance imaging
MRAP	mean right atrial pressure		
MRAS	main renal artery stenosis	M & R I & O	measure and record input and output
MRC	Master of Rehabilitation Counseling	MRL	minimal response level moderate rubra lochia
MRCA	magnetic resonance coronary angiography	MRLVD	maximum residue limits of veterinary drugs
MRCC	metastatic renal cell carcinoma	MRLT	mesalamine-related lung toxicity
MRCP	magnetic resonance cholangiopancreatography	MRM	modified radical mastectomy
	Member of the Royal College of Physicians	MRN	magnetic resonance neurography
	mental retardation, cerebral palsy		medical record number medical resident's note
MRCPs	movement-related cortical potentials	mRNA	messenger ribonucleic acid
MRCS	Member of the Royal College of Surgeons	MROU	medial rectus, both eyes
MRD	margin reflex distance	MRP	multidrug resistance associated protein
	Medical Records Department	MP-RAGE	magnetization prepared rapid acquisition gradient-echo
	Minimal Record of Disability		
	minimal residual disease	MRPN	medical resident progress note
MRDD	maximum recommended daily dose	MRS	magnetic resonance spectroscopy
	Mental Retardation and Development Disabilities		mental retardation syndrome
	mentally retarded and developmentally disabled		methicillin-resistant *Staphylococcus aureus*
		MRSA	methicillin-resistant *Staphylococcus aureus*
MRDM	malnutrition-related diabetes mellitus	MRSE	methicillin-resistant *Staphylococcus epidermidis*
MRE	manual resistance exercise		
	most recent episode	MRSI	magnetic resonance spectroscopic imaging
MRFC	mouse rosette-forming cells	MRSS	methicillin-resistant *Staphylococcus* species
MR FIT	Multiple Risk Factor Intervention Trial	MRT	magnetic resonance tomography
MRG	murmurs, rubs, and gallops		malignant rhabdoid tumor
MRH	Maddox rod hyperphoria		modified rhyme test

MRTA	magnetic resonance tomographic angiography	MSB	mainstem bronchus
		MSBOS	maximum surgical blood order schedule
MRU	medical resource utilization	MSBP	Munchausen syndrome by proxy
MRV®	mixed respiratory vaccine	MSC	major symptom complex
MRX	*Moraxella catarrhalis* vaccine		midsystolic click
			MS Contin®
MR × 1	may repeat once	MSCA	McCarthy Scales of Children's Abilities
MS	mass spectroscopy		
	Master of Science	MSCC	midstream clean-catch (urine culture)
	medical student		
	mental status	MSCCC	Master Sciences, Certified Clinical Competence
	milk shake		
	minimal support	MSCs	mesenchymal stem cells
	mitral sounds	MSCU	medical special care unit
	mitral stenosis	MSCWP	musculoskeletal chest wall pain
	moderately susceptible		
	morning stiffness	MSD	male sexual dysfunction
	morphine sulfate		microsurgical diskectomy
	motile sperm		midsleep disturbance
	multiple sclerosis	MSDBP	mean sitting diastolic blood pressure
	muscle spasm		
	muscle strength	MSDS	material safety data sheet
	musculoskeletal		
M & S	microculture and sensitivity	MSE	Mental Status Examination
3MS	Modified Mini-Mental Status (examination)	Msec	milliseconds
		MSEL	myasthenic syndrome of Eaton-Lambert
MS III	third-year medical student		
MSA	Medical Savings Accounts	MSER	mean systolic ejection rate
	membrane-stabilizing activity		Mental Status Examination Record
	metropolitan statistical area	MSF	meconium-stained fluid
	microsomal autoantibodies		megakaryocyte stimulating factor
	multiple system atrophy	MSG	massage
MSAF	meconium-stained amniotic fluid		methysergide (Sansert)
			monosodium glutamate
MSAFP	maternal serum alpha-fetoprotein	MSH	melanocyte-stimulating hormone
MSAP	mean systemic arterial pressure	MSHA	mannose-sensitive hemagglutinin
MSAS	Mandel Social Adjustment Scale	MSI	magnetic source imaging
			mass sociogenic illness
MSAS-SF	Memorial Symptom Assessment Scale – short form		microsatellite instability
			multiple subcortical infarction

	musculoskeletal impairment
MSIR®	morphine sulfate immediate release tablets
MSIS	Multiple Severity of Illness System
MSK	medullary sponge kidney musculoskeletal
MSKCC	Memorial Sloan-Kettering Cancer Center
MSL	midsternal line multiple symmetrical lipomatosis
MSLT	multiple sleep latency test
MSM	magnetic starch microspheres men who have sex with men methsuximide (Celontin) methylsulfonylmethane midsystolic murmur
MSN	Master of Science in Nursing
MSNA	muscle sympathetic nerve activity
MSO	managed services organization mentally stable and oriented mental status, oriented most significant other
MSO₄	morphine sulfate (this is a dangerous abbreviation)
MSOF	multisystem organ failure
MSPN	medical student progress notes
MSPU	medical short procedure unit
MSQ	Mental Status Questionnaire meters squared
MSR	muscle stretch reflexes
MSRPP	Multidimensional Scale for Rating Psychiatric Patients
MSS	Marital Satisfaction Scale mean sac size microsatellite stable

	minor surgery suite
MSSA	methicillin-susceptible *Staphylococcus aureus*
MSS-CR	mean sac size and crown-rump length
MSSP	Maternal Support Services Program
MSSU	midstream specimen of urine
MST	maladies sexuellement transmissibles (French–sexually transmitted diseases) mean survival time median survival time mental stress test multiple subpial transection
MSTA®	mumps skin test antigen
MSTI	multiple soft tissue injuries
MSU	maple syrup urine midstream urine monosodium urate
MSUD	maple-syrup urine disease
MSUs	midstream specimens of urine
mSv	millisievert (radiation unit)
MSW	Master of Social Work multiple stab wounds
MT	empty macular target maggot therapy maintenance therapy malaria therapy malignant teratoma Medical Technologist metatarsal middle turbinate monitor technician muscles and tendons muscle tone music therapy (Therapist) myringotomy tube(s)
M/T	masses of tenderness myringotomy with tubes
M & T	*Monilia* and *Trichomonas* muscles and tendons

	myringotomy and tubes	MTHFR	methylene tetrahydrofolate reductase
MTA	Medical Technical Assistant		
	metatarsal adduction	MTI	magnetization transfer imaging
	multi-targeted antifolate		malignant teratoma intermediate
MTAD	tympanic membrane of the right ear		
MT/AK	music therapy/ audiokinetics	MTJ	midtarsal joint
MTAS	tympanic membrane of the left ear	MTL	Metropolitan Life (Insurance Company) Table (for desirable weight)
MTAU	tympanic membranes of both ears		
		MTLE	medial (mesial) temporal-lobe epilepsy
MTB	*Mycobacterium tuberculosis*	MTM	modified Thayer-Martin medium
MTBC	Music Therapist-Board Certified		mouth-to-mouth (resuscitation)
MTBE	methyl tert-butyl ether		
MTC	magnetization transfer contrast	MTP	master treatment plan
			medical termination of pregnancy
	medullary thyroid carcinoma		metatarsophalangeal
	metoclopramide		microsomal triglyceride transfer protein
	mitomycin		
MTD	maximum tolerated dose	MTR _	mother
	metastatic trophoblastic disease	MTR-O	no masses, tenderness, or rebound
	minimum toxic dose	MTRS	Licensed Master Therapeutic Recreation Specialist
	Monroe tidal drainage		
	Mycobacterium tuberculosis direct (test)	MTS	mesial temporal sclerosis
MTDDA	Minnesota Test for Differential Diagnosis of Aphasia	MTST	maximal treadmill stress test
MTDI	maximum tolerable daily intake	MTT	mamillothalamic tract
			mean transit time
MTDT	*Mycobacterium tuberculosis* direct test		methylthiotetrazole
MTE	multiple trace elements	MTU	malignant teratoma undifferentiated
MTE-4®	trace metal elements injection (there is also a #5, #6, and #7)		methylthiouracil
		MTX	methotrexate
		MTZ	mirtazapine (Remeron)
MTET	modified treadmill exercise testing		mitoxantrone (Novantrone)
MTF	medical treatment facility	MU	million units
			Murphy unit
MTG	middle temporal gyrus (gyri)	mU	milliunits
	midthigh girth	MUA	manipulation under anesthesia

MUAC	middle upper arm circumference		millivolts
			minute volume
MUD	matched-unrelated donor		mitoxantrone and etoposide
MUDDLES	miosis, urination, diarrhea, diaphoresis, lacrimation, excitation of central nervous system, and salivation (effects of cholinesterase inhibitors)		mitral valve
			mixed venous
			multivesicular
		MVA	malignant vertricular arrhythmias
			manual vacuum aspiration
			mitral valve area
MUDPILES	methanol, metformin; uremia; diabetic ketoacidosis; phenformin, paraldehyde; iron, isoniazid, ibuprofen; lactic acidosis; ethanol, ethylene glycol; and salicylates, sepsis (causes of metabolic acidosis)		motor vehicle accident
		M-VAC	methotrexate, vinblastine doxorubicin (Adriamycin), and cisplatin
		MVB	methotrexate and vinblastine
			mixed venous blood
		MVC	maximal voluntary contraction
MUE	medication use evaluation		motor vehicle collision (crash)
MUFA	monounsaturated fatty acid	MVc	mitral valve closure
MUGA	multigated (radionuclide) angiogram	MVD	microvascular decompression
	multiple gated acquisition (scan)		microvessel density
			mitral valve disease
MUGX	multiple gated acquisition exercise		multivessel disease
		MVE	mitral valve (leaflet) excursion
MULE	microcomputer upper limb exerciser		Murray Valley encephalitis
MuLV	murine leukemia virus	MV Grad	mitral valve gradient
MUM	mumps virus vaccine	MVI	multiple vitamin injection
MUNSH	Memorial University of Newfoundland Scale of Happiness	MVI®	brand name for parenteral multivitamins
MUO	metastasis of unknown origin	MVI 12®	brand name for parenteral multivitamins
MUPAT	multiple-site perineal applicator technique	MVO	mixed venous oxygen saturation
MUSE®	Medicated Urethral System for Erection (alprostadil urethral suppository)	MVO_2	myocardial oxygen consumption
		MVP	mean venous pressure
			mitomycin, vinblastine, and cisplatin (Platinol AQ)
mus-lig	musculoligamentous		
MUU	mouse uterine units		
MV	mechanical ventilation		mitral valve prolapse

MVPP	mechlorethamine, vinblastine, procarbazine, and prednisone	MYR	myringotomy
		MYS	medium yellow soft (stools)
MVPS	mitral valve prolapse syndrome	MZ	monozygotic
MVR	massive vitreous retraction	MZL	marginal zone lymphocyte
	micro-vitreoretinal (blade)	MZT	monozygotic twins
	mitral valve regurgitation		
	mitral valve replacement		
MVRI	mixed vaccine respiratory infections		
MVS	mitral valve stenosis		
	motor, vascular, and sensory		
MVT	movement		
	multiform ventricular tachycardia		
	multivitamin		
MVU	Montevideo units		
MVV	maximum ventilatory volume		
	maximum voluntary ventilation		
	mixed vespid venom		
MWB	minimal weight bearing		
MWD	maximum walking distance		
	microwave diathermy		
M-W-F	Monday-Wednesday-Friday		
MWI	Medical Walk-In (Clinic)		
MWS	Mickety-Wilson syndrome		
MWT	maintenance of wakefulness test		
	Mallory-Weiss tear		
	malpositioned wisdom teeth		
Mx	manifest refraction		
	mastectomy		
	maxilla		
	movement		
	myringotomy		
My	myopia		
MYD	mydriatic		
myelo	myelocytes		
	myelogram		
MyG	myasthenia gravis		
MYOP	myopia		

N

			not applicable
			not available
			nurse aide
			nurse's aid
			Nurse Anesthetist
N	nausea		nursing assistant
	negative	N & A	normal and active
	Negro	NAA	N-acetylaspartate
	Neisseria		neutron activation analysis
	nerve		no apparent abnormalities
	neutrophil		nucleic acid amplification
	never	NAAC	no apparent anesthesia
	newton		complications
	night	NAA/Cr	N-acetylaspartate/creatine
	nipple		ratio
	nitrogen	NAAT	nucleic acid amplification
	no		techniques (testing)
	nodes	NAATPT	not available at the
	nonalcoholic		present time
	none	NAB	not at bedside
	normal	NABS	normoactive bowel
	North (as in the location		sounds
	2N, would be second	NABX	needle aspiration biopsy
	floor, North wing)	NAC	acetylcysteine (N-
	not		acetylcysteine;
	notified		Mucomyst)
	noun		neoadjuvant
	NPH insulin		chemotherapy
	size of sample		no acute changes
N I	first through twelfth	NACD	no anatomical cause of
N XII	cranial nerves		death
O.1 N	tenth-normal	NaClO	sodium hypochlorite
N_2	nitrogen	NaCl	sodium chloride (salt)
N 2.5	phenylephrine HCl 2.5%	NaCMC	sodium carboxymethyl
	ophthalmic solution		cellulose
	(Neo-Synephrine)	NACS	Neurologic and Adaptive
n-3	omega-3		Capacity Score
5'-N	5'-nucleotidase	NACT	neoadjuvant
Na	sodium		chemotherapy
Na^+	sodium	NAD	nicotinamide adenine
NA	Narcotics Anonymous		dinucleotide
	Native American		no active disease
	Negro adult		no acute distress
	new admission		no apparent distress
	nicotinic acid		no appreciable disease
	nonalcoholic		normal axis deviation
	norethindrone acetate		nothing abnormal detected
	normal axis	NADA	New Animal Drug
	not admitted		Application

NADE	New Animal Drug Evaluation	NAPD	no active pulmonary disease
NADPH	nicotinamide adenine dinucleotide phosphate	Na Pent	Pentothal Sodium
		NAR	no action required
NADSIC	no apparent active disease seen in chest		no adverse reaction
			nonambulatory restraint
NaE	exchangeable sodium		not at risk
NaF	sodium fluoride		
NAF	nafcillin	NARC	narcotic(s)
	Native-American female	NaRI	noradrenaline reuptake inhibitor
	Negro adult female		
	normal adult female	NART	National Adult Reading Test (United Kingdom)
	Notice of Adverse Findings (FDA post-audit letter)	NAS	nasal
			neonatal abstinence syndrome
NAFLD	nonalcoholic fatty liver disease		no abnormality seen
			no added salt
NAG	narrow angle glaucoma	NASBA	nucleic-acid sequencing based amplification
NaHCO₃	sodium bicarbonate		
NAI	no action indicated	NASH	nonalcoholic steatohepatitis
	no acute inflammation		
	nonaccidental injury	NAS-NRC	National Academy of Sciences – National Research Council
	Nuremberg Aging Inventory		
NaI	sodium iodide	NaSSA	noradrenergic and specific serotonergic antidepresssant
NAION	nonarteritic ischemic optic neuropathy		
		NASTT	nonspecific abnormality of ST segment and T wave
NAIT	neonatal alloimmune thrombocytopenia		
		NAT	N-acetyltransferase
NAL	nasal angiocentric lymphoma		no action taken
			no acute trauma
NAM	nail-apparatus melanoma		nonaccidental trauma
			nonspecific abnormality of T wave
	Native-American male		
	normal adult male		nucleic acid test
NANB	non-A, non-B (hepatitis) (hepatitis C)	Na⁹⁹ᵐ Tc0₄⁻	sodium pertechnetate Tc 99m
NANBH	non-A, non-B hepatitis (hepatitis C)	NAUC	normalized area under the curve
NANC	nonadrenergic, noncholinergic	NAW	nasal antral window
NANDA	North American Nursing Diagnosis Association (taxonomy)	NAWM	normal-appearing white matter
		NB	nail bed
NAP	narrative, assessment, and plan		needle biopsy
			neuroblastomas
	nosocomial acquired pneumonia		newborn
NAPA	N-acetyl procainamide		

nitrogen balance
note well
NBC newborn center
nonbed care
NBCCS nevoid basal-cell carcinoma syndrome
NBD neurologic bladder dysfunction
no brain damage
NBF not breast fed
NBH new bag (bottle) hung
NBHH newborn helpful hints
NBI no bone injury
NBICU newborn intensive care unit
nBiPAP nasal bilevel (biphasic) positive airway pressure
NBL/OM neuroblastoma and opsoclonus-myoclonus
NBM no bowel movement
normal bone marrow
normal bowel movement
nothing by mouth
NBN newborn nursery
NBP needle biopsy of prostate
no bone pathology
NBQC narrow base quad cane
NBR no blood return
NBS newborn screen (serum thyroxine and phenylketonuria)
Nijmegen breakage syndrome
no bacteria seen
normal bowel sounds
NBT nitroblue tetrazolium reduction (tests)
normal breast tissue
NBTE nonbacterial thrombotic endocarditis
NBTNF newborn, term, normal female
NBTNM newborn, term, normal, male
NBW normal birth weight (2,500–3,999 g)
NC nasal cannula
Negro child
neurologic check

no change
no charge
no complaints
noncontributory
normocephalic
nose clamp
nose clips
not classified
not completed
not cultured
9 NC rubitecan (9-nitrocamptothecin)
NCA neurocirculatory asthenia
no congenital abnormalities
N/CAN nasal cannula
NCAP nasal continuous airway pressure
NCAS zinostatin (neocarzinostatin)
NC/AT normocephalic atraumatic
NCB natural childbirth
no code blue
NCC no concentrated carbohydrates
nursing care card
NCCAM National Center for Complementary and Alternative Medicine (NIH)
NCCLS National Committee for Clinical Laboratory Standards
NCCN National Comprehensive Cancer Network
NCCP noncardiac chest pain
NCCTG North Central Cancer Treatment Group
NCCU neurosurgical continuous care unit
NCD neck-capsule distance
no congenital deformities
normal childhood diseases
not considered disabling
not considered disqualifying
Nursing-Care Dependency (scale)

NCDB	National Cancer Data Base	NCQA	National Commission for Quality Assurance
NCE	new chemical entity	nCR	nodular complete response
NCEP	National Cholesterol Education Program	NCRA	National Cancer Registrars Association
NCF	neutrophilic chemotactic factor	NCRC	nonchild-resistant container
NCHS	National Center for Health Statistics	NCRR	National Center for Research Resources (NIH)
NCI	National Cancer Institute		
NCIC	National Cancer Institute of Canada	NCS	nerve conduction studies no concentrated sweets noncontact supervision not clinically significant zinostatin (neocarzinostatin)
NCI-CTC	National Cancer Institute Common Toxicity Criteria		
NCIC-CTG	National Cancer Institute of Canada Clinical Trials Group	NCSE	nonconvulsive status epilepticus
NCIS	nursing care information sheet	NCT	neoadjuvant chemotherapy neutron capture therapy noncontact tonometry Nursing Care Technician
NCIT	Nursing Care Intervention Tool		
NCJ	needle catheter jejunostomy	NCV	nerve conduction velocity nuclear venogram
NCL	neuronal ceroid lipofuscinosis nuclear cardiology laboratory	ND	Doctor of Naturopathy (Naturopathic Physician) nasal deformity nasoduodenal natural death neck dissection neonatal death neurological development neurotic depression Newcastle disease no data no disease nondisabling nondistended none detectable normal delivery normal development nose drops not detected not diagnosed not done nothing done Nursing Doctorate
NCLD	neonatal chronic lung disease		
NCM	nailfold capillary microscope nonclinical manager		
NCNC	normochromic, normocytic		
NCO	no complaints offered noncommissioned officer		
NCOG	North California Oncology Group		
NCP	no caffeine or pepper nursing care plan		
NCPAP	nasal continuous positive airway pressure		
NCPB	neurolytic celiac plexus block		
NcpPCu	nonceruloplasmin plasma copper		
NCPR	no cardiopulmonary resuscitation	N&D	nodular and diffuse

Nd	neodymium		norethindrone
NDA	New Drug Application		norepinephrine
	no data available		not elevated
	no demonstrable		not examined
	antibodies	NEAA	nonessential amino acids
	no detectable activity	NEAC	norethindrone acetate
NDC	National Drug Code	NEAD	nonepileptic attack
NDD	no dialysis days		disorder
NDE	near-death experience	NEAT	nonexercise activity
NDEA	no deviation of electrical		thermogenesis
	axis	NEB	hand-held nebulizer
NDF	neutral density filter (test)	NEC	necrotizing entercolitis
	no disease found		noise equivalent counts
NDGA	nordihydroguaiaretic acid		nonesterified cholesterol
NDI	National Death Index		not elsewhere classified
	nephrogenic diabetes	NED	no evidence of disease
	insipidus	NEEG	normal
NDIR	nondispersive infrared		electroencephalogram
NDIRS	nondispersive infrared	NEEP	negative end-expiratory
	spectrometer		pressure
NDM	neonatal diabetes mellitus	NEF	negative expiratory force
Nd/NT	nondistended, nontender	NEFA	nonesterified fatty acids
NDP	nedaplatin	NEFG	normal external female
	net dietary protein		genitalia
	Nurse Discharge Planner	NEFT	nasoenteric feeding tube
NDR	neurotic depressive	NEG	negative
	reaction		neglect
	normal detrusor reflex	NEI	National Eye Institute
NDS	Neurologic Disability		(NIH)
	Score	NEJM	*New England Journal of*
NDST	neurodevelopmental		*Medicine*
	screening test	NEM	neurotrophic enhancing
NDT	nasal duodenostomy tube		molecule
	neurodevelopmental		no evidence of
	techniques		malignancy
	neurodevelopmental	NEMD	nonexudative macular
	treatment		degeneration
	noise detection threshold		nonspecific esophageal
NDV	Newcastle disease virus		motility disorder
Nd:YAG	neodymium:yttrium-	NENT	nasal endotracheal tube
	aluminum-garnet (laser)	NEO	necrotizing external otitis
Nd:YLF	neodymium: yttrium-	NEOH	neonatal high risk
	lithium-fluoride (laser)	NEOM	neonatal medium risk
NE	nausea and emesis	NEP	needle-exchange program
	nephropathica epidemica		neutral endopeptidase
	neurological examination		no evidence of pathology
	never exposed	NEPD	no evidence of pulmonary
	no effect		disease
	no enlargement	NEPHRO	nephrogram

NEPPK	nonepidermolytic palmoplantar keratoderma	NFP	natural family planning
			no family physician
			not for publication
NER	no evidence of recurrence	NFT	no further treatment
NERD	no evidence of recurrent disease	NFTD	normal full-term delivery
		NFTE	not found this examination
NES	nonepileptic seizure		
	nonstandard electrolyte solution	NFTs	neurofibrillary tangles
		NFTSD	normal full-term spontaneous delivery
	not elsewhere specified		
NESP	novel erythropoiesis stimulating protein	NFTT	nonorganic failure to thrive
NET	choroidal or subretinal neovascularization	NFW	nursed fairly well
		NG	nanogram (ng) $(10^{-9}$ gram)
	Internet		
	naso-endotracheal tube		nasogastric
	neuroectodermal tumor		night guard
NETA	norethindrone acetate (Aygestin)		nitroglycerin
			no growth
NETT	nasal endotracheal tube		norgestrel
NEX	nose-to-ear-to-xiphoid	ng	nanogram
	number of excitations	NGB	neurogenic bladder
NETZ	needle (diathermy) excision of the transformation zone	NGF	nerve growth factor
		n giv	not given
		NGJ	nasogastro-jejunostomy
NF	necrotizing fasciitis	NGM	norgestimate
	Negro female	NGOs	nongovernmental organizations
	neurofibromatosis		
	night frequency (of voiding)	NGR	nasogastric replacement
		NGRI	not guilty by reason of insanity
	none found		
	not found	NGSF	nothing grown so far
	nursed fair	NGT	nasogastric tube
	nursing facility		normal glucose tolerance
NF1	neurofibromatosis type 1	NgTD	negative to date
NF2	neurofibromatous type 2	NGU	nongonococcal urethritis
NFA	Nerve Fiber Analyzer®	NH	nursing home
NFALO	Nerve Fiber Analyzer laser oththalmoscope	NHA	no histologic abnormalities
NFAP	nursing facility-acquired pneumonia	NHB	nonheart beating (donor)
NFAR	no further action required	NHC	neighborhood health center
NFD	no family doctor		
NFFD	not fit for duty		neonatal hypocalcemia
NFI	nerve-function impairment		nursing home care
	no-fault insurance	NH3	ammonia
	no further information	NH4Cl	ammonium chloride
NFL	nerve fiber layer	NHCU	nursing home care unit
NFLX	norfloxacin (Noroxin)	NHD	normal hair distribution

NHE	sodium/hydrogen exchanger
NHGRI	National Human Genome Research Institute (NIH)
NHL	nodular histiocytic lymphoma
	non-Hodgkin's lymphomas
nHL	normalized hearing level
NHLBI	National Heart, Lung, and Blood Institute (NIH)
NHLPP	hereditary neuropathy with liability for pressure palsy
NHM	no heroic measures
NHO	notify house officer
NHP	Nottingham Health Profile
	nursing home placement
NHS	National Health Service (UK)
NHT	neoadjuvant hormonal therapy
	nursing home transfer
NHTR	nonhemolytic transfusion reaction
NHW	nonhealing wound
NI	neurological improvement
	no improvement
	no information
	none indicated
	not identified
	not isolated
NIA	National Institute on Aging (NIH)
	no information available
NIAAA	National Institute on Alcohol Abuse and Alcoholism (NIH)
NIAID	National Institute of Allergy and Infectious Diseases (NIH)
NIAL	not in active labor
NIAMS	National Institute of Arthritis and Musculoskeletal and Skin Diseases (NIH)

NIA-RI	National Institute on Aging–Reagan Institute
NIBP	noninvasive blood pressure
NIBPM	noninvasive blood pressure measurement
NICC	neonatal intensive care center
	noninfectious chronic cystitis
NICE	National Institute for Clinical Excellence (United Kingdom)
	new, interesting, and challenging experiences
NICHD	National Institute of Child Health and Human Development (NIH)
NICO	noninvasive cardiac output (monitor)
NICS	noninvasive carotid studies
NICU	neonatal intensive care unit
	neurosurgical intensive care unit
NID	no identifiable disease
	not in distress
NIDA	National Institute of Drug Abuse (NIH)
NIDA five	National Institute on Drug Abuse screen for cannabinoids, cocaine metabolite, amphetamine/methamphetamine, opiates, and phencyclidine
NIDCD	National Institute of Deafness and other Communication Disorders (NIH)
NIDCR	National Institute of Dental and Craniofacial Research (NIH)
NIDD	noninsulin-dependent diabetes

NIDDK	National Institute of Diabetes and Digestive and Kidney Diseases (NIH)	NIOPCs	no intraoperative complications
NIDDM	noninsulin-dependent diabetes mellitus	NIOSH	National Institute of Occupational Safety and Health (NIH)
NIDR	National Institute of Dental Research (NIH)	NIP	catnip no infection present no inflammation present
NIEHS	National Institute of Environmental Health Sciences (NIH)	NIPAs	noninherited paternal antigens
NIF	negative inspiratory force neutrophil inhibitory factor not in file	NIPD	nocturnal intermittent peritoneal dialysis
		NIPPV	noninvasive positive-pressure ventilation
NIFS	noninvasive flow studies	NIPS	Neonatal Infant Pain Scale
NIG	NSAIA (nonsteroidal anti-inflamatory agent) induced gastropathy	NIP/S	noninvasive programming stimulation
		NIR	near infrared
NIGMS	National Institute of General Medical Sciences (NIH)	NIRCA	nonisotopic RNase cleavage assay
NIH	National Institutes of Health	NISH	nonradioactive *in situ* hybridization
NIHD	noise-induced hearing damage	NISS	New Injury Severity Score
NIHL	noise-induced hearing loss	NISs	no-impact sports
		NISV	nonionic surfactant vesicle
NIID	neuronal intranuclear inclusion disease	NITD	neuroleptic-induced tardive dyskinesia
NIL	not in labor	Nitro	nitroglycerin (this is a dangerous abbreviation) sodium nitroprusside (this is a dangerous abbreviation)
NIMAs	noninherited maternal antigens		
NIMH	National Institute of Mental Health (NIH)		
NIMHDIS	National Institute for Mental Health Diagnostic Interview Schedule (NIH)	NIV	noninvasive ventilation
		NIVLS	noninvasive vascular laboratory studies
NINDS	National Institute of Neurological Disorders and Stroke (NIH)	NJ	nasojejunal
		NK	natural killer (cells) not known
NINR	National Institute for Nursing Research (NIH)	NKA	no known allergies
		nkat	nanokatal (nanomole/sec)
NINU	neuro intermediate nursing unit	NKB	no known basis not keeping baby neurokinin B
		NKC	nonketotic coma
		NKD	no known diseases
NINVS	noninvasive neurovascular studies	NKDA	no known drug allergies
		NKFA	no known food allergies

NKH	nonketotic hyperglycemia	NM	nanometer (nm) (10^{-9} meters)
NKHA	nonketotic hyperosmolar acidosis		Negro male
			neuromuscular
NKHHC	nonketotic hyperglycemic-hyperosmolar coma		neuronal microdysgenesis
			nodular melanoma
NKHOC	nonketotic hyperosmolar coma		nonmalignant
			not measurable
NKHS	nonketotic hyperosmolar syndrome		not measured
			not mentioned
NKMA	no known medication (medical) allergies		nuclear medicine
			nurse manager
NL	nasolacrimal	N & M	nerves and muscles
	nonlatex		night and morning
	normal	NMBA	neuromuscular blocking agent
NLB	needle liver biopsy		
NLC	nocturnal leg cramps	NMC	no malignant cells
NLC & C	normal libido, coitus, and climax	NMD	Doctor of Naturopathic Medicine
NLD	nasolacrimal duct		neuromuscular disorders
	necrobiosis lipoidica diabeticorum		neuronal migration disorders
	no local doctor		Normosol M and 5% Dextrose®
NLDO	nasolacrimal duct obstruction		
		NMDA	N-methyl-D-aspartate
NLE	neonatal lupus erythematosus	NMDP	National Marrow Donor Pool
	nursing late entry	NME	new molecular entity
NLEA	Nutrition Labeling and Education Act of 1990	NMES	neuromuscular electrical stimulation
NLF	nasolabial fold	NMF	neuromuscular facilitation
	nelfinavir (Viracept)	NMH	neurally mediated hypotension
NLFGNR	nonlactose fermenting gram-negative rod		
		NMHH	no medical health history
NLM	National Library of Medicine	NMI	no manifest improvement
			no mental illness
	no limitation of motion		no middle initial
NLMC	nocturnal leg muscle cramp		no more information
			normal male infant
NLN	no longer needed	NMJ	neuromuscular junction
NLO	nasolacrimal occlusion	NMKB	not married, keeping baby
NLP	natural language processing	NMM	nodular malignant melanoma
	nodular liquifying panniculitis	NMN	no middle name
	no light perception	NMNKB	not married, not keeping baby
NLS	neonatal lupus syndrome	nmol	nanomole (one billionth [10^{-9}] of a mole)
NLT	not later than		
	not less than		
NLV	nelfinavir (Viracept)	NMOH	no medical ocular history

NMP	normal menstrual period	NNP	Neonatal Nurse Practitioner
NMR	nuclear magnetic resonance (same as magnetic resonance imaging)		non-nociceptive pain
		N:NPK	grams of nitrogen to non-protein kilocalories
NMRS	nuclear magnetic resonance spectroscopy	NNR	not necessary to return
		NNRTI	non-nucleoside reverse transcriptase inhibitor
NMRT (R)	Nuclear Medicine Radiologic Technologist (Registered)	NNS	neonatal screen (hematocrit, total bilirubin, and total protein)
NMS	neonatal morphine solution		
	neuroleptic malignant syndrome		nicotine nasal spray
			non-nutritive sucking
NMSC	nonmelanoma skin cancer	NNT	number needed to treat
NMSE	normalized mean square root		
		NNU	net nitrogen utilization
NMSIDS	near-miss sudden infant death syndrome	NO	nasal oxygen
			nitric oxide
NMT	nebulized mist treatment		nitroglycerin ointment
	no more than		none obtained
NMTB	neuromuscular transmission blockade		nonobese
			number (no.)
NMTCB	Nuclear Medicine Technology Certification Board		nursing office
		N$_2$O	nitrous oxide
		NOAEL	no observed adverse effect level
NMT(R)	Nuclear Medicine Technologist Registered	N$_2$O:O$_2$	nitrous oxide to oxygen ratio
NN	narrative notes		
	Navajo neuropathy	noc.	night
	neonatal	noct	nocturnal
	neural network	NOD	nonobese diabetic
	normal nursery		notice of disagreement
	nurses' notes		notify of death
N/N	negative/negative	NOED	no observed effect dose
NNB	normal newborn	NOEL	no observable effect level
NNBC	node-negative breast cancer	NOFT	nonorganic failure to thrive
NND	neonatal death	NOFTT	nonorganic failure to thrive
NNE	neonatal necrotizing enterocolitis		
		NOH	neurogenic orthostatic hypotension
NNIS	National Nosocomial Infections Surveillance	NOI	nature of illness
NNM	Nicolle-Novy-MacNeal (media)	NOK	next of kin
		NOL	not on label
NNL	no new laboratory (test orders)	NOM	nonsuppurative otitis media
NNN	normal newborn nursery	NOMI	nonocclusive mesenteric infarction
NNO	no new orders		

NOMS	not on my shift	NOV L	human insulin zinc suspension (Novolin L)
NO/N₂	nitric oxide; nitrogen		
NONMEM	non-linear mixed-effects model (modeling)	NOV N	human insulin isophane suspension (Novolin N)
non pal	not palpable		
non-REM	nonrapid eye movement (sleep)	NOV R	human insulin regular (Novolin R)
non rep	do not repeat	NP	nasal prongs
NON VIZ	not visualized		nasopharyngeal
NOOB	not out of bed		near point
NOP	not on patient		neutrogenic precautions
NOR	norethynodrel		neurophysin
	normal		neuropsychiatric
	nortriptyline		newly presented
NOR-EPI	norepinephrine		nonpalpable
norm	normal		no pain
NOS	neonatal opium solution (diluted deodorized tincture of opium)		not performed
			not pregnant
			not present
	new-onset seizures		nuclear pharmacist
	nitric oxide synthase		nuclear pharmacy
	no organisms seen		nursed poorly
	not on staff		nurse practitioner
	not otherwise specified	NPA	nasal pharyngeal airway
NOSI	nitric oxide synthase inhibitors		near point of accommodation
			no previous admission
NOSIE	Nurse's Observation Scale (Schedule) for Inpatient Evaluation	NPAT	nonparoxysmal atrial tachycardia
		NPBC	node-positive breast cancer
NOSPECS	categories for classifying eye changes in Graves' ophthalmopathy: **n**o signs or symptoms, **o**nly signs, **s**oft tissue involvement with symptoms and signs, **p**roptosis, **e**xtraocular muscle involvement, **c**orneal involvement, and **s**ight loss (visual acuity)	NPC	nasopharyngeal carcinoma
			near point convergence
			Niemann-Pick disease Type C (sphingomyelin lipidosis)
			nodal premature contractions
			nonpatient contact
			nonproductive cough
			nonprotein calorie
			no prenatal care
NOT	nocturnal oxygen therapy		no previous complaint(s)
NOU	not on unit	NPCC	nonprotein carbohydrate calories
NOV 70/30	human insulin, regular 30 units/mL with human insulin isophane suspension 70 units/mL (Novolin 70/30)		
		NPCPAP	nasopharyngeal continuous positive airway pressure
		NPD	Niemann-Pick disease

227

	nonprescription drugs	NPP	normal postpartum
	no pathological diagnosis	NPPNG	nonpenicillinase-producing *Neisseria gonorrhoeae*
NPDL	nodular poorly differentiated lymphocytic		
		NPPV	noninvasive positive-pressure ventilation
NPDR	nonproliferative diabetic retinopathy	NPR	normal pulse rate
NPE	neurogenic pulmonary edema		nothing per rectum
		NPRL	normal pupillary reaction to light
	neuropsychologic examination	NPS	new patient set-up
	no palpable enlargement	NPSA	nonphysician surgical assistant
	normal pelvic examination	NPSD	nonpotassium-sparing diuretics
NPEM	nocturnal penile erection monitoring	NPSF	National Patient Safety Foundation
NPF	nasopharyngeal fiberscope	NPSG	nocturnal polysomnography
	no predisposing factor	NPT	near-patient tests
N-PFMSO₄	nebulized preservative-free morphine sulfate		neopyrithiamin hydrochloride
NPG	nonpregnant		
NPH	isophane insulin (neutral protamine Hagedorn)		nocturnal penile tumescence
			no prior tracings
	no previous history		normal pressure and temperature
	normal pressure hydrocephalus		
		NPU	net protein utilization
NPhx	nasopharynx	NPV	negative predictive value
NPI	Neuropsychiatric Inventory		nothing per vagina
		NPY	neuropeptide Y
	no present illness	NPZ	neuropsychologic text z
	Nottingham Prognostic Index	NQECN	nonqueratinizing epidermoid carcinoma
NPIS	Numeric Pain Intensity Scale	NQMI	non-Q wave myocardial infarction
NPJT	nonparoxysmal junctional tachycardia	NQWMI	non-Q wave myocardial infarction
NPL	insulin lispro protamine component suspension	NR	do not repeat
NPLSM	neoplasm		newly reformulated
NPK	nonprotein kilocalories		none reported
NPM	nothing per mouth		nonreactive
NPN	nonprotein nitrogen		nonrebreathing
NPNC	no prenatal care		no refills
NPNT	nonpalpable, nontender		no report
NPO	nothing by mouth		no response
NPOC	nonpurgeable organic carbon		no return
			normal range
NPOD	Neuropsychiatric Officer of the Day		normal reaction

	not reached		nicotine-replacement therapy
	not reacting		
	not remarkable	NRTs	nitron radical traps
	not resolved	NS	nephrotic syndrome
	number		neurological signs
NRAF	nonrheumatic atrial fibrillation		neurosurgery
			nipple stimulation
NRB	Noninstitutional Review Board		nodular sclerosis
			no-show
	nonrebreather (oxygen mask)		nonsmoker
			normal saline solution
NRBC	normal red blood cell		(0.9% sodium chloride solution)
	nucleated red blood cell		
			normospermic
NRBS	nonrebreathing system		no sample
NRC	National Research Council		not seen
			not significant
	normal retinal correspondence		nuclear sclerosis
			nursing service
	Nuclear Regulatory Commission		nutritive sucking
			nylon suture
NREM	nonrapid eye movement	NSA	normal serum albumin
NREMS	nonrapid eye movement sleep		(albumin, human)
			no salt added
NREMT-P	National Registry of Emergency Medical Technicians–Paramedic level		no significant abnormalities
		NSAA	nonsteroidal antiandrogen
		NSABP	National Surgical Adjuvant Breast Project
NRF	normal renal function		
NRI	nerve root involvement	NSAD	no signs of acute disease
	nerve root irritation	NSAIA	nonsteroidal anti-inflammatory agent
	no recent illnesses		
	norepinephrine reuptake inhibitor	NSAID	nonsteroidal anti-inflammatory drug
N-RLX	nonrelaxed		
NRM	nonrebreathing mask	NSAP	nonspecific abdominal pain
	no regular medicines		
	normal range of motion	NSBGP	nonspecific bowel gas pattern
	normal retinal movement		
NRN	no return necessary	NSC	no significant change
NRO	neurology		nonservice-connected
NROM	normal range of motion	NSCC	nonsmall cell carcinoma
NRP	nonreassuring patterns	NSCD	nonservice-connected disability
NRPR	nonbreathing pressure relieving		
		NSCFPT	no significant change from previous tracing
NRS	Neurobehavioral Rating Scale		
		NSCIDRC	National Spinal Cord Injury Data Research Center
NRT	neuromuscular reeducation techniques		

NSCLC	nonsmall-cell–lung cancer	NSPs	nonstarch polysaccharides
NSCST	nipple stimulation contraction stress test	NSPVT	nonsustained polymorphic ventricular tachycardia
NSD	nasal septal deviation	NSR	nasoseptal repair
	no significant disease (difference, defect, deviation)		nonspecific reaction
			normal sinus rhythm
			not seen regularly
	nominal standard dose	NSRP	nerve-sparing radical prostatectomy
	normal spontaneous delivery	NSS	neurological signs stable
NSDA	nonsteroid dependent asthmatic		normal size and shape
			not statistically significant
NSDU	neonatal stepdown unit		nutritional support service
NSE	neuron-specific enolase		sodium chloride 0.9% (normal saline solution)
	normal saline enema (0.9% sodium chloride)	1/2 NSS	sodium chloride 0.45% (1/2 normal saline solution)
N s̄ E	nausea without emesis		
NSF	no significant findings	NSSC	normal size, shape and consistency (uterus)
NSFTD	normal spontaneous full-term delivery	NSSL	normal size, shape, and location
NSG	nursing		
NSGCT	nonseminomatous germ-cell tumors	NSSP	normal size, shape, and position
NSGCTT	nonseminomatous germ-cell tumor of the testis	NSSTT	nonspecific ST and T (wave)
NSGT	nonseminomatous germ-cell tumor	NSST-TWCs	nonspecific ST-T wave changes
NSHD	nodular sclerosing Hodgkin's disease	NST	nonstress test
			normal sphincter tone
NSI	negative self-image		not sooner than
	no signs of infection		nutritional support team
	no signs of inflammation	NSTD	nonsexually transmitted disease
NSICU	neurosurgery intensive care unit	NSTGCT	nonseminomatous testicular germ cell tumor
NSILA	nonsuppressible insulin-like activity		
NSIP	nonspecific interstitial pneumonia	NSTI	necrotizing soft-tissue infection
NSMMVT	nonsustained monomorphic ventricular tachycardia	NSTT	nonseminomatous testicular tumors
		NSU	neurosurgical unit
NSN	Neo-Synephrine		nonspecific urethritis
	nephrotoxic serum nephritis	NSV	nonspecific vaginitis
		NSVD	normal spontaneous vaginal delivery
NSO	Neosporin® ointment		
NSOM	near field scanning optical microscope	NSVT	nonsustained ventricular tachycardia
NSP	neck and shoulder pain	NSX	neurosurgical examination

NSY	nursery	NTM	nocturnal tumescence monitor
NT	nasotracheal		nontuberculous mycobacterium
	next time	NTMB	nontuberculous myobacteria
	Nordic Track®		
	normal temperature	NTMI	nontransmural myocardial infarction
	normotensive		
	nortriptyline	NTND	not tender, not distended
	not tender	NTP	narcotic treatment program
	not tested		
	nourishment taken		Nitropaste® (nitroglycerin ointment)
	numbness and tingling		
	nursing technician		nonthrombocytopenic preterm (infant)
N&T	nose and throat		
	numbness and tingling		normal temperature and pressure
N Tachy	nodal tachycardia		
NT-ANP	N-terminal atrial natriuretic peptide		sodium nitroprusside
		NTPD	nocturnal tidal peritoneal dialysis
NTBR	not to be resuscitated		
NTC	neurotrauma center	NTS	nasotracheal suction
NTCS	no tumor cells seen		nicotine transdermal system
NTD	negative to date		
	neural-tube defects		nontyphoidal salmonellae
	nitroblue tetrazolium dye (test)		nucleus tractus solitarii
NTE	neutral thermal environment	NTT	nasotracheal tube
			nonthrombocytopenic term (infant)
	not to exceed		
NTED	neonatal toxic-shock-syndrome-like exanthematous disease	NTU	nephelometric turbidity units
		NTX	naltrexone (ReVia)
NTF	normal throat flora	NTZ	nitazoxanide
NTG	nitroglycerin	NTZ Long-acting®	oxymetazoline nasal spray
	nontoxic goiter		
	nontreatment group	NU	name unknown
	normal tension glaucoma	NUD	nonulcer dyspepsia
NTGO	nitroglycerin ointment	NUG	necrotizing ulcerative gingivitis
NTI	narrow therapeutic index		
	no treatment indicated	nullip	nullipara
NTIS	National Technical Information Service (U.S. Department of Commerce)	NUN	nonurea nitrogen
		NV	naked vision
			nausea and vomiting
NTL	nectar-thick liquid (diet consistency)		near vision
			negative variation
	nortriptyline		neovascularization
	no time limit		neurovascular
NTLE	neocortical temporal-lobe epilepsy		new vessel
			next visit

N

nonvenereal
nonveteran
normal value
not vaccinated
not verified

N&V nausea and vomiting
NVA near visual acuity
NVAF nonvalvular atrial fibrillation
NVB Navelbine (vinorelbine tartrate)
NVC neurovascular checks
nvCJD new-variant Creutzfeldt-Jakob disease
NVD nausea, vomiting, and diarrhea
neck vein distention
neovascularization of the (optic) disk
neurovesicle dysfunction
normal vaginal delivery
no venereal disease
no venous distention
nonvalvular disease
NVDC nausea, vomiting, diarrhea, and constipation
NVE native
native valve endocarditis
neovascularization elsewhere
NVG neovascular glaucoma
neoviridogrisein
NVL neurovascular laboratory
NVM neovascular membrane
NVP nausea and vomiting of pregnancy
nevirapine (Viramune)
NVS neurological vital signs
neurovascular status
NVSS normal variant short stature
NW naked weight
nasal wash
not weighed
NWB nonweight bearing
NWBL nonweight bearing, left
NWBR nonweight bearing, right

NWC number of words chosen
NWD neuroleptic withdrawal
normal well developed
NWS New World screwworm (*Cochliomyia hominivorax* [Coquerel])
NWTS National Wilms' Tumor Study (rating scale)
NWTSG National Wilms' Tumor Study Group
Nx nephrectomy
next
NYD not yet diagnosed
NYHA New York Heart Association (classification of heart disease)
nyst nystagmus
NZ enzyme

O

O	eye
	objective findings
	obvious
	occlusal
	often
	open
	oral
	ortho
	other
	oxygen
	pint
	zero
$\bar{o}$	negative
	no
	none
	pint
	without
O+	blood type O positive
O−	blood type O negative
Ⓞ	orally (by mouth)
$_1O_2$	singlet oxygen
O_2	both eyes
	oxygen
O_2^-	superoxide
O_3	ozone
O157	*Escherichia coli* O157
OA	occipital artery
	occipitoatlantal
	occiput anterior
	old age
	on admission
	on arrival
	ophthalmic artery
	oral airway
	oral alimentation
	osteoarthritis
	Overeaters Anonymous
O/A	on or about
O & A	observation and assessment
	odontectomy and alveoloplasty
OAA	Old Age Assistance

OAA/S	Observer's Assessment of Alertness/Sedation
OAB	overactive bladder
OAC	omeprazole, amoxicillin, and clarithromycin
	oral anticoagulant(s)
	overaction
OAD	obstructive airway disease
	occlusive arterial disease
	overall diameter
OAE	otoacoustic emissions
OAF	oral anal fistula
	osteoclast activating factor
OAG	open angle glaucoma
OAP	old age pension
OAS	Older Adult Services
	oral allergy syndrome
	organic anxiety syndrome
	outpatient assessment service
	overall survival
	Overt Aggression Scale
OASDHI	Old Age, Survivors, Disability, and Health Insurance
OASI	Old Age and Survivors Insurance
OASIS	Outcomes and Assessment Information Set
OASO	overactive superior oblique
OASR	overactive superior rectus
OASS	Overt Agitation Severity Scale
OAT	ornithine aminotransferase
OATS	osteochondral autograft transfer system
OAV	oculoauriculovertebral (dysplasia)
OAW	oral airway
OB	obese
	obesity
	obstetrics
	occult blood
	osteoblast
OBA	office-based anesthesia
OB-A	obstetrics-aborted
OB-Del	obstetrics-delivered
OBE	out-of-body experience

OBE-CALP	placebo capsule or tablet	Occup Rx	occupational therapy
OBG	obstetrics and gynecology	OCD	obsessive-compulsive disorder
Ob-Gyn	obstetrics and gynecology		osteochondritis dissecans
Obj	objective	OCE	outpatient code editor
obl	oblique	OCG	oral cholecystogram
OB marg	obtuse marginal	OCI	Obsessive-Compulsive Inventory
OB-ND	obstetrics-not delivered		
OBP	office blood pressure	OCL®	oral colonic lavage
OBRR	obstetric recovery room	OCN	obsessive-compulsive neurosis
OBS	obstetrical service		
	organic brain syndrome		Oncology Certified Nurse
OBT	obtained	OCNS	Obsessive-Compulsive Neurosis Scale
OBTM	omeprazole, bismuth subcitrate, tetracycline, and metronidazole		
		O-CNV	occult choroidal neovascularization
OBUS	obstetrical ultrasound	OCOR	on-call to operating room
OBW	open bed warmer		
OC	obstetrical conjugate	OCP	ocular cicatricial pemphigoid
	office call		
	on call		oral contraceptive pills
	only child		ova, cysts, parasites
	open cholecystectomy	OCR	oculocephalic reflex
	optical chromatography		optical character recognition
	oral care		
	oral contraceptive	OCS	Obsessive-Compulsive Scale
	osteocalcin		
	osteoclast		oral cancer screening
O & C	onset and course	11-OCS	11-oxycorticosteroid
OCA	oculocutaneous albinism	OCT	octreotide (Sandostatin)
	open care area		optical coherence tomograph (tomography)
	oral contraceptive agent		
OCAD	occlusive carotid artery disease		oral cavity tumors
			ornithine carbamyl transferase
OCBZ	oxcarbazepine (Trileptal)		
OCC	occasionally		oxytocin challenge test
	occlusal	OCU	observation care unit
	old chart called	OCVM	occult cerebrovascular malformations
OCCC	open chest cardiac compression		
		OCX	oral cancer examination
	ovarian clear cell carcinoma	OD	Doctor of Optometry
			Officer-of-the-Day
occl	occlusion		once daily (this is a dangerous abbreviation as it is read as right eye)
OCCM	open chest cardiac massage		
OCC PR	open chest cardiopulmonary resuscitation		
			on duty
OCC Th	occupational therapy		optic disk

	oral-duodenal	O-E	standard observed minus expected
	outdoor	O&E	observation and examination
	outside diameter		
	ovarian dysgerminoma	OEC	outer ear canal
	overdose	OEI	opioid escalation index
	right eye	O_2EI	oxygen extraction index
Δ OD 450	deviation of optical density at 450	OENT	oral endotracheal tube
		OEP	oil of evening primrose (evening primrose oil)
ODA	occipitodextra anterior		
	once-daily aminoglycoside	OEPA	vincristine (Oncovin), etoposide, prednisone, and doxorubicin (Adriamycin)
	osmotic driving agent		
ODAC	Oncologic Drugs Advisory Committee (of the US Food and Drug Administration)		
		OER	oxygen extraction ratios
		O_2ER	oxygen extraction ratio
	on demand analgesia computer	OERR	order entry/results-reports (Veterans Administration's physician computer order entry system)
ODAT	one day at a time		
ODC	oral disease control		
	ornithine decarboxylase		
	outpatient diagnostic center	OET	oral esophageal tube
ODCH	ordinary diseases of childhood	OETT	oral endotracheal tube
		OF	occipital-frontal
ODD	oculodentodigital (dysplasia)		optic fundi
			osteitis fibrosa
	opposition defiance disorder	OFC	occipital-frontal circumference
OD'd	overdosed		orbitofacial cleft
ODed	overdosed	OFF	shoes off during weighing
ODM	occlusion dose monitor	OFI	other febrile illness
	ophthalmodynamometry	OFLOX	ofloxacin (Floxin)
ODN	optokinetic nystagmus	OFLX	ofloxacin (Floxin)
ODP	occipitodextra posterior	OFM	open face mask
	offspring of diabetic parents	OFNE	oxygenated fluorocarbon nutrient emulsion
OD/P	right eye patched	OFPF	optic fundi and peripheral fields
ODQ	on direct questioning		
ODS	organized delivery system	OFR	oxygen-free radicals
ODSS	Office of Disability Support Services	OFTT	organic failure to thrive
		OG	Obstetrics-Gynecology
ODSU	oncology day stay unit		orogastric (feeding)
	One Day Surgery Unit		outcome goal (long-term goal)
ODT	occipitodextra transverse		
		OGC	oculogyric crisis
	orally disintegrating tablet	OGCT	ovarian germ cell tumor
OE	on examination	OGD	Office of Generic Drugs (of the Food and Drug Administration)
	orthopedic examination		
	otitis externa		

OGT	orogastric tube		overhead trapeze
OGTT	oral glucose tolerance test	OHTN	ocular hypertension
OH	occupational history	OHTx	orthotopic heart transplantation
	ocular history	OI	opportunistic infection
	on hand		osteogenesis imperfecta
	open-heart		otitis interna
	oral hygiene	OIF	oil-immersion field
	orthostatic hypotension	OIG	Office of the Inspector General
	outside hospital		
17-OH	17-hydroxycorticosteroids	OIH	orthoiodohippurate
OHA	oral hypoglycemic agents	OIHA	orthoiodohippuric acid
OHC	outer hair cell (in cochlea)	OINT	ointment
OH Cbl	hydroxycobalamine	OIRDA	occipital intermittent rhythmical delta activity
17-OHCS	17-hydroxycorticosteroids		
OHD	hydroxy vitamin D	OIS	optical intrinsic signal (imaging)
	organic heart disease		
25(OH)D₃	25-hydroxy vitamin D (calcifediol, Calderol)		optimum information size
		OIT	ovarian immature teratoma
OHF	old healed fracture		
	Omsk hemorrhagic fever	OIU	optical internal urethrotomy
	overhead frame		
OHFA	hydroxy fatty acid	OJ	orange juice (this is a dangerous abbreviation as it is read as OS-left eye)
OHFT	overhead frame and trapeze		
OHG	oral hypoglycemic		
OHI	oral hygiene instructions		orthoplast jacket
OHIAA	hydroxyindolacetic acid	OK	all right
OHL	oral hairy leukoplakia		approved
OHNS	Otolaryngology, Head, and Neck Surgery (Dept.)		correct
		OKAN	optokinetic after nystagmus
OHP	obese hypertensive patient	OKN	optokinetic nystagmus
		OKT	Ortho Kung T cell, designation for a series of antigens
	oxygen under hyperbaric pressure		
17 OHP	17-hydroxyprogesterone	OL	left eye
OHRP	open-heart rehabilitation program		open label (study)
		OLA	occiput left anterior
OHRR	open-heart recovery room		occipitolaevoanterior
OHS	occupational health service	OLB	open liver biopsy
			open lung biopsy
	ocular histoplasmosis syndrome	OLD	obstructive lung disease
		OLF	ouabain-like factor
	ocular hypoperfusion syndrome	OLM	ocular larva migrans
			ophthalmic laser microendoscope
	open-heart surgery		
OHSS	ovarian hyperstimulation syndrome	OLNM	occult lymph node metastases
OHT	ocular hypertension		

O

OLP	abnormal lipoprotein
OLR	optic labyrinthine righting
	otology, laryngology, and rhinology
OLS	ordinary least squares
	ouabain-like substance
OLT	occipitolaevoposterior
	orthotopic liver transplantation
OLTP	online transaction processing
OLTx	orthotopic liver transplantation
OLV	one-lung ventilation
OLZ	olanzapine (Zyprexa)
OM	every morning (this is a dangerous abbreviation)
	obtuse marginal
	ocular melanoma
	oral motor
	oral mucositis
	organomegaly
	osteomalacia
	osteomyelitis
	otitis media
O_2M	oxygen mask
OM_1	first obtuse marginal (branch)
OM_2	second obtuse marginal (branch)
OMA	older maternal age
OMAC	otitis media, acute, catarrhal
OMAS	otitis media, acute, suppurating
OMB	obtuse marginal branch
OMB_1	first obtuse marginal branch
OMB_2	second obtuse marginal branch
OMC	open mitral commissuortomy
OMCA	otitis media, catarrhalis, acute
OMCC	otitis media, catarrhalis, chronic
OMD	organic mental disorder
OME	Office of Medical Examiner
	otitis media with effusion
7-OMEN	menogaril
OMFS	oral and maxillofacial surgery
OMG	ocular myasthenia gravis
OMI	old myocardial infarct
OMP	oculomotor (third nerve) palsy
OMPA	otitis media, purulent, acute
OMPC	otitis media, purulent, chronic
OMR	operative mortality rate
OMS	oral morphine sulfate
	organic mental syndrome
	organic mood syndrome
OMSA	otitis media secretory (or suppurative) acute
OMSC	otitis media secretory (or suppurative) chronic
OMT	oral mucosal transudate
	Osteopathic manipulative technique
OMVC	open mitral valve commissurotomy
OMVD	optimized microvessel density (analysis)
OMVI	operating motor vehicle intoxicated
ON	every night (this is a dangerous abbreviation)
	optic nerve
	optic neurophathy
	oronasal
	Ortho-Novum®
	overnight
ONC	over-the-needle catheter
	vincristine (Oncovin)
OND	ondansetron (Zofran)
	other neurologic disorder(s)
ONH	optic nerve head
	optic nerve hypoplasia
ONM	ocular neuromyotonia
ON RR	overnight recovery room
ONS	Office for National Statistics (United Kingdom)

ONSD	optic nerve sheath decompression	open
		operation
ONSF	optic nerve sheath fenestration	organophosphorous
		oropharynx
ONTR	orders not to resuscitate	oscillatory potentials
OO	ophthalmic ointment	osteoporosis
	oral order	outpatient
	other	overpressure
	out of	O&P	ova and parasites (stool examination)
o/o	on account of	
O&O	off and on	OPA	oral pharyngeal airway
OOB	out of bed		outpatient anesthesia
OOBL	out of bilirubin light	OPAC	opacity (opacification)
OOBBRP	out of bed with bathroom privileges	OPAT	outpatient parenteral antibiotic therapy
OOC	onset of contractions	OPB	outpatient basis
	out of cast	OPC	operable pancreatic carcinoma
	out of control		
OO Con	out of control		oropharyngeal candidiasis
OOD	outer orbital diameter		outpatient care
	out of doors		outpatient catheterization
OOF	out of facility		outpatient clinic
OOH	out of hospital	OPCA	olivopontocerebellar atrophy
OOH&NS	ophthalmology, otorhinolaryngology, and head and neck surgery	OPCAB	off-pump coronary artery bypass (grafting)
		op cit	in the work cited
OOI	out of isolette	OPCS-4	Classification of Surgical Operations and Procedures (4th revision)
OOL	onset of labor		
OOLR	ophthalmology, otology, laryngology, and rhinology		
		OPD	oropharyngeal dysphagia
OOM	onset of menarche		Orphan Products Development (office of)
OOP	out of pelvis		
	out of plaster		outpatient department
	out on pass	O'p'-DDD	mitotane (Lysodren)
OOPS	out of program status	OPDUR	on-line prospective drug utilization review
OOR	out of room		
OORW	out of radiant warmer	OPE	oral peripheral examination
OOS	out of sequence		
	out of specification (deviation from standard)		outpatient evaluation
		OPEN	vincristine (Oncovin), prednisone, etoposide, and mitoxantrone (Novantrone)
	out of splint		
	out of stock		
OOT	out of town	OPERA	outpatient endometrial resection/ablation
OOW	out of wedlock		
OP	oblique presentation	OPG	ocular plethysmography
	occiput posterior		osteoprotegerin

OPL	oral premalignant lesion other party liability	OR	odds ratio oil retention open reduction operating room Orthodox own recognizance
OPLL	ossification of posterior latitudinal ligament		
OPM	occult primary malignancy		
OPN	osteopontin	ORA	occiput right anterior
OPO	organ procurement organizations	ORC	outpatient rehabilitation centers
OPOC	oral pharynx, oral cavity	ORCH	orchiectomy
OPP	opposite	ORD	orderly
OPPG	oculopneumoplethysmography	OREF	open reduction, external fixation
OPPOS	opposition	ORF	open reading frame
OPPS	Outpatient Prospective Payment System	OR&F	open reduction and fixation
OPQRST	onset, provocation, quality, radiation, severity, and time (an EMT mnemonic used in initial patient questioning)	ORIF	open reduction internal fixation
		ORL	oblique retinacular ligament otorhinolaryngology (otology, rhinology and laryngology)
OPRDU	outpatient renal dialysis unit	ORMF	open reduction metallic fixation
OPS	Objective Pain Scores operations Orpington prognostic scale outpatient surgery	ORN	operating room nurse osteoradionecrosis
		OROS	ostomotic release oral system
OPSI	overwhelming postsplenectomy infection	ORP	occiput right posterior
		ORS	olfactory reference syndrome oral rehydration salts
OPSU	outpatient surgical unit		
O PSY	open psychiatry	ORT	oestrogen (estrogen)-replacement therapy operating room technician oral rehydration therapy Registered Occupational Therapist
OPT	optimum outpatient treatment		
OPT c CA	Ohio pediatric tent with compressed air		
OPT c O$_2$	Ohio pediatric tent with oxygen		
OPTN	Organ Procurement and Transplantation Network	OR XI	oriented to time
		OR X2	oriented to time and place
OPT-NSC	outpatient treatment, nonservice-connected	OR X3	oriented to time, place, and person
OPT-SC	outpatient treatment, service-connected	OR X4	oriented to time, place, person, and objects (watch, pen, book)
OPV	oral polio vaccine outpatient visit	OS	left eye

	mouth (this is a dangerous abbreviation as it is read as left eye)		occupational therapy
			old tuberculin
			oral transmucosal
	occipitosacral		orotracheal
	oligospermic		outlier threshold
	opening snap		oxytocin (Pitocin)
	ophthalmic solution (this is a dangerous abbreviation as it is read as left eye)	O/T	oral temperature
		OTA	open to air
		OTC	ornithine transcarbamoylase
	oral surgery		Orthopedic Technician, Certified
	Osgood-Schlatter (disease)		
	osmium		over the counter (sold without prescription)
	osteosarcoma		
	overall survival	OTCD	ornithine-transcarbamylase deficiency
OSA	obstructive sleep apnea		
	off-site anesthesia		
	osteosarcoma	OTD	optimal therapeutic dose
OSA/HS	obstructive sleep apnea/hypopnea syndrome		organ tolerance dose
			out-the-door
		OTE	(McMaster) Overall Treatment Evaluation
OSAS	obstructive sleep apnea syndrome		
		OTFC	oral transmucosal fentanyl citrate (Fentanyl Oralet)
OSCAR	On-line Survey Certification and Reporting		
		OTH	other
		OTHS	occupational therapy home service
OSCC	oral squamous cell carcinoma		
		OTIS	Organization of Teratology Information Services
OSCE	Objective Structured Clinical Examination		
OSD	Osgood-Schlatter disease	OTO	one-time only
	overseas duty		otolaryngology
	overside drainage		otology
OSE	ovarian surface epithelium	OTPT	oral triphasic tablets (contraceptive)
OSESC	opening snap ejection systolic click		
		OTR	Occupational Therapist, Registered
OSFT	outstretched fingertips		
OSH	outside hospital	OTRL	Occupational Therapist, Registered Licensed
OSHA	Occupational Safety & Health Administration		
		OT/RT	occupational therapy/recreational therapy
OSM S	osmolarity serum		
OSM U	osmolarity urine	OTS	orotracheal suction
OSN	off-service note	OTT	orotracheal tube
OSP	outside pass	OTW	off-the-wall
OS/P	left eye patched	OU	each eye
OSS	osseous	OUES	oxygen uptake efficiency slope
	over-shoulder strap		
OST	optimal sampling theory	OULQ	outer upper left quadrant
OT	occiput transverse	OU/P	both eyes patched

OURQ	outer upper right quadrant	
OUS	obstetric ultrasound	
OV	office visit	
	ovary	
	ovum	
OVAL	ovalocytes	
OVF	Octopus® visual field	
OVR	Office of Vocational Rehabilitation	
OVS	obstructive voiding symptoms (syndrome)	
OW	once weekly (this is a dangerous abbreviation)	
	open wound	
	outer wall	
	out of wedlock	
	ova weight	
O/W	oil in water	
	otherwise	
OWL	out of wedlock	
OWNK	out of wedlock not keeping (baby)	
OWR	Osler-Weber-Rendu (disease)	
OWT	zero work tolerance	
OX	oximeter	
O×1	oriented to time	
O×2	oriented to time and place	
O×3	oriented to time, place, and person	
O×4	oriented to time, place, person, and objects (watch, pen, book)	
OXA	oxacillinase	
	oxaliplatin	
OXC	oxcarbazepine (Trileptal)	
Oxi	oximeter (oximetry)	
Ox-LDL	oxidized low-density lipoprotein	
OXPHOS	oxidative phosphorylation	
OxPt	oxaliplatin	
OXM	pulse oximeter	
Oxy-5®	benzoyl peroxide	
OXZ	oxazepam (Serax)	
OZ	optical zone	
	ounce	

P

P	para
	peripheral
	phosphorus
	pint
	plan
	poor
	protein
	Protestant
	pulse
	pupil
$\bar{p}$	after
/P	partial lower denture
P/	partial upper denture
P1	pilocarpine 1% ophthalmic solution
P$_2$	pulmonic second heart sound
P20	Ocusert® P20
^{32}P	radioactive phosphorus
P40	Ocusert® P40
PA	panic attack
	paranoid
	periapical (x-ray)
	pernicious anemia
	phenol alcohol
	Physician Assistant
	pineapple
	platelet aggregometry
	posterior-anterior (posteroanterior) (x-ray)
	presents again
	professional association (similar to a corporation)
	Pseudomonas aeruginosa
	psychiatric aide
	psychoanalysis
	pulmonary artery
Pa	pascal
P&A	percussion and auscultation
	phenol and alcohol (procedure for of toenail)

P

position and alignment

$P_2 > A_2$ pulmonic second heart sound greater than aortic second heart sound

PAB premature atrial beat
pulmonary artery banding

PABA aminobenzoic acid (para-aminobenzoic acid)

PABD preoperative autologous blood donation

PAC cisplatin (Platinol), doxorubicin (Adriamycin), and cylcophosphamide
phenacemide
Physical Assessment Center
Physician Assistant, Certified
picture archiving communication (system)
Port-a-cath®
premature atrial contraction
prophylactic anticonvulsants
pulmonary artery catheter

PA-C Physician Assistant, Certified

PACATH pulmonary artery catheter

PACE population-adjusted clinical epidemiology

PACG primary angle-closure glaucoma

PACH pipers to after coming head

PACI partial anterior cerebral infarct

PACO$_2$ partial pressure (tension) of carbon dioxide, alveolar

PaCO$_2$ partial pressure (tension) of carbon dioxide, artery

PACS picture archiving and communications systems

PACT prism and alternate cover test
Program of Assertive Community Treatment

PAC-V cisplatin (Platinol), doxorubicin (Adriamycin), and cyclophosphamide

PACU postanesthesia care unit

PAD pelvic adhesive disease
peripheral artery disease
pharmacologic atrial defibrillator
preliminary anatomic diagnosis
preoperative autologous donation
primary affective disorder

PADP pulmonary arterial diastolic pressure
pulmonary artery diastolic pressure

PADS Post Anesthesia Discharge Scoring System

PAE postanoxic encephalopathy
postantibiotic effect
pre-admission evaluation
progressive assistive exercise

PAEDP pulmonary artery and end-diastole pressure

PAF paroxysmal atrial fibrillation
platelet activating factor

PA&F percussion, auscultation, and fremitus

PAGA premature appropriate for gestational age

PAGE polyacrylamide gel electrophoresis

PAH para-aminohippurate
phenylalanine hydroxylase
polycyclic aromatic hydrocarbons
polynuclear aromatic hydrocarbon

	predicted adult height		polyarteritis nodosa
	pulmonary arterial hypertension	PANDAS	pediatric autoimmune neuropsychiatric disorders associated with streptococcal infections
PAHO	Pan American Health Organization		
PAI	plasminogen activator inhibitor	PANENDO	panendoscopy
		PANESS	physical and neurological examination for soft signs
	platelet accumulation index		
PAIDS	pediatric acquired immunodeficiency syndrome	PANP	pelvic autonomic nerve preservation
		PANSS	Positive and Negative Syndrome Scale
PAIgG	platelet-associated immunoglobulin G	PAO	peak acid output
			peripheral arterial occlusion
PAIVMs	passive accessory intervertebral movements	PAO_2	alveolar oxygen pressure (tension)
PAIVS	pulmonary atresia with intact ventricle septum	PaO_2	arterial oxygen pressure (tension)
PAK	pancreas and kidney	PAOD	peripheral arterial occlusive disease
PAL	posterior axillary line		
	posteroanterior and lateral	PAOP	pulmonary artery occlusion pressure
PALA	N-phosphoacetate-L aspartate	PAP	passive aggressive personality
Pa Line	pulmonary artery line		peroxidase-anti-peroxidase
PALN	para-aortic lymph node		pokeweed antiviral protein
PALP	palpation		positive airway pressure
PALS	pediatric advanced life support		primary atypical pneumonia
			prostatic acid phosphatase
	periarterial lymphatic sheath		pulmonary alveolar proteinosis
PAM	partial allosteric modulators		pulmonary artery pressure
	potential acuity meter	Pap smear	Papanicolaou's smear
	primary acquired melanosis	PA/PS	pulmonary atresia/ pulmonary stenosis
	primary amebic meningoencephalitis	PAPVC	partial anomalous pulmonary venous connection
2-PAM	pralidoxime (Protopam)		
PAMP	pulmonary arterial (artery) mean pressure	PAPVR	partial anomalous pulmonary venous return
PAN	pancreas		
	pancreatic	PAQLQ	Pediatric Asthma Quality of Life Questionnaire
	pancuronium (Pavulon)		
	panoral x-ray examination	PAR	parafin
	periodic alternating nystagmus		
	polyacrylonitrile (filter)		

P

	parainfluenza (paramyxovirus) vaccine	PASA	aminosalicylic acid (para-aminosalicylic acid)
	parallel	PA/S/D	pulmonary artery systolic/diastolic
	perennial allergic rhinitis	Pas Ex	passive exercise
	platelet aggregate ratio	PASG	pneumatic antishock garment
	possible allergic reaction	PASI	Psoriasis Area and Severity Index
	postanesthetic recovery		
	procedures, alternatives, and risks	PASK	peripheral anterior stromal keratopathy
	pulmonary arteriolar resistance	PASP	pulmonary artery systolic pressure
PARA	number of pregnancies producing viable offspring	PASS	Pain Anxiety Symptoms Scale
	paraplegic	PAT	paroxysmal atrial tachycardia
	parathyroid		passive alloimmune thrombocytopenia
PARA 1	having borne one child		
Paraflu	Parainfluenza		patella
PARC	perennial allergic rhinoconjunctivitis		patient
			percent acceleration time
PAROM	passive assistance range of motion		peripheral arterial tone
			platelet aggregation test
PARR	postanesthesia recovery room		preadmission testing
			pregnancy at term
PARS	postanesthesia recovery score	PATH	pituitary adrenotropic hormone
PARU	postanesthetic recovery unit		pathology
PAS	aminosalicylic acid (para-aminosalicylic acid)	PATP	preadmission testing program
	periodic acid-Schiff (reagent)	PATS	payment at time of service
	peripheral anterior synechia	PAV	Pavulon (pancuronium bromide)
	physician-assisted suicide	PAVe	procarbazine, melphalan (Alkeran), and vinblastine (Velban)
	pneumatic antiembolic stocking		
	postanesthesia score	PAVF	pulmonary arteriovenous fistula
	premature auricular systole	PAVM	pulmonary arteriovenous malformation
	Professional Activities Study	PAVNRT	paroxysmal atrial ventricular nodal re-entrant tachycardia
	pulmonary artery stenosis		
	pulsatile antiembolism system (stockings)	PAWP	pulmonary artery wedge pressure
PA-S	Physician Assistant, Student	PAX	periapical x-ray
		PB	barometric pressure

P

British Pharmacopeia
parafin bath
phenylbutyrate
piggyback
powder board
power building
premature beat
Presbyterian
protein-bound
pudendal block
pyridostigmine bromide
(Mestinon)

Pb lead
phenobarbital

p/b postburn

P&B pain and burning
Papanicolaou and breast
(examinations)
phenobarbital and
belladonna

PBA percutaneous bladder
aspiration

PBAL protected bronchoalveolar
lavage

PbB whole blood lead

PBC point of basal
convergence
prebed care
primary biliary cirrhosis

PBD percutaneous biliary
drainage
postburn day
proliferative breast
disease

PBE partial breech extraction
power building exercise

PBF placental blood flow
pulmonary blood flow

PBFS penile blood flow study

PBG porphobilinogen

PBI protein-bound iodine

PBK pseudophakic bullous
keratopathy

PBL peripheral blood
lymphocyte
primary brain lymphoma

PBLC premature birth live child

PBM pharmacy benefit
management (manager)

PBMC peripheral blood
mononuclear cell

PBMNC peripheral blood
mononuclear cell

PBN polymyxin B sulfate,
bacitracin, and
neomycin

PB:ND problem: nursing
diagnosis

PBNS percutaneous bladder neck
stabilization

PBO placebo

PBP phantom breast pain
protein-bound
polysaccharide

PBPC peripheral blood
progenitor cell

PBPCT peripheral blood
progenitor cell
transplant

PBPI penile-brachial pulse
index

PBPs penicillin-binding proteins

PBS phosphate-buffered saline
prune-belly syndrome

PBSC peripheral blood stem
cells

PBT primary brain tumor

PBT$_4$ protein-bound thyroxine

PbtO$_2$ brain tissue partial
pressure of oxygen

PBV percutaneous balloon
valvuloplasty

PBZ phenoxybenzamine
phenylbutazone
pyribenzamine

ΦBZ phenylbutazone

PC after meals
cisplatin (Platinol) and
cyclophosphamide
packed cells
pancreatic carcinoma
pathologic consultation
photocoagulation
placebo-controlled (study)
platelet concentrate
Pneumocystis carinii
poor condition
popliteal cyst

	posterior chamber		pneumatosis cystoides coli
	premature contractions		poison control center
	present complaint		precipitated calcium carbonate
	productive cough		
	professional corporation		progressive cardiac care
	psychiatric counselor	PCCC	pediatric critical care center
	pubococcygeus (muscle)		
PCA	passive cutaneous anaphylaxis	PCCI	penetrating craniocerebral injuries
	patient care assistant (aide)	PCCM	primary care case management
	patient-controlled analgesia	PCCU	postcoronary care unit
	penicillamine	PCD	pacer-cardioverter-defibrillator
	porous coated anatomic (joint replacement)		paroxysmal cerebral dysrhythmia
	postcardiac arrest		plasma cell dyscrasias
	postciliary artery		postmortem cesarean delivery
	postconceptional age		
	posterior cerebral artery		primary ciliary dyskinesia
	posterior communicating artery		programmed cell death
	procainamide		
	procoagulation activity	PCDAI	Pediatric Crohn's Disease Activity Index
	prostate cancer		
PCa	prostate cancer	PCE	physical capacities evaluation
PCAC	Physical Care Assessment Center		potentially compensable event
PCASSO	patient-centered access to secure systems online		pseudophakic corneal edema
PCB	pancuronium bromide	PCE®	erythromycin particles in tablets
	para cervical block		
	placebo	PCEA	patient-controlled epidural analgesia
	postcoital bleeding		
	prepared childbirth	PCEC	purified chick embryo cell (culture)
	procarbazine (Matulane)		
	Pseudomonas cepacia bacteremia	PCF	pharyngeal conjunctival fever
PCBH	personal care boarding home	PCFT	platelet complement fixation test
PCBMN	palmar cutaneous branch of the median nerve	PCG	phonocardiogram
			pubococcygeus (muscle)
PCBs	polychlorinated biphenyls	PCGG	percutaneous coagulation of gasserian ganglion
PCBUN	palmar cutaneous branch of the ulnar nerve	PCGLV	poorly contractile globular left ventricle
PCC	patient care coordinator		
	petrous carotid canal	PCH	paroxysmal cold hemoglobinuria
	pheochromocytoma		

	periocular capillary hemangioma	PCNSL	primary central nervous system lymphoma
	personal care home	PCNT	percutaneous nephrostomy tube
PCHI	permanent childhood hearing impairment	PCO	patient complains of
PCHL	permanent childhood hearing loss		polycystic ovary
PC&HS	after meals and at bedtime		posterior capsular opacification
PCI	percutaneous coronary intervention	PCO_2	partial pressure (tension) of carbon dioxide, artery
	pneumatosis cystoides intestinalis	PCOD	polycystic ovarian disease
	prophylactic cranial irradiation	PCOE	prescriber (physician) computer order entry
PCINA	patient-controlled intranasal analgesia	P COMM A	posterior communicating artery
PCIOL	posterior chamber intraocular lens	PCOS	polycystic ovary syndrome
PC-IRV	pressure-controlled inverse-ratio ventilation	PCP	patient care plan
			phencyclidine (phenylcyclohexyl piperidine)
PCKD	polycystic kidney disease		
PCL	pacing cycle length		*Pneumocystis carinii* pneumonia
	plasma cell leukemia		
	posterior chamber lens		primary care person
	posterior cruciate ligament		primary care physician
	proximal collateral ligament		primary care provider
			prochlorperazine (Compazine)
PCLI	plasma cell labeling index		
PCLN	psychiatric consultation liaison nurse		pulmonary capillary pressure
PCLR	paid claims loss ratio	PCR	patient care report
PCM	primary cutaneous melanoma		percutaneous coronary revascularization
	protein-calorie malnutrition		polymerase chain reaction
	pubococcygeal muscle		protein catabolic rate
PC-MRI	phase-contrast magnetic resonance imaging	PCr	plasma creatinine
		PCRA	pure red-cell aplasia
PCMX	chloroxylenol	PCR/PSA	polymerase chain reaction analysis of prostate-specific antigen
PCN	penicillin		
	percutaneous nephrostomy	PCS	patient care system
	primary care nursing		patient-controlled sedation
PCNA	proliferating cell nuclear antigen		personal care service
			portable cervical spine
PCNL	percutaneous nephrostolithotomy		portacaval shunt
			postconcussion syndrome
PCNs	posterior cervical nodes	P c/s	primary cesarean section

P

247

PC-SPES	an herbal refined powder preparation of eight medicinal plants	2PD	two point discriminatory test
PCT	percent	^{103}Pd	palladium 103
	porphyria cutanea tarda	PDA	parenteral drug abuser
	postcoital test		patent ductus arteriosus
	posterior chest tube		poorly differentiated adenocarcinoma
	primary chemotherapy		posterior descending (coronary) artery
	progesterone challenge test		property damage accident
PCTA	percutaneous transluminal angioplasty	PDAF	platelet-derived angiogenesis factor
PCU	palliative care unit	PDAP	peritoneal dialysis-associated peritonitis
	primary care unit		
	progressive care unit	PDB	preperitoneal distention balloon
	protective care unit		
PCV	packed cell volume	PDC	patient denies complaints
	polycythemia vera		poorly differentiated carcinoma
	pressure-controlled ventilation		private diagnostic clinic
	procarbazine, lomustine (CCNU [Cee Nu]), and vincristine		property damage collision (crash)
			pyruvate dehydogenase complex
PCVC	percutaneous central venous catheter	PD&C	postural drainage and clapping
PCWP	pulmonary capillary wedge pressure	PDCA	Plan-Do-Check-Act (process improvement)
PCX	paracervical	PDD	cisplatin
PCXR	portable chest radiograph		pervasive developmental disorder
PCZ	procarbazine (Matulane)		premenstrual dysphoric disorder
	prochlorperazine (Compazine)		primary degenerative dementia
PD	interpupillary distance	PDE	paroxysmal dyspnea on exertion
	Paget's disease		
	pancreaticoduodenectomy		pulsed Doppler echocardiography
	panic disorder		
	Parkinson's disease	PDE 5	phosphodiesterase type 5
	percutaneous drain	PDEGF	platelet-derived epidermal growth factor
	peritoneal dialysis		
	personality disorder		
	pharmacodynamics	PDF	Portable Document Format
	pocket depth (dental)		
	poorly differentiated	PDFC	premature dead female child
	postural drainage		
	pressure dressing		
	prism diopter	PDGF	platelet-derived growth factor
	progressive disease		
	pupillary distance		
P/D	packs per day (cigarettes)		

PDGXT	predischarge graded exercise test		Progressive Deterioration Scale
PDH	past dental history	PDT	percutaneous dilatational tracheostomy
	pyruvate dehydrogenase		photodynamic therapy
PDI	Pain Disability Index		postdisaster trauma
	phasic detrusor instability	PDTC	pyrrolidine dithiocarbamate
PDIGC	patient dismissed in good condition	PDU	pulsed Doppler ultrasonography
PDL	periodontal ligament	PDUFA	Prescription Drug User Fee Act (1992)
	poorly differentiated lymphocytic		
	postures of daily living	PDW	platelet distribution width
	progressively diffused leukoencephalopathy	PDWHF	platelet-derived wound healing factors
	pulsed-dye laser	PDx	principal diagnosis
PDL-D	poorly differentiated lymphocytic-diffuse	pDXA	peripheral dual energy x-ray absorptiometry
PDL-N	poorly differentiated lymphocytic-nodular	PE	cisplatin (Platinol AQ) and etoposide
PDMC	premature dead male child		pedal edema
PDN	Paget's disease of the nipple		pelvic examination
			phenytoin equivalent (150 mg of fosphenytoin sodium is equivalent to 100 mg of phenytoin sodium)
	prednisone		
	private duty nurse		
	prosthetic disk nucleus		
PDOX	pegylated doxorubicin		
PDP	peak diastolic pressure		physical education (gym)
PD & P	postural drainage and percussion		physical examination
			physical exercise
PDPH	postdural puncture headache		plasma exchange
			pleural effusion
PDQ	pretty damn quick (at once)		pneumatic equalization
			polyethylene
PDR	patients' dining room		preeclampsia
	Physicians' Desk Reference		premature ejaculation
			pressure equalization
	postdelivery room		pulmonary edema
	proliferative diabetic retinopathy		pulmonary embolism
	prospective drug review	P_1E_1®	epinephrine 1%, pilocarpine 1% ophthalmic solution
PDRcVH	proliferative diabetic retinopathy with vitreous hemorrhage	P&E	prep and enema
		PE24	Preemie Enfamil 24
PDRP	proliferative diabetic retinopathy	PEA	pelvic examination under anesthesia
PDS	pain dysfunction syndrome		pre-emptive analgesia
	polydioxanone suture		pulseless electrical activity

P

PEARL	physiologic endometrial ablation/resection loop
	pupils equal accommodation, reactive to light
	pupils equal and reactive to light
PEARLA	pupils equal and react to light and accommodation
PEB	cisplatin, etoposide, and bleomycin
PEC	pectoralis
	pulmonary ejection click
PECCE	planned extracapsular cataract extraction
PECHO	prostatic echogram
PECHR	peripheral exudative choroidal hemorrhagic retinopathy
$PECO_2$	mixed expired carbon dioxide tension
PED	paroxysmal exertion-induced dyskinesia
	pediatrics
	pigment epithelial detachments
PEDD	proton-electron dipole-dipole
PEDI-DEG	pediatric deglycerolized red blood cells
Peds	pediatrics
PEE	punctate epithelial erosion
PEEP	positive end-expiratory pressure
PEF	cisplatin (Platinol AQ), epirubicin, and fluorouracil
	peak expiratory flow
PEFR	peak expiratory flow rate
PEFSR	partial expiratory flow static recoil curve
PEG	pegylated
	percutaneous endoscopic gastrostomy
	pneumoencephalogram
	polyethylene glycol

PEG-ELS	polyethylene glycol and iso-osmolar electrolyte solution
PEGG	Parent Education and Guidance Group
PEG-J	percutaneous endoscopic gastrojejunostomy
PEG-JET	percutaneous endoscopic gastrostomy with jejunal extension tube
PEG-SOD	polyethylene glycol-conjugated superoxide dismutase (pegorgotein)
PEI	cisplatin (Platinol AQ), etoposide, and ifosfamide
	percutaneous ethanol injection
	phosphate excretion index
	physical efficiency index
	polyethylenimine
PEJ	percutaneous endoscopic jejunostomy
PEK	punctate epithelial keratopathy
PEL	permissible exposure limits
	primary effusion lymphomas
PELD	percutaneous endoscopic lumbar diskectomy
PELV	pelvimetry
PEM	prescription event monitoring
	protein-energy malnutrition
PEMA	phenylethylmalonamide
PEMS	physical, emotional, mental, and safety
PEN	parenteral and enteral nutrition
	Pharmacy Equivalent Name
PENS	percutaneous electrical nerve stimulation
	percutaneous epidural nerve stimulator
PEO	progressive external ophthalmoplegia

PEP	patient education program	PERT	pancreatic enzyme replacement therapy
	pharmacologic erection program		program evaluation and review technique
	postexposure prophylaxis	PERV	porcine endogenous retroviruses
	preejection period		
	protein electrophoresis	PER$_w$	pertussis, whole-cell antigens, vaccine
PEPI	preejection period index		
PEPP	payment error prevention program	PES	polyethersulfone
			preexcitation syndrome
PER	by		programmed electrical stimulation
	pediatric emergency room		
	pertussis (whooping cough) vaccine, antigens not otherwise unspecified		pseudoexfoliation syndrome
		peSPL	peak equivalent sound pressure level
	protein efficiency ratio	PET	poor exercise tolerance
PER$_a$	pertussis, acellular antigen(s), vaccine		positron-emission tomography
PERC	perceptual		preeclamptic toxemia
	percutaneous		pressure equalizing tubes
PERF	perfect		problem elicitation technique
	perforation		
Peri Care	perineum care	PETN	pentaerythritol tetranitrate
PERIO	periodontal disease	PEx	physical examination
	periodontitis	PEX# 3	plasma exchange number three
peri-pads	perineal pads		
PERL	pupils equal, reactive to light	PF	patellofemoral
			peak flow
PERLA	pupils equally reactive to light and accommodation		peripheral fields
			plantar flexion
			power factor
per os	by mouth (this is a dangerous abbreviation as it is read as left eye)		preservative free
			prostatic fluid
			pulmonary fibrosis
PERR	pattern evoked retinal response		push fluids
PERRL	pupils equal, round, and reactive to light	PF3	platelet factor 3
		PF4	platelet factor 4
PERRLA	pupils equal, round, reactive to light and accommodation	16PF	The Sixteen Personality Factors test
		PFA	foscarnet (phosphonoformatic acid) (Foscavir)
PERR-LADC	pupils equal, round, reactive to light and accommodation directly and consensually		platelet function analysis
			psychological first aid
			pure free acid
PERRRLA	pupils equal, round, regular, react to light and accommodation	PFB	potential for breakdown
			pseudofolliculitis barbae
		PFC	patient-focused care

P

	perfluorochemical	PFT
	permanent flexure contracture	
	persistent fetal circulation	PFTC
	prolonged febrile convulsions	
P̄ FEEDS	after feedings	PFU
PFFD	proximal femoral focal deficiency (defect)	PFW
PFFFP	Pall filtered fresh frozen plasma	PFWB
PFGE	pulsed field gel electrophoresis	PG
PfHRP-2	*Plasmodium falciparum* histidine-rich protein 2	
PFHx	positive family history	
PFI	progression-free interval	
PFJ	patellofemoral joint	
PFJS	patellofemoral joint syndrome	
PFL	cisplatin (Platinol AQ), fluorouracil, and leucovorin	
PFL+IFN	cisplatin (Platinol AQ), fluorouracil, leucovorin, and interferon alfa 2b	PGA
PFM	porcelain fused to metal primary fibromyalgia	
PFME	pelvic floor muscle exercise	
PFO	patent foramen ovale	PGCs
PFP	progression free probability	PGE
PFPC	Pall filtered packed cells	PGE₁
PFPS	patellofemoral pain syndrome	
PFR	parotid flow rate peak flow rate	PGE₂
PFRC	plasma-free red cells	PGF
PFROM	pain-free range of motion	PGF₂∝
PFS	patellar femoral syndrome	
	prefilled syringe	PGGF
	preservative-free solution (system)	PGGM
	primary fibromyalgia syndrome	PGH
	progression-free survival	PGI
	pulmonary function studies (study)	PGI₂

PFT	parafascicular thalamotomy
	pulmonary function test
PFTC	primary fallopian tube carcinoma
PFU	plaque-forming unit
PFW	pHisoHex® face wash
PFWB	Pall filtered whole blood
	Psychological General Well-Being (index)
PG	paged in hospital
	paregoric
	performance goal (short-term goal)
	phosphatidylglycerol
	picogram (pg) (10^{-12} gram)
	placental grade (biophysical profile)
	polygalacturonate
	pregnant
	prostaglandin
	pyoderma gangrenosum
PGA	prostaglandin A
	prothrombin time, **g**amma-glutamyl transpeptidase activity, and serum **a**polipoprotein AI concentration
PGCs	primordial germ cells
PGE	posterior gastroenterostomy
	proximal gastric exclusion
PGE₁	alprostadil (prostaglandin E₁)
PGE₂	dinoprostone (prostaglandin E₂)
PGF	paternal grandfather
PGF₂∝	dinoprost (prostaglandin F₂∝)
PGGF	paternal great-grandfather
PGGM	paternal great-grandmother
PGH	pituitary growth hormones
PGI	potassium, glucose, and insulin
PGI₂	epoprostenol (Prostacyclin)

PGL	persistent generalized lymphadenopathy		pharynx
		Pharm	Pharmacy
	primary gastric lymphoma	PharmD	Doctor of Pharmacy
PGM	paternal grandmother	PHb	pyridoxylated hemoglobin
	phosphoglucomutase	PHC	posthospital care
PGP	paternal grandparent		primary health care
Pgp	P-glycoprotein		primary hepatocellular carcinoma
PGR	pulse generated runoff		
PgR	progesterone receptor	PHCA	profound hypothermic cardiac arrest
P-graph	penile plethysmograph		
PGS	Persian Gulf syndrome	PHD	paroxysmal hypnogenic dyskinesia
PGT	play-group therapy		
P±GTC	partial seizures with or without generalized tonic-clonic seizures		Public Health Department
		PhD	Doctor of Philosophy
		PHE	periodic health examination
PG-TXL	poly (L-glutamic acid)-paclitaxel		
		PHEN-FEN	phentermine and fenfluramine
PGU	postgonococcal urethritis		
PGW	person gametocyte week	PHEO	pheochromocytoma
PGY-1	postgraduate year one (first year resident)	PHEP	progressive home exercise program
		PHF	paired helical filament
pH	hydrogen ion concentration	PHG	portal hypertensive gastropathy
PH	past history	PHH	paraesophageal hiatus hernia
	personal history		
	pinhole		posthemorrhagic hydrocephalus
	poor health		
	pubic hair	PHHI	persistent hyperinsulinemic hypoglycemia of infancy
	public health		
	pulmonary hypertension		
P&H	physical and history		
Ph¹	Philadelphia chromosome		
PHA	arterial pH	PHI	phosphohexose isomerase
	passive hemagglutinating		prehospital index
	peripheral hyperalimentation	PHIS	posthead injury syndrome
		PHL	Philadelphia (chromosome)
	phenylalanine		
	phytohemagglutinin antigen	PHLS	Public Health Laboratory Service (United Kingdom)
	postoperative holding area		
PHACO	phacoemulsification	PHMB	polyhexamethylene biguanine
PHACO OD	phacoemulsification of the right eye		
		PHMD	polyhexamethylene (Baquacil, a pool cleaner)
PHACO OS	phacoemulsification of the left eye		
PHAL	peripheral hyperalimentation	PHN	postherpetic neuralgia
			public health nurse
PHAR	pharmacist		Puritan® heated nebulizer
	pharmacy		

PHNC	public health nurse coordinator	physically impaired
		poison ivy
PHNI	pinhole no improvement	postincident
PHO	Physician/Hospital Organization	postinjury
		premature infant
PHOB	phobic anxiety	present illness
PHP	pooled human plasma	principal investigator
	postheparin plasma	protease inhibitor
	prepaid health plan	pulmonary infarction
	pseudohypoparathy-	pulmonic insufficiency
	roidism	PI-3 parainfluenza 3 virus
	pyridoxalated hemoglobin	P & I probe and irrigation
	polyoxyethylene	PIA personal injury accident
	conjugate	PIAT Peabody Individual
PHPT	primary	Achievement Test
	hyperparathyroidism	PIB professional information
PHPV	persistent hyperplastic	brochure
	primary vitreous	PIBD paucity of interlobular
PHR	peak heart rate	bile ducts
PhRMA	Pharmaceutical Research	PIC penicillin-inhibitor
	and Manufacturers of	combinations
	America (Formerly the	peripherally inserted
	Pharmaceutical	catheter
	Manufacturers	personal injury collision
	Association)	(crash)
PHS	partial hospitalization	polysaccharide-iron
	program	complex
	US Public Health Service	postintercourse
PHT	phenytoin (Dilantin)	PICA Porch Index of
	portal hypertension	Communicative
	postmenopausal hormone	Ability
	therapy	posterior inferior
	primary hyperthyroidism	cerebellar artery
	pulmonary hypertension	posterior inferior
PHV	peak height velocity	communicating artery
PHVA	pinhole visual acuity	PICC peripherally inserted
PHVD	posthemorrhagic	central catheter
	ventricular dilatation	PICHI pulse-inversion contrast
PHx	past history	harmonic imaging
Phx	pharynx	PICT pancreatic islet cell
PHY	physician	transplantation
PhyO	physician's orders	PICU pediatric intensive care
PI	package insert	unit
	pallidal index	psychiatric intensive care
	pancreatic insufficiency	unit
	Pearl Index	PICVC peripherally inserted
	performance improvement	central venous catheter
	peripheral iridectomy	PID pelvic inflammatory
	persistent illness	disease

P

	prolapsed intervertebral disk	PIND	progressive intellectual and neurological deterioration
	proportional-integral-derivative (controller)	PIO	pemoline (Cylert)
PIE	pulmonary infiltration with eosinophilia	PIO$_2$	partial pressure of inspired oxygen
	pulmonary interstitial emphysema	PIOK	poikilocytosis
PIEE	pulsed irrigation for enhanced evacuation	PIP	peak inspiratory pressure
			postictal psychosis
PIF	peak inspiratory flow		postinfusion phlebitis
PIFG	poor intrauterine fetal growth		proximal interphalangeal (joint)
PIG	pertussis immune globulin		pulmonary immaturity of prematurity
PIGI	pregnancy-induced glucose intolerance		pulmonary insufficiency of the premature
PIGN	postinfectious glomerulonephritis	PIPB	performance index phonetic balance
PIH	pregnancy induced hypertension	PI-PB	performance intensity-phonemically balanced
	preventricular intraventricular hemorrhage	PIPIDA	N-para-isopropyl-acetanilide-iminodiacetic acid
	prolactin inhibiting hormone	PIPJ	proximal interphalangeal joint
PIIID	peripheral indwelling intermediate infusion device	PIP/TZ	piperacillin-tazobactam (Zosyn)
PIIIP	aminoterminal type three procollagen propeptide	PIQ	Performance Intelligence Quotient (part of Wechsler tests)
PIIS	posterior inferior iliac spine	PIS	pregnancy interruption service
PIL	patient information leaflet	PISA	phase invariant signature algorithm
PILO	pilocarpine		
PIM	pulse-inversion mode (ultrasound)		proximal isovelocity surface area
PIMIA	potentiometric ionophore mediated immunoassay	PIT	patellar inhibition test
			peak isometric torque
PIMS	programmable implantable medication system		Pitocin (oxytocin)
PIN	pain in (the) neck (no place for such a term in a written document)		Pitressin (vasopressin) (this is a dangerous abbreviation)
			pituitary
	personal identification number		pulsed inotrope therapy
	posterior interosseous nerve	PITP	pseudo-idiopathic thrombocytopenic purpura
	prostatic intraepithelial neoplasia	PITR	plasma iron turnover rate
		PIV	peripheral intravenous

P

PIV-3	parainfluenza virus type 3
PIVD	protruded intervertebral disk
PIVH	periventricular-intraventricular hemorrhage
PIVKA	proteins induced in vitamin K absence
PIWT	partially impacted wisdom teeth
PJ	procelin jacket (crown)
PJB	premature junctional beat
PJC	premature junctional contractions
PJI	prosthetic joint infection
PJRT	permanent form of junctional reciprocating tachycardia
PJS	peritoneojugular shunt
	Peutz-Jeghers syndrome
PJT	paroxysmal junctional tachycardia
PJVT	paroxysmal junctional-ventricular tachycardia
PK	penetrating keratoplasty
	pharmacokinetics
	plasma potassium
	pyruvate kinase
PKB	prone knee bend
PKC	protein kinase C
PKD	paroxysmal kinesigenic dyskinesia
	polycystic kidney disease
PKND	paroxysmal nonkinesigenic dyskinesia
PKP	penetrating keratoplasty
PKR	phased knee rehabilitation
PK Test	Prausnitz-Küstner transfer test
PKU	phenylketonuria
pk yrs	pack-years (smoking one pack of cigarettes a day for one year is termed 1 pack-year of smoking, thus 2 packs a day for 20 years would be 40 pack-years)
PL	light perception

	palmaris longus
	place
	placebo
	plantar
	plethoric (infant color)
	transpulmonary pressure
PLA	placebo
	Plasma-Lyte A
	posterolateral (coronary) artery
	potentially lethal arrhythmia
	Product License Application
	pulpolinguoaxial
PLAD	proximal left anterior descending (artery)
Plan B®	levonorgestrel (a progestogen emergency contraceptive)
PLAP	placental alkaline phosphatase
PLAT C	platelet concentration
PLAT P	platelet pheresis
PLAX	parasternal long axis
PLB	phospholamban
	placebo
	posterolateral branch
PLBO	placebo
PLC	peripheral lymphocyte count
	pityriasis lichenoides chronica
PLD	partial lower denture
	percutaneous laser diskectomy
PLDD	percutaneous laser disk decompression
PLE	polymorphic light eruption
	protein-losing enteropathy
PLED	periodic lateralizing epileptiform discharge
PLEVA	pityriasis lichenoides et varioliformis acuta
PLF	prior level of function
PLFC	premature living female child

PLG	plague (*Yersinia pestis*) (*la Peste*) vaccine	PLT	platelet
		PLT EST	platelet estimate
PLH	paroxysmal localized hyperhidrosis	PLTF	plaintiff
		PLTS	platelets
PLIF	posterior lumbar interbody fusion	PLUG	plug the lung until it grows
PLL	prolymphocytic leukemia	PLV	posterior left ventricular
PLLA	poly-l-lactic acid	PLX	plexus
PLM	periodic leg movement	PLYO	plyometric
	Plasma-Lyte M	PLZF	promyelocytic leukemia zinc finger
	polarized-light microscope	PM	afternoon
	precise lesion measuring (device)		evening
			pacemaker
	product-line manager		particulate matter
PLMC	premature living male child		petit mal
			physical medicine
PLMD	periodic limb movement disorder		pneumomediastinum
			poliomyelitis
PLMS	periodic limb movements during sleep		polymyositis
			poor metabolizers
PLN	pelvic lymph node		postmenopausal
	popliteal lymph node		postmortem
PLND	pelvic lymph node dissection		presents mainly
			pretibial myxedema
PLO	pluronic lecithin organogels		primary motivation
			prostatic massage
PLOF	previous level of functioning		pulpomesial
PLOSA	physiologic low stress angioplasty	PM_{10}	particulate matter greater than 10 micrometers diameter
PLP	partial laryngopharyngectomy	PMA	positive mental attitude
	phantom limb pain		premarket approval (application) (for medical devices)
	protolipid protein		
PLPH	postlumbar puncture headache		premenstrual asthma
PLR	pupillary light reflex		Prinzmetal's angina
PLS	Papillon-Lefèvre syndrome		progress myoclonic ataxia
	plastic surgery	PMAA	Premarket Approval Application (medical devices)
	point locator stimulator		
	Preschool Language Scale	PMB	polymorphonuclear basophil (leukocytes)
	primary lateral sclerosis		
PLs	premalignant lesions		polymyxin B
PLSO	posterior leafspring orthosis		postmenopausal bleeding
		PMC	premature mitral closure
PLST	progressively lowered stress threshold		pseudomembranous colitis
PLSURG	plastic surgery	PMCP	para-monochlorophenol

	perinatal mortality counseling program	PMMA	polymethyl methacrylate
PMCT	perinatal mortality counseling team	PMMF	pectoralis major myocutaneous flap
PMD	perceptual motor development	PMN	polymodal nociceptors
	primary myocardial disease		polymorphonuclear leukocyte
	primidone (Mysoline)		Premarket Notification (medical devices)
	private medical doctor	PMNL	polymorphonuclear leukocyte
	progressive muscular dystrophy	PMNN	polymorphonuclear neutrophil
PMDD	premenstrual dysphoric disorder	PMNS	postmalarial neurological syndrome
PM/DM	polymyositis and dermatomyositis	PMO	postmenopausal osteoporosis
PME	pelvic muscle exercise	pmol	picomole
	polymorphonuclear esosinophil (leukocytes)	PMP	pain management program
	postmenopausal estrogen		previous menstrual period
PMEALS	after meals		psychotropic medication plan
PMEC	pseudomembranous enterocolitis	PMPA	tenofovir
PMF	progressive massive fibrosis	PMPM	per member, per month
	pupils mid-position, fixed	PMPO	postmenopausal palpable ovary
PMH	past medical history	PMPY	per member, per year
PMHx	past medical history	PMR	pacemaker rhythm
PMI	Pain Management Index		percutaneous revascularization
	past medical illness		polymorphic reticulosis
	patient medication instructions		polymyalgia rheumatica
	plea of mental incompetence		premedication regimen
	point of maximal impulse		prior medical record
	posterior myocardial infarction		progressive muscle relaxation
PMID	PubMed Unique Identifier (National Library of Medicine)		proportional mortality ratios
		PM&R	physical medicine and rehabilitation
PML	polymorphonuclear leukocytes	PMS	performance measurement system
	posterior mitral leaflet		periodic movements of sleep
	premature labor		poor miserable soul
	progressive multifocal leukoencephalopathy		postmarketing surveillance
	promyelocytic leukemia		postmenopausal syndrome
PMLCL	primary mediastinal large-cell lymphoma		premenstrual syndrome
			pulse, motor, and sensory

PMT	pacemaker-mediated tachycardia		premature nodal contraction
	point of maximum tenderness		prenatal care
			prenatal course
	premenstrual tension		Psychiatric Nurse Clinician
PMTS	premenstrual tension syndrome	PND	paroxysmal nocturnal dyspnea
PMV	prolapse of mitral valve		pelvic node dissection
PMW	pacemaker wires		postnasal drip
PMZ	postmenopausal zest		pregnancy, not delivered
PN	parenteral nutrition	PNE	peripheral neuroepithelioma
	percussion note		
	percutaneous nephrosonogram		primary nocturnal enuresis
	percutaneous nucleotomy	PNET	primitive neuroectodermal tumors
	periarteritis nodosa		
	peripheral neuropathy	PNET-MB	primitive neuroectodermal tumors-medulloblastoma
	pneumonia		
	polyarteritis nodosa		
	poorly nourished	PNEUMO	pneumothorax
	positional nystagmus	PNF	primary nonfunction
	postnasal		proprioceptive neuromuscular fasciculation (reaction)
	postnatal		
	practical nurse		
	premie nipple	PNH	paroxysmal nocturnal hemoglobinuria
	primary nurse		
	progress note		polynitroxyl-hemoglobin
	pyelonephritis	PNI	peripheral nerve injury
P & N	pins and needles		Prognostic Nutrition Index
	psychiatry and neurology		
PN_2	partial pressure of nitrogen	PNKD	paroxysmal nonkinesigenic dyskinesia
PNA	Pediatric Nurse Associate		
	polynitroxyl albumin	PNL	percutaneous nephrolithotomy
PNa	plasma sodium		
PNAB	percutaneous needle aspiration biopsy	PNMG	persistent neonatal myasthenia gravis
PNAC	parenteral nutrition associated cholestasis	PNMT	phenylethanolamine-N-methyltransferase
PNAS	prudent no added salt	PNNP	Perinatal Nurse Practitioner
PNB	percutaneous needle biopsy	PNP	peak negative pressure
	popliteal nerve block		Pediatric Nurse Practitioner
	premature newborn		
	premature nodal beat		progressive nuclear palsy
	prostate needle biopsy		purine nucleoside phosphorylase
PNC	penicillin		
	peripheral nerve conduction	PNR	physician's nutritional recommendation

PNRB	partial non-rebreather (oxygen mask)
PNS	partial nonprogressing stroke
	peripheral nerve stimulator
	peripheral nervous system
	practical nursing student
PNSP	penicillin-nonsusceptible *S. pneumoniae*
PNT	percutaneous nephrostomy tube
	percutaneous neuromodulatory therapy
pnthx	pneumothorax
PNTML	pudendal-nerve terminal motor latency
PNU	pneumococcal (*Streptococcus pneumoniae*) vaccine, not otherwise specified
	protein nitrogen units
PNU$_{cn}$	pneumococcal (*Streptococcus pneumoniae*) conjugate vaccine
PNU$_{ps}$	pneumococcal (*Streptococcus pneumoniae*) polysaccharide vaccine
PNV	postoperative nausea and vomiting
	prenatal vitamins
Pnx	pneumonectomy
	pneumothorax
PO	by mouth (*per os*)
	phone order
	postoperative
P&O	parasites and ova
	prosthetics and orthotics
P$_{O2}$	partial pressure (tension) of oxygen, artery
PO$_4$	phosphate
POA	pancreatic oncofetal antigen
	power of attorney
	primary optic atrophy

POACH	prednisone, vincristine (Oncovin), doxorubicin (Adriamycin), cyclophosphamide, and cytarabine
POAG	primary open-angle glaucoma
POB	phenoxybenzamine (Dibenzyline)
	place of birth
POBC	primary operable breast cancer
POC	plans of care
	point-of-care
	position of comfort
	postoperative care
	product of conception
POD	pacing on demand
	place of death
	Podiatry
	polycystic ovarian disease
POD 1	postoperative day one
PODx	preoperative diagnosis
POE	patient-oriented evidence
	point (portal, port) of entry
	position of ease
	provider order entry
POEM	Patient-Oriented Evidence That Matters
POEMS	plasma cell dyscrasia with polyneuropathy, organomegaly, endocrinopathy, monoclonal protein (M-protein), and skin changes
POEx	postoperative exercise
POF	physician's order form
	position of function
	premature ovarian failure
P of I	proof of illness
POG	Pediatric Oncology Group
	Penthrane,® oxygen, and gas (nitrous oxide)
	products of gestation
POH	perillyl alcohol
	personal oral hygiene

	presumed ocular histoplasmosis	POOH	postoperative open heart (surgery)
POHA	preoperative holding area	POP	pain on palpation
POHI	physically or otherwise health impaired		persistent occipitoposterior
POHS	presumed ocular histoplasmosis syndrome		plaster of paris
			popiliteal
			posterior oral pharynx
POI	Personal Orientation Inventory		postoperative
		POPC	Pediatric Overall Performance Category (scale)
	postoperative instructions		
POIB	place outpatient in inpatient bed	poplit	popliteal
		POPs	progesterone-only pills
POIK	poikilocytosis	POR	physician of record
POL	physician's office laboratory		problem-oriented record
		PORP	partial ossicular replacement prosthesis
	poliovirus vaccine, not otherwise specified	PORR	postoperative recovery room
	premature onset of labor		
POLS	postoperative length of stay	PORT	perioperative respiratory therapy
POLY	polychromic erythrocytes		portable
	polymorphonuclear leukocyte		postoperative radiotherapy
			postoperative respiratory therapy
POLY-CHR	polychromatophilia		
POM	pain on motion	POS	parosteal osteosarcoma
	polyoximethylene		physician's order sheet
	prescription-only medication		point-of-service
			positive
POMA	Performance-Oriented Mobility Assessment	POSHPATE	problem, onset, associated symptoms, previous history, precipitating factors, alleviating/ aggravation factors, timing, an etiology (prompts for taking history and chief complaint)
POMC	pro-opiomelanocortin		
POMP	prednisone, vincristine (Oncovin), methotrexate, and mercaptopurine (Purinthol)		
POMR	problem-oriented medical record		
		poss	possible
POMS	Profile of Mood States	post	posterior
POMS-FI	Fatigue-Inertia Subscale of the Profile of Mood States		postmortem examination (autopsy)
		PostC	posterior chamber
		PostCap	posterior capsule
PON	postoperative note	Post-M	urine specimen after prostate massage
PONI	postoperative narcotic infusion		
		post op	postoperative
PONV	postoperative nausea and vomiting	Post Sag D	posterior sagittal diameter

POp — postoperative

P

post tib	posterial tibial	PIIIP	aminoterminal type three protocollegan propeptide
PostVD	posterior vitreous detachment		
POSYC	Pain Observation Scale for Young Children	PPIX	protoporphyrin nine
POT	peak occupancy time	PPA	palpation, percussion, and auscultation
	plans of treatment		phenylpropanolamine
	potassium		phenylpyruvic acid
	potential		postpartum amenorrhea
POTS	postural tachycardia syndrome	PP&A	palpation, percussion, and auscultation
POU	placenta, ovaries, and uterus	$PPAR_g$	peroxisome-proliferator-activated receptor gamma
POV	privately owned vehicle	PPARs	peroxisome proliferator-activated receptors
POW	prisoner of war		
POWSBP	pulse oximetry waveform systolic blood pressure	PPAS	postpolio atrophy syndrome
POX	pulse oximeter (reading)	PPB	parts per billion
			pleuropulmonary blastoma
PP	near point of accommodation		positive pressure breathing
			prostate puncture biopsy
	paradoxical pulse	PPBE	postpartum breast engorgment
	partial upper and lower dentures		
		PPBS	postprandial blood sugar
	pedal pulse	PPC	plaster of paris cast
	per protocol		progressive patient care
	periodontal pockets		
	peripheral pulses	PPCD	posterior polymorphous corneal dystrophy
	pin prick		
	pink puffer (emphysema)	PPCF	plasma prothrombin conversion factor
	Planned Parenthood		
	plasmapheresis	PPD	packs per day
	plaster of paris		posterior polymorphous dystrophy
	poor person		
	posterior pituitary		postpartum day
	postpartum		probing pocket depth (dental)
	postprandial		
	presenting part		purified protein derivative (of tuberculin)
	private patient		
	prophylactics		pylorus-sparing pancreaticoduodenectomy
	protoporphyria		
	proximal phalanx	P & PD	percussion & postural drainage
	pulse pressure		
	push pills	PPD-B	purified protein derivative, Battey
P-P	probability-probability (plots)		
		PPDR	preproliferative diabetic retinopathy
P&P	pins and plaster		
	policy and procedure	PPD-S	purified protein derivative, standard

PPE	palmar-plantar erythrodysesthesia (syndrome)	PPLOV	painless progressive loss of vision
	personal protective equipment	PPM	parts per million
			permanent pacemaker
	professional performance evaluation		persistent pupillary membrane
	pruritic papular eruption		physician practice management
PPES	palmar-plantar erythrodysesthesia syndrome	PPMA	postpoliomyelitis muscular atrophy
	pedal pulses equal and strong	PPMS	psychophysiologic musculoskeletal (reaction)
PPF	pellagra preventive factor	PPN	peripheral parenteral nutrition
	plasma protein fraction		
PPG	photoplethysmography	PPNAD	primary pigmented nodular adrenocortical disease
	postprandial glucose		
	pylorus-preserving gastrectomy	PPNG	penicillinase producing *Neisseria gonorrhoeae*
PPGI	psychophysiologic gastrointestinal (reaction)	PPO	prefered provider organization
PPH	postpartum hemorrhage	PPOB	postpartum obstetrics
	primary postpartum hemorrhage	PPP	patient prepped and positioned
	primary pulmonary hypertension		pearly penile papules
PPHN	persistent pulmonary hypertension of the newborn		pedal pulse present
			peripheral pulses palpable (present)
PPHx	previous psychiatric history		platelet-poor plasma
			postpartum psychosis
PPIX	protoporphyrin nine		preferred practice patterns
PPI	patient package insert		proportional pulse pressure (SBP minus DBP)/SBP
	permanent pacemaker insertion		
	prepulse inhibition		protamine paracoagulation phenomenon
	Present Pain Intensity	PPPBL	peripheral pulses palpable both legs
	proton-pump inhibitor		
PPIVMs	passive physiological intervertebral movements	PPPD	pylorus-preserving pancreatoduodenectomy
PPJ	pure pancreatic juice	PPPG	postprandial plasma glucose
PPK	population pharmacokinetics	PPPM	Parents' Postoperative Pain Measure
PPL	pars plana lensectomy		per patient, per month
Ppl	pleural pressure	PPQ	Postoperative Pain Questionnaire
PPLO	pleuropneumonia-like organisms	PPR	patient progress record

P

PPr	periodontal prophylactics	patient relations
PPRC	Physician Payment Review Commission	per rectum
		pityriasis rosea
PPROM	prolonged premature rupture of membranes	premature
		profile
pPROM	premature rupture of the membranes before 37 weeks gestation	progressive resistance
		prolonged remission
		prone
PPS	peripheral pulmonary stenosis	Protestant
		Puerto Rican
	postpartum sterilization	pulmonic regurgitation
	postperfusion syndrome	pulse rate
	postpoliomyelitis syndrome	P=R pupils equal in size and reaction
	postpump syndrome	P & R pelvic and rectal
	prospective payment system	pulse and respiration
		PR-2 Bennett pressure ventilator
	pulses per second	
PPSS	peripheral protein sparing solution	PRA panel reactive antibodies (organ transplants)
PPT	person, place, and time	percent reactive antibody
	Physical Performance Test	
	posterior pelvic tilt	plasma renin activity
PPTL	postpartum tubal ligation	PRAFO pressure relief ankle-foot orthosis
PPU	perforated peptic ulcer	
PPV	pars plana vitrectomy	PRAT platelet radioactive antiglobulin test
	patent processus vaginalis	PRBC packed red blood cells
	pneumococcal polysaccharide vaccine	PRC packed red cells
	positive predictive value	peer review committee
	positive-pressure ventilation	PRCA pure red cell aplasia
		PrCa prostate cancer
PPVT	Peabody Picture Vocabulary Test	PRD polycystic renal disease
		PRE passive resistance exercises
PPW	plantar puncture wound	
PPY	packs per year (cigarettes)	progressive resistive exercise
PQ	pronator quadratus	
pQCT	peripheral quantitative computed tomography	proton relaxation enhancement
PQOCN	Psychiatric Questionnaire Obsessive-Compulsive Neurosis	Pred prednisone
		PREG Pregestimil® (infant formula)
PQRI	Product Quality Research Initiative	Pre-M urine specimen before prostate massage
PR	far point of accommodation	PREMIE premature infant
		pre-op before surgery
	pack removal	prep prepare for surgery
	partial remission	preposition

PRERLA	pupils round, equal, react to light and accommodation		protein
			prothrombin
		prob	probable
prev	prevent	PROCTO	procotoscopic
	previous		proctology
PRFD	percutaneous radio-frequency denervation	PROG	prognathism
			prognosis
PRFNB	percutaneous radio-frequency facet nerve block		program
			progressive
		PROM	passive range of motion
PRG	phleborheogram		premature rupture of membranes
PRH	past relevant history		
	postocclusive reactive hyperemia	ProMACE	prednisone, methotrexate, calcium leucovorin, doxorubicin (Adriamycin), cyclophosphamide, and etoposide
	preretinal hemorrhage		
PRI	Pain Rating Index		
	Patient Review Instrument		
prim	primary		
PRIMIP	primipara (1st pregnancy)	PROMM	passive range of motion machine
PR interval	part of the electrocardio-graphic cycle from onset of atrial depolarization on onset of ventricular depolarization		
		Promy	promyelocyte
		PRO MYELO	promyelocytes
		PRON	pronation
		PROS	prostate
PRISM	Pediatric Risk of Mortality Score		prosthesis
		PROT REL	protrusive relationship
PRIT®	pretargeted radioimmunotherapy	prov	provisional
		PROVIMI	proteins, vitamins, and minerals
PRK	photorefractive keratectomy		
		PROX	proximal
PRL	prolactin	PRP	panretinal photocoagulation
PRLA	pupils react to light and accommodation		
			patient recovery plan
PRM	partial rebreathing mask		penicllinase-resistant penicillin
	passive range of motion		
	phosphoribomutase		penicillin-resistant pneumococci
	photoreceptor membrane		
	prematurely ruptured membrane		pityriasis rubra pilaris
			platelet rich plasma
	primidone		polyribose ribitol phosphate
PRMF	preretinal macular fibrosis		
PRM-SDX	pyrimethamine; sulfadoxine (Fansidar)		poor progression of R wave in precordial leads
PRN	as occasion requires		
PRO	Professional Review Organization		progressive rubella panencephalitis
	proline		
	pronation	PrP	prion protein

P

PRP-D	*Haemophilus influenzae,* type b diphtheria conjugate vaccine		pressure sore pressure support protective services
PRPP	5-phosphoribosyl-1-pyrophosphate		pulmonary stenosis pyloric stenosis
PRP-T	polysaccharide tetanus conjugate vaccine		pyrimethamine; sulfadoxine (Fansidar)
PRRE	pupils round, regular, and equal		serum from pregnant women
PRRERLA	pupils round, regular, equal; react to light and accommodation	P/S	polyunsaturated to saturated fatty acids ratio
PRS	prolonged respiratory support	P & S	pain and suffering paracentesis and suction
PRSL	potential renal solute load		permanent and stationary
PRSP	penicillinase-resistant synthetic penicillins penicillin-resistant *Streptococcus pneumoniae*	PS I	healthy patient with localized pathological process
		PS II	a patient with mild to moderate systemic disease
PRSs	positive rolandic spikes		
PRST	Blood Pressure, Heart Rate, Sweating, and Tears (scale to assess analgesic needs)	PS III	a patient with severe systemic disease limiting activity but not incapacitating
PRT	pelvic radiation therapy protamine response test	PS IV	a patient with incapacitating systemic disease
PRTCA	percutaneous rotational transluminal coronary angioplasty	PS V	moribund patient not expected to live (These are American
PRTH-C	prothrombin time control		Society of
PRV	polycythemia rubra vera		Anesthesiologists'
PRVEP	pattern reversal visual evoked potentials		physical status patient classifications.
PRW	past relevant work polymerized ragweed		Emergency operations are designated by "E"
PRX	panoramic facial x-ray		after the classification.)
PRZF	pyrazofurin		
PS	paradoxic sleep	PSA	polysubstance abuse
	paranoid schizophrenia		product selection allowed
	pathologic stage		prostate-specific antigen
	patient's serum	PsA	psoriatic arthritis
	performance status	PSAB	pretreatment prostate-specific antigen
	peripheral smear		
	physical status	PSAD	prostate-specific antigen density
	plastic surgery (surgeon)		
	polysulfone (filter)	PSADT	prostate-specific antigen doubling time
	posterior synechiae		
	posterior synechiotomy	PSAG	*Pseudomonas aeruginosa*

PSAV	prostate-specific antigen velocity	PSIC	pediatric surgical intensive care
PSBO	partial small bowel obstruction	PSIG	pounds per square inch gauge
PSC	Pediatric Symptom Checklist	PSIS	posterior superior iliac spine
	percutaneous suprapubic cystostomy	PSM	presystolic murmur
	posterior subcapsular cataract	PSMA	personal self-maintenance activities
	primary sclerosing cholangitis		progressive spinal muscular atrophy
	pronation spring control		prostate-specific membrane antigen
	pubosacrococcygeal (diameter)	PSMF	protein-sparing modified fasting (Blackburn diet)
PSCC	posterior subcapsular cataract	PSM-R	Optimism-Pessimism Scale, revised
PSC Cat	posterior subcapsular cataract	PSMS	Physical Self Maintenance Scale
PSCH	peripheral stem cell harvest	PSNP	progressive supranuclear palsy
PSCP	posterior subcapsular precipitates	PSO	pelvic stabilization orthosis
PSCT	peripheral stem cell transplant		physician supplemental order
PSCU	pediatric special care unit		Polysporin ointment
PSD	pilonidal sinus disease		proximal subungual onychomycosis
	poststroke depression		
	power spectral density	pSO_2	arterial oxygen saturation
	psychosomatic disease	P/sore	pressure sore
PSDS	palmar surface desensitization	PSP	pancreatic spasmolytic peptide
PSE	portal systemic encephalopathy		phenolsulfonphthalein
	pseudoephedrine		photostimulable phosphor
PSF	posterior spinal fusion		progressive supranuclear palsy
PSG	peak systolic gradient		
	polysomnogram	PSPDV	posterior superior pancreaticoduodenal vein
	portosystemic gradient		
PSGN	poststreptococcal glomerulonephritis	PSR	Psychiatric Status Rating (scale)
PSH	past surgical history	PSRA	pressure sore risk assessment
	postspinal headache		
PSHx	past surgical history	PSRBOW	premature spontaneous rupture of bag of waters
PSI	Physiologic Stability Index	PSReA	poststreptococcal reactive arthritis
	pounds per square inch	PSRT	photostress recovery test
	punctate subepithelial infiltrate	PSS	painful shoulder syndrome

P

pediatric surgical service

physiologic saline solution (0.9% sodium chloride)

progressive systemic sclerosis

PSSP penicillin-sensitive *Streptococcus pneumoniae*

PST paroxysmal supraventricular tachycardia
Patient Service Technician
platelet survival time
postural stress test

PSTT placental site trophoblastic tumor

PSU pseudomonas (*P. aeruginosa*) vaccine

PSUD psychoactive substance use disorder

PSUR periodic safety update reporting

PSV peak systolic velocity
pressure supported ventilation

PSVT paroxysmal supraventricular tachycardia

PSW psychiatric social worker

PSWF positive sharp wave fibrillations (electromyograph)

PSY presexual youth

PSZ pseudoseizures

PT cisplatin (Platinol AQ)
parathormone
parathyroid
paroxysmal tachycardia
patient
phage type
phenytoin (Dilantin)
phototoxicity
physical therapy
pine tar
pint
posterior tibial
preterm
pronator teres
prothrombin time

Pt platinum

P/T pain and tenderness
piperacillin/tazobactam (Zosyn®)

P1/2T pressure one-half time

P&T pain and tenderness
paracentesis and tubing (of ears)
peak and trough
permanent and total
Pharmacy and Therapeutics (Committee)

PTA patellar tendon autograft
percutaneous transluminal angioplasty
Physical Therapy Assistant
plasma thromboplastin antecedent
post-traumatic amnesia
pretreatment anxiety
prior to admission
pure-tone average

PTAB popliteal-tibial artery bypass

PTAS percutaneous transluminal angioplasty with stent placement

PTB patellar tendon bearing
prior to birth
pulmonary tuberculosis

PTBA percutaneous transluminal balloon angioplasty

PTBD percutaneous transhepatic biliary drain (drainage)

PTBD-EF percutaneous transhepatic biliary drainage—enteric feeding

PTBS post-traumatic brain syndrome

PTB-SC-SP patellar tendon bearing-supracondylar-suprapatellar

PTC patient to call
percutaneous transhepatic cholangiography
plasma thromboplastin components

	post-tetanic count	PTER	percutaneous transluminal endomyocardial revascularization
	premature tricuspid closure		
	prior to conception	PTF	patient transfer form
	pseudotumor cerebri		pentoxifylline
PT-C	prothrombin time control		post-tetanic facilitation
PTCA	percutaneous transluminal coronary angioplasty	PTFE	polytetrafluoroethylene
		PTG	parathyroid gland
PTCDLF	pregnancy, term, complicated delivered, living female		photoplethysmogram
		PTGBD	percutaneous transhepatic gallbladder drainage
PTCDLM	pregnancy, term, complicated delivered, living male	PTH	parathyroid hormone
			post-transfusion hepatitis
			prior to hospitalization
PTCL	peripheral T-cell lymphoma	PTHC	percutaneous transhepatic cholangiography
PTCR	percutaneous transluminal coronary recanalization	PTHrP	parathyroid hormone-related protein
		PTHS	post-traumatic hyperirritability syndrome
PTCRA	percutaneous transluminal coronary rotational atherectomy		
		PTI	pressure-time integral
PTD	percutaneous transpedicular diskectomy	PTJV	percutaneous transtracheal jet ventilation
		PTK	phototherapeutic keratectomy
	period to discharge		
	permanent and total disability	PTL	preterm labor
			pudding-thick liquid (diet consistency)
	persistent trophoblastic disease		Sodium Pentothal
		PTLD	post-transplantation lymphoproliferative disorder (disease)
	pharmacy to dose		
	pharyngotracheal duct		
	prior to delivery	PTM	patient monitored
PTDM	post-transplant diabetes mellitus		posterior trabecular meshwork
PTDP	permanent transvenous demand pacemaker	PTMC	percutaneous transvenous mitral commissurotomy
PTE	pretibial edema	PTMDF	pupils, tension, media, disk, and fundus
	proximal tibial epiphysis		
		PTMR	percutaneous transmyocardial revascularization
	pulmonary thromboembolectomy		
	pulmonary thromboembolism	PT-NANB	post-transfusion non-A, non-B (hepatitis C)
PTE-4®	trace metal elements injection (there is also a #5 and #6)	PTNB	preterm newborn
		pTNM	postsurgical resection-pathologic staging of cancer
PTED	pulmonary thromboembolic disease		

P

269

PTO	part-time occlusion (eye patch)	PTV	posterior tibial vein
	please turn over	PTWTKG	patient's weight in kilograms
	proximal tubal obstruction	PTX	paclitaxel (Taxol)
PTP	posterior tibial pulse		parathyroidectomy
	post-transfusion purpura		pelvic traction
PTPM	post-traumatic progressive myelopathy		pentoxifylline (Trental)
			phototherapy
PTPN	peripheral (vein) total parenteral nutrition		pneumothorax
		PTZ	pentylenetetrazol
P to P	point to point		phenothiazine
PTR	paratesticular rhabdomyosarcoma	PU	pelvic-ureteric
			pelviureteral
	patella tendon reflex		peptic ulcer
	patient to return		pregnancy urine
	prothrombin time ratio	P & U	Pharmacia & Upjohn Company
PT-R	prothrombin time ratio		
PTRA	percutaneous transluminal renal angioplasty	PUA	pelvic (examination) under anesthesia
PTS	patellar tendon suspension	PUB	pubic
	Pediatric Trauma Score	PUBS	percutaneous umbilical blood sampling
	permanent threshold shift		
	prior to surgery	PUC	pediatric urine collector
PTSD	post-traumatic stress disorder	PUD	partial upper denture
			peptic ulcer disease
PTT	partial thromboplastin time		percutaneous ureteral dilatation
	platelet transfusion therapy	PUE	pyrexia of unknown etiology
	protein truncation testing	PUF	pure ultrafiltration
PTT-C	partial thromboplastin time control	PUFA	polyunsaturated fatty acids
PTTG	pituitary tumor transforming gene	PUFFA	polyunsaturated free fatty acids
PTTW	patient tolerated traction well	pul.	pulmonary
		PULP	pulpotomy
PTU	pain treatment unit	Pulse A	pulse apical
	pregnancy, term, uncomplicated	PULSE OX	pulse oximetry
	propylthiouracil	Pulse R	pulse radial
PTUCA	percutaneous transluminal ultrasonic coronary angioplasty	PULSES	(physical profile) physical condition, upper limb functions, lower limb functions, sensory components, excretory functions, and support factors
PTUDLF	pregnancy, term, uncomplicated delivered, living female		
PTUDLM	pregnancy, term, uncomplicated delivered, living male	PUN	plasma urea nitrogen

PUND	pregnancy, uterine, not delivered
PUNL	percutaneous ultrasonic nephrolithotripsy
PUO	pyrexia of unknown origin
PUP	percutaneous ultrasonic pyelolithotomy
PU/PL	partial upper and lower dentures
PUPPP	pruritic urticarial papules and plaque of pregnancy
PUS	percutaneous ureteral stent preoperative ultrasound
PUU	Puumala hantavirus
PUV	posterior urethral valves
PUVA	psoralen-ultraviolet-light (treatment)
PUW	pick-up walker
PV	papillomavirus
	Parvovirus
	per vagina
	plasma volume
	polio vaccine
	polycythemia vera
	popliteal vein
	portal vein
	postvoiding
	prenatal vitamins
	projectile vomiting
	pulmonary vein
P & V	peak and valley (this is a dangerous abbreviation, use peak and trough)
	pyloroplasty and vagotomy
PVA	polyvinyl alcohol
	Prinzmetal's variant angina
PVAD	prolonged venous access devices
PVAM	potential visual acuity meter
PVAR	pulmonary vein atrial reversal
PVB	cisplatin, (Platinol AQ) vinblastine, and bleomycin

	paravertebral block
	porcelain veneer bridge
	premature ventricular beat
PVC	paclitaxel, vinblastine, and cisplatin
	polyethylene vacuum cup
	polyvinyl chloride
	porcelain veneer crown
	postvoiding cystogram
	premature ventricular contraction
	pulmonary venous congestion
$Pv\text{co}_2$	partial pressure (tension) of carbon dioxide, vein
PVD	patient very disturbed
	peripheral vascular disease
	posterior vitreous detachment
	premature ventricular depolarization
PVDA	prednisone, vincristine, daunorubicin, and asparaginase
PVDF	polyvinyl difluoride
PVE	perivenous encephalomyelitis
	premature ventricular extrasystole
	prosthetic value endocarditis
P vera	polycythemia vera
PVF	peripheral visual field
PVFS	postviral fatigue syndrome
PVGM	perifoveolar vitreoglial membrane
PVH	periventricular hemorrhage
	periventricular hyperintensity
	pulmonary vascular hypertension
PVI	pelvic venous incompetence
	peripheral vascular insufficiency
	portal-vein infusion
PVK	penicillin V potassium

P

PVL	peripheral vascular laboratory		peripheral vascular surgery
	periventricular leukomalacia		peritoneovenous shunt
PVM	paraverteabral muscle		persistent vegetative state
	proteins, vitamins, and minerals		Plummer-Vinson syndrome
PVMS	paravertebral muscle spasms		pulmonic valve stenosis
		PVT	paroxysmal ventricular tachycardia
PVN	peripheral venous nutrition		previous trouble
PVNS	pigmented villonodular synovitis		private
			proximal vein thrombosis
PVO	peripheral vascular occlusion	PVTT	tumor thrombus in the portal vein
	portal vein occlusion	PVV	persistent varicose veins
	pulmonary venous occlusion	PW	pacing wires
PVo	pulmonary valve opening		patient waiting
Pvo$_2$	partial pressure (tension) of oxygen, vein		plantar wart
	peripheral vascular occlusive disease		posterior wall
			pulse width
			puncture wound
PVOD	pulmonary vascular obstructive disease	P&W	pressures and waves
		PWA	persons with AIDS
PVP	cisplatin (Platinol AQ) and etoposide (Ve Pesid)	P wave	part of the electrocardiographic cycle representing atrial depolarization
	penicillin V potassium	PWB	partial weight bearing
	peripheral venous pressure		Positive Well-being (scale)
	polyvinylpyrrolidone		psychological well-being
	posteroventral pallidotomy	PWBL	partial weight bearing, left
P-VP-B	cisplatin (Platinol AQ), etoposide (VP-16), and bleomycin	PWBR	partial weight bearing, right
PVR	peripheral vascular resistance	PWCA	personal watercraft accident
	perspective volume rendering	PWD	patients with diabetes
	postvoiding residual		person(s) with a disability
	proliferative vitreoretinopathy		powder
		PWE	people with epilepsy
	pulmonary vascular resistance	PWI	pediatric walk-in clinic
	pulse-volume recording		perfusion-weighted (magnetic resonance) imaging
PVRI	pulmonary vascular resistance index		posterior wall infarct
PVS	percussion, vibration and suction	PWLV	posterior wall of left ventricle
		PWM	pokeweed mitogens

PWMI	posterior wall myocardial infarction		**Q**
PWO	persistent withdrawal occlusion		
PWP	pulmonary wedge pressure	Q	every
PWS	port-wine stain		quadriceps
	Prader-Willi syndrome	QA	quality assurance
PWTd	posterior wall thickness at end-diastole	QAC	before every meal (this is a dangerous abbreviation)
PWV	polistes wasp venom	QALE	quality-adjusted life expectancy
	pulse-wave velocity	QALYs	quality-adjusted life years
Px	physical exam	QAM	every morning (this is a dangerous abbreviation)
	pneumothorax		
	prognosis	QAS	quality-adjusted survival
	prophylaxis	QB	blood flow
PXAT	paroxysmal atrial tachycardia	QC	quad cane
			quality control
PXE	pseudoxanthoma elasticum		quick catheter
PXF	pseudoexfoliation	QCA	quantitative coronary angiography
PXL	paclitaxel (Taxol)		
PXS	dental prophylaxis (cleaning)	Q compound	Chinese cucumber
PY	pack years (see pk yrs)	QCT	quantitative computed tomography
PYE	person-years of exposure		
PYHx	packs per year history	QD	dialysate flow
PYLL	potential years of life lost		every day (this is a dangerous abbreviation as it is read as four times daily-QID)
PYP	pyrophosphate		
PYP®	technetium Tc 99m pyrophosphate kit		
PZ	peripheral zone	QDAM	once daily in the morning
PZA	pyrazinamide	QDPM	once daily in the evening
	pyrazoloacridine (a drug class of sidatine/hyponotics)	QDS	United Kingdom abbreviation for four times a day
PZD	partial zona drilling	QE	quinidine effect
	partial zonal dissection	QED	every even day (this is a dangerous abbreviation as it will be read as four times daily-QID)
PZI	protamine zinc insulin		
			quick and early diagnosis
		QEE	quadriceps extension exercise
		QFV	Q fever (*Coxiella burnetii*) vaccine
		q4h	every four hours
		qh	every hour

qhs	every night (this is a dangerous abbreviation as it is read as every hour-QHR and four times daily-QID)	qohs	every other night (this is a dangerous abbreviation as it is not recognized)
		QOL	quality of life
QIAD	Quantitative Inventory of Alcohol Disorders	QOLIE-31	quality of life in epilepsy
		QOM	quality of motion
QID	four times daily	QON	every other night (this is a dangerous abbreviation)
QIDM	four times daily with meals and at bedtime	qpm	every evening (this is a dangerous abbreviation)
QIG	quantitative immunoglobulins	QPOS	Quality Point of Service
		QP/QS	ratio of pulmonary blood to systemic blood flow
QIW	four times a week (this is a dangerous abbreviation)	*QQH*	United Kingdom abbreviation for every four hours
QJ	quadriceps jerk	QR	quiet room
QKD interval	Korotkoff sounds	QRC	qualitative radiocardiography
QL	quality of life	QRE	quality-related event
QLI	Quality of Life Index	QRNG	quinolone-resistant *N. gonorrhoeae*
QLS	quality of life score		
QM	every morning (this is a dangerous abbreviation as it will not be understood)	QRS	part of electrocardiographic wave representing ventricular depolarization
QMB	qualified Medicare beneficiary	QS	every shift quadriceps set quadrilateral socket sufficient quantity
QMI	Q wave myocardial infarction		
QMRP	qualified mental retardation professional	*qs ad*	a sufficient quantity to make
QMT	quantitative muscle testing	QS&L	quarters, subsistence, and laundry
q.n.	every night (this is a dangerous abbreviation as it is read as every hour)	Qs/Qt	intrapulmonary shunt fraction
		QSP	physiological shunt fraction
q.n.s.	quantity not sufficient	qt	quart
qod	every other day (this is a dangerous abbreviation as it is read as every day or four times a day-QID)	QTB	quadriceps tendon bearing
		QTC	quantitative tip cultures
		QTL	quantitative trait locus
		Q-TWiST	quality-adjusted time without symptoms (of disease) and toxicity
qoh	every other hour (this is a dangerous abbreviation as it is read as every day or four times a day-QID)	QUAD	quadrant quadriceps quadriplegic
		QU	quiet

QUART	quadrantectomy, axillary dissection, and radiotherapy
QUS	quantitative (bone) ultrasound
QW	every week (this is a dangerous abbreviation)
QWB	Quality of Well-Being (scale)
QWE	every weekend (this is a dangerous abbreviation)
QWK	once a week (this is a dangerous abbreviation)
Q4wk	every four weeks (this is a dangerous abbreviation)

R

R	radial
	rate
	ratio
	reacting
	rectal
	rectum
	regular
	regular insulin
	resistant
	respiration
	reticulocyte
	retinoscopy
	right
	roentgen
	rub
r	recombinant
(R)	registered trademark
	right
−R	Rinne's test, negative
+R	Rinne's test, positive
RA	radiographic absorptiometry
	rales
	readmission
	renal artery
	repeat action
	retinoic acid
	rheumatoid arthritis
	right arm
	right atrium
	right auricle
	room air
	rotational atherectomy
RAA	renin-angiotensin-aldosterone
	right atrial abnormality
RAAS	renin-angiotensin-aldosterone system
RAB	rabies vaccine, not otherwise specified
	rice (rice cereal), applesauce, and banana (diet)

275

RAB_DEV	rabies vaccine, duck embryo culture	RAIT	radioimmunotherapy
		RAIU	radioactive iodine uptake
RAB_FRhL-2	rabies vaccine, diploid fetal-rhesus-lung-2 cell line	RALT	routine admission laboratory tests
		RAM	radioactive material
RABG	room air blood gas		rapid alternating movements
RAB_HDCV	rabies vaccine, human diploid cell culture		rectus abdominis myocutaneous
RAB_PCEC	rabies vaccine, purified chick embryo cell culture	RAN	resident's admission notes
RAC	right antecubital right atrial catheter	R₂AN	second year resident's admission notes
RACCO	right anterior caudocranial oblique	RANTES	regulated upon activation, normal T cell expressed and secreted
RACT	recalcified whole-blood activated clotting time	RAO	right anterior oblique
RAD	ionizing radiation unit radical radiology reactive airway disease right axis deviation	RAP	right abdominal pain right atrial pressure
		RAPA	radial artery pseudoaneurysm
		RAQ	right anterior quadrant
RADCA	right anterior descending coronary artery	RAP	recurrent abdominal pain Resident Assessment Protocol
RADISH	rheumatoid arthritis diffuse idiopathic skeletal hyperostosis	RAPD	random amplified polymorphic DNA relative afferent pupillary defect
RADS	ionizing radiation units rapid assay delivery systems reactive airway disease syndrome	RAPs	Resident Assessment Protocols
		RAR	right arm, reclining
RAE	right atrial enlargement	RARs	retinoic acid receptors
RAEB	refractory anemia, erythroblastic	RAS	recurrent aphthous stomatitis renal artery stenosis renin-angiotensin system reticular activating system right arm, sitting
RAEB-T	refractory anemia with excess blasts in transition		
RAF	rapid atrial fibrillation		
RAFF	rectus abdominis free flap	RASE	rapid-acquisition spin echo
RAFT	Rehabilitative Addicted Family Treatment	RAST	radioallergosorbent test
RAG	room air gas	RAT	right anterior thigh
RAH	right atrial hypertrophy	RA test	test for rheumatoid factor
RAHB	right anterior hemiblock	RATG	rabbit antithymocyte globulin
rAHF	antihemophilic factor (recombinant)	RATx	radiation therapy
RAI	Resident Assessment Instrument	RAU	recurrent aphthous ulcers
RAID	radioimmunodetection	RAVLT	Rey Auditory Verbal Learning Test

R

276

R(AW)	airway resistance	
RB	relieved by	
	retinoblastoma	
	retrobulbar	
	right breast	
	right buttock	
R & B	right and below	
RBA	right basilar artery	
	right brachial artery	
	risks, benefits, and alternatives (discussion with patient)	
RBB	right breast biopsy	
RBBB	right bundle branch block	
RBBX	right breast biopsy examination	
RBC	ranitidine bismuth citrate	
	red blood cell (count)	
RBCD	right border cardiac dullness	
RBCM	red blood cell mass	
RBC s/f	red blood cells spun filtration	
RBCV	red blood cell volume	
RBD	REM (rapid eye movement sleep) behavior disorder	
	right border of dullness	
RBE	relative biologic effectiveness	
RBF	renal blood flow	
RBG	random blood glucose	
RBILD	respiratory bronchiolitis-associated interstitial lung disease	
RBL	Roche Biomedical Laboratory	
RBON	retrobulbar optic neuritis	
RBOW	rupture bag of water	
RBP	retinol-binding protein	
RBRVS	Medicare resource-based relative-value scale	
RBS	random blood sugar	
RBT	rational behavior therapy	
RBV	right brachial vein	
RBVO	right brachial vein occlusion	
RC	race	

	radiocarpal (joint)
	Red Cross
	report called
	retrograde cystogram
	retruded contact (position)
	right coronary
	Roman Catholic
	root canal
	rotator cuff
R/C	reclining chair
R & C	reasonable and customary
RCA	radiographic contrast agent
	radionuclide cerebral angiogram
	right carotid artery
	right coronary artery
	root cause analysis
RCBF	regional cerebral blood flow
RCC	rape crisis center
	renal cell carcinoma
	Roman Catholic Church
RCCA	right common carotid artery
RCCT	randomized controlled clinical trial
RCD	relative cardiac dullness
RCE	right carotid endarterectomy
RCF	Reiter complement fixation
RCF®	enteral nutrition product
RCFA	right common femoral angioplasty
	right common femoral artery
RCFE	residential care facility for the elderly
RCH	residential care home
RCHF	right-sided congestive heart failure
RCIP	rape crisis intervention program
RCL	range of comfortable loudness
RCM	radiographic contrast media
	restricted cardiomyopathy

R

	retinal capillary microaneurysm		Registered Dental Assistant
	right costal margin		representational difference analysis
RCOG	Royal College of Obstetricians and Gynaecologists	RDB	randomized double-blind (trial)
RCP	respiratory care plan	RDCS	Registered Diagnostic Cardiac Sonographer
	retrograde cerebral perfusion	RDD	renal dose dopamine
	Royal College of Physicians	RDE	remote data entry
RCPM	raven colored progressive matrices	RDEA	right deviation of electrical axis
RCPT	Registered Cardiopulmonary Technician	RDG	right dorsogluteal
		RDH	Registered Dental Hygienist
RCR	replication-competent retrovirus (assay)	RDI	respiratory disturbance index
	rotator cuff repair	RDIH	right direct inguinal hernia
RCS	repeat cesarean section	RDLBBB	rate-dependent left bundle branch block
	reticulum cell sarcoma		
	Royal College of Surgeons	RDM	right deltoid muscle
RCT	randomized clinical trial	RDMS	Registered Diagnostic Medical Sonographer
	Registered Care Technologist	RDMs	reactive drug metabolites
	root canal therapy	RDOD	retinal detachment, right eye
	Rorschach Content Test		
RCU	respiratory care unit	RDOS	retinal detachment, left eye
RCV	red cell volume		
	right colic vein	RDP	random donor platelets
RCX	ramus circumflexus		right dorsoposterior
RD	radial deviation	RDPE	reticular degeneration of the pigment epithelium
	Raynaud's disease		
	reaction of degeneration	RDS	research diagnostic criteria
	reflex decay		respiratory distress syndrome
	Registered Dietitian		
	renal disease	RDT	regular dialysis (hemodialysis) treatment
	respiratory disease		
	respiratory distress		
	restricted duty	RDTD	referral, diagnosis, treatment, and discharge
	retinal detachment		
	Reye's disease		
	rhabdomyosarcoma	RDU	recreational drug use
	right deltoid	RDVT	recurrent deep vein thrombosis
	ruptured disk		
RDA	recommended daily allowance	RDW	red (cell) distribution width

R

RE	concerning	regurg	regurgitation
	Rasmussen's encephalitis	rehab	rehabilitation
	rectal examination	REL	relative
	reflux esophagitis		religion
	regarding	RELE	resistive exercise, lower
	regional enteritis		extremities
	reticuloendothelial	REM	rapid eye movement
	retinol equivalents		recent event memory
	right ear		remarried
	right eye		remission
	rowing ergometer		roentgen equivalent unit
^{186}Re	rhenium 186	REMS	rapid eye movement sleep
R & E	rest and exercise	REO	respiratory and enteric
	round and equal		orphan (viruses)
R ↑ E	right upper extremity	REP	rapid electrophoresis
R ↓ E	right lower extremity		repair
RE✓	recheck		repeat
READM	readmission		report
REAL	Revised European	REP CK	rapid electrophoresis
	American Lymphoma		creatine kinase
	(classification)	REPL	recurrent early pregnancy
REALM	Rapid Estimation of Adult		loss
	Literacy in Medicine	repol	repolarization
REC	rear end collision	REPS	repetitions
	recommend	REPT	Registered Evoked
	record		Potential Technologist
	recovery	RER	renal excretion rate
	recreation	RER+	replication error positive
	recur	RES	recurrent erosion
RECA	right external carotid		syndrome
	artery		resection
RECT	rectum		resident
REDs	reproductive endocrine		reticuloendothelial system
	diseases	RESC	resuscitation
RED SUBS	reducing substances	RESP	respirations
REE	resting energy expenditure		respiratory
RE-ED	re-education	REST	restoration
R-EEG	resting		restriction of
	electroencephalogram		environmental
REEGT	Registered		stimulation therapy
	Electroencephalogram	RET	retention
	Technologist		reticulocyte
REF	referred		retina
	refused		retired
	renal erythropoietic factor		return
ref→	refer to		right esotropia
REG	radioencephalogram	ret detach	retinal detachment
	regression analysis	retic	reticulocyte
Reg block	regional block anesthesia	RETRO	retrograde

R

RETRX	retractions	RFLF	retained fetal lung fluid
REUE	resistive exercise, upper extremities	RFLP	restriction fragment length polymorphism (patterns)
REV	reverse	RFM	rifampin (Rifadin)
	review	RFP	Renal function panel (see page 358)
	revolutions		request for payment
RF	radiofrequency		request for proposal
	reduction fixation		right frontoposterior
	renal failure	RFS	rapid frozen section
	respiratory failure		refeeding syndrome
	restricted fluids		relapse-free survival
	rheumatic fever	RFT	right frontotransverse
	rheumatoid factor		routine fever therapy
	right foot	RFTC	radiofrequency thermocoagulation
	risk factor		
	radiofrequency	RFUT	radioactive fibrinogen uptake
R/F	retroflexed		
R&F	radiographic and fluoroscopic	RFV	reason for visit
			right femoral vein
RFA	radio-frequency ablation	RG	regurgitated (infant feeding)
	right femoral artery		
	right forearm		right (upper outer) gluteus
	right frontoanterior	R/G	red/green
RFB	retained foreign body	RGA	right gastroepiploic artery
	radial flow chromatography		
		RGM	recurrent glioblastoma multiforme
	residual functional capacity		
RFC	reduced folate carrier		right gluteus medius
RFD	residue-free diet	RGO	reciprocating gait orthosis
RFDT	Reach in Four Directions Test	RGP	rigid gas-permeable (contact lens)
RFE	return flow enema	Rh	Rhesus factor in blood
RFFIT	rapid fluorescent focus inhibition test	RH	reduced haloperidol
			relative humidity
rFVIII FS	antihemophilic factor (recombinant), formulated with sucrose (Kogenate)		rest home
			retinal hemorrhage
			right hand
			right hemisphere
RFg	visual fields by Goldmann-type perimeter		right hyperphoria
			room humidifier
RFIPC	Rating Form of IBD (inflammatory bowel disease) Patient Concerns	Rh+	Rhesus positive
		Rh−	Rhesus negative
		RHA	rheumatoid arthritis (therapeutic) vaccine
RFL	radionuclide functional lymphoscintigraphy		right hepatic artery
		rHA	recombinant human albumin
	right frontolateral		

R

rhAPC	recombinant human activated protein C	RHV	right hepatic vein
		RHW	radiant heat warmer
RHB	raise head of bed	RI	ramus intermedius
	right heart border		(coronary artery)
RH/BSO	radial hysterectomy and bilateral salpingo-oophorectomy		refractive index
			regular insulin
			relapse incidence
RHC	respiration has ceased		renal insufficiency
	right heart catheterization		respiratory illness
	right hemicolectomy		rooming in
	routine health care	RIA	radioimmunoassay
RHD	radial head dislocation	RIAT	radioimmune antiglobulin test
	relative hepatic dullness		
	rheumatic heart disease	RIBA	recombinant immunoblot assay
	right-hand dominant		
rh-DNase	dornase alfa (Pulmozyme)	RIC	right iliac crest
RHF	rheumatic fever vaccine		right internal carotid (artery)
	right heart failure		
RHG	right hand grip	RICA	right internal carotid artery
r-hGH(m)	mammalian-cell–derived recombinant human growth hormone (Serostim)		
		RICE	rest, ice, compression, and elevation
		RICM	right intercostal margin
RHH	right homonymous hemianopsia	RICS	right intercostal space
		RICU	respiratory intensive care unit
RHIA	Registered Health Information Administrator		
		RID	radial immunodiffusion
RHINO	rhinoplasty		ruptured intervertebral disk
RHIT	Registered Health Information Technician		
		RIE	radiation induced emesis
RHL	right hemisphere lesions		rocket immunoelectrophoresis
	right heptic lobe		
rhm	roentgens per hour at one meter	RIF	rifampin
			right iliac fossa
RHO	right heel off		right index finger
Rho(D)	immune globulin to an Rh-negative woman		rigid internal fixation
		RIG	rabies immune globulin
RhoGAM®	Rh$_O$ (D) immune globulin	RIGS	radioimmunoguided surgery
RHP	resting head pressure		
rhPDGF	recombinant human platelet-derived growth factor	RIH	right inguinal hernia
		RIJ	right internal jugular
		RIMA	reversible inhibitor of monoamine oxidase-type A
RHR	resting heart rate		
RHS	right hand side		right internal mammary anastamosis
RHT	right hypertropia		
rHuEPO	recombinant human erythropoietin		right internal mammary artery

R

RIND	reversible ischemic neurologic defect		right lateral border
		RLBCD	right lower border of cardiac dullness
RINV	radiation-induced nausea and vomiting	RLC	residual lung capacity
RIO	right inferior oblique (muscle)	RLD	related living donor
			right lateral decubitus
RIOJ	recurrent intrahepatic obstructive jaundice		ruptured lumbar disk
		RLDP	right lateral decubital position
R-IOL	remove intraocular lens		
RIP	radioimmunoprecipitin test	RLE	right lower extremity
		RLF	retrolental fibroplasia
	rapid infusion pump		right lateral femoral
	respiratory inductance plethysmograph	RLFP	Remaining Lifetime Fracture Probability
	rhythmic inhibitory pattern	RLG	right lateral gaze
		RLGS	restriction landmark genomic scanning
RIPA	ristocetin-induced platelet agglutination	RLH	reactive lymphoid hyperplasia
RIR	right inferior rectus		
RIS	responding to internal stimuli	RLL	right liver lobe
			right lower lid
RISA	radioactive iodinated serum albumin		right lower lobe
		RLN	recurrent laryngeal nerve
RIST	radioimmunosorbent test		regional lymph node(s)
RIT	radioimmunotherapy	RLND	regional lymph node dissection
	ritonavir (Norvir)		
	Rorschach Inkblot Test	RLQ	right lower quadrant
RITA	right internal thoracic artery	RLQD	right lower quadrant defect
RIVD	ruptured intervertebral disk	RLR	right lateral rectus
		RLRTD	recurrent lower respiratory tract disease
RIX	radiation-induced xerostomia	RLS	restless legs syndrome
RJ	radial jerk (reflex)		Ringer's lactate solution
	right jugular		stammerer who has difficulty in enunciating R, L, and S
RK	radial keratotomy		
	right kidney		
RKS	renal kidney stone	RLSB	right lower scapular border
RKT	Registered Kinesiotherapist		right lower sternal border
RL	right lateral	RLT	right lateral thigh
	right leg	RLTCS	repeat low transverse cesarean section
	right lower		
	right lung	RLUs	relative light units
	Ringer's lactate	RLWD	routine laboratory work done
	rotation left		
R → L	right to left	RLX	right lower extremity
RLA	right lower arm	RM	radical mastectomy
RLB	right lateral bending		repetitions maximum

	respiratory movement		repetitive motion
	risk manager		syndrome
	(management)		rhabdomyosarcoma
	risk model		Rocky Mountain spotted
	room		fever vaccine
R&M	routine and microscopic	RMS®	rectal morphine sulfate
1-RM	single repetition		(suppository)
	maximum lift	RMSB	right middle sternal
RMA	Registered Medical		border
	Assistant	RMSE	root mean square error
	right mentoanterior	RMSF	Rocky Mountain spotted
	Rivermead motor		fever
	assessment	RMT	Registered Music
RMB	right main bronchus		Therapist
RMBPC	Revise Memory and		right mentotransverse
	Behavior Problems	RMV	respiratory minute volume
	Checklist	RN	Registered Nurse
RMCA	right main coronary artery		right nostril (nare)
	right middle cerebral	Rn	radon
	artery	R/N	renew
RMCAT	right middle cerebral	RNA	radionuclide angiography
	artery thrombosis		ribonucleic acid
RMCL	right midclavicular line	RNC	Registered Nurse,
RMD	rippling muscle disease		Certified
RME	resting metabolic	RNCD	Registered Nurse,
	expenditure		Chemical Dependency
	right mediolateral	RNCNA	Registered Nurse
	episiotomy		Certified in Nursing
RMEE	right middle ear		Administration
	exploration	RNCNAA	Registered Nurse
rMET	recombinant		Certified in Nursing
	methioninase		Administration
RMF	right middle finger		Advanced
RMK #1	remark number 1	RNCS	Registered Nurse
RML	right mediolateral		Certified Specialist
	right middle lobe	RND	radical neck dissection
RMLE	right mediolateral	RNEF	resting (radio-) nuclide
	episiotomy		ejection fraction
RMO	responsible medical	RNF	regular nursing floor
	officer	RNFL	retinal nerve fiber layer
RMP	right mentoposterior	RNI	reactive nitrogen
RMR	resting metabolic rate		intermediates
	right medial rectus	RNLP	Registered Nurse, license
	root mean square residue		pending
RMRM	right modified radical	RNP	Registered Nurse
	mastectomy		Practitioner
RMS	red-man syndrome		restorative nursing
	Rehabilitation Medicine		program
	Service		ribonucleoprotein

R

RNS	replacement normal saline (0.9% sodium chloride)	ROMCP	range of motion complete and painfree
RNST	reactive nonstress test	ROMI	rule out myocardial infarction
RNUD	recurrent nonulcer dyspepsia	ROMSA	right otitis media, suppurative, acute
RO	reality orientation	ROMSC	right otitis media, suppurative, chronic
	relative odds	ROMWNL	range of motion within normal limits
	report of		
	reverse osmosis	ROP	retinopathy of prematurity
	routine order(s)		right occiput posterior
	Russian Orthodox	ROR	the French acronym for measles-mumps-rubella vaccine
R/O	rule out		
ROA	right occiput anterior		
ROAC	repeated oral doses of activated charcoal	R or L	right or left
		RoRx	radiation therapy
ROAD	reversible obstructive airway disease	ROS	review of systems
			rod outer segments
ROC	receiver operating characteristic	ROSA	rank-order stability analysis
	record of contact	ROSC	restoration of spontaneous circulation
	resident on call		
	residual organic carbon	ROSS	review of signs and symptoms
ROCF	Rey-Osterrieth complex figure	ROT	remedial occupational therapy
ROD	rapid opioid detoxification		right occipital transverse
			rotator
RODA	rapid opiate detoxification under anesthesia	ROU	recurrent oral ulcer
		ROUL	rouleaux (rouleau)
ROE	report of event	ROW	rest of (the) week
	right otitis externa	RP	radial pulse
ROF	review of outside films		radical prostatectomy
ROG	rogletimide		radiopharmaceutical
ROH	rubbing alcohol		Raynaud's phenomenon
ROI	region of interest		responsible party
	release of information		resting position
ROIDS	hemorrhoids		restorative proctocolectomy
ROIH	right oblique inguinal hernia		retinitis pigmentosa
			retrograde pyelogram
ROJM	range of joint motion		root plane
ROL	right occipitolateral	RPA	radial photon absorptiometry
ROLC	roentgenologically occult lung cancer		Registered Physician's Assistant
ROM	range of motion		
	rifampicin 600 mg, ofloxacin 400 mg, and minocycline 100 mg		restenosis postangioplasty
	right otitis media		
	rupture of membranes		
Romb	Romberg		

	ribonuclease protection assay	RPO	right posterior oblique
RPAC	right pulmonary artery	RPP	radical perineal prostatectomy
	Registered Physician's Assistant Certified		rate-pressure product
RPC	root planing and curettage		retropubic prostatectomy
RPCF	Reiter protein complement fixation	RPPS	retropatellar pain syndrome
RPD	removable partial denture	RPR	rapid plasma reagin (test for syphilis)
RPE	rating of perceived exertion		
	retinal pigment epithelium		Reiter protein reagin
RPED	retinal pigment epithelium detachment	RPT	Registered Physical Therapist
RPEP	rabies postexposure prophylaxis	RPTA	Registered Physical Therapist Assistant
	right pre-ejection period	RPU	retropubic urethropexy
RPF	relaxed pelvic floor	RPV	right portal vein
	renal plasma flow		right pulmonary vein
	retroperitoneal fibrosis	RQ	respiratory quotient
RPFT	Registered Pulmonary Function Technologist	RQLQ	Respiratory Quality of Life Questionnaire
RPG	retrograde percutaneous gastrostomy	RR	recovery room
			regular rate
	retrograde pyelogram		regular respirations
RPGN	rapidly progressive glomerulonephritis		relative risk
			respiratory rate
RPH	retroperitoneal hemorrhage		response rate
			retinal reflex
RPh	Registered Pharmacist		rotation right
RPHA	reverse passive hemagglutination	R/R	rales-rhonchi
		R&R	rate and rhythm
RPI	resting pressure index		recent and remote
	reticulocyte production index		recession and resection
RPICA	right posterior internal carotid artery		resect and recess (muscle surgery)
RPICCE	round pupil intracapsular cataract extraction		rest and recuperation
			remove and replace
RPL	retroperitoneal lymphadenectomy	RRA	radioreceptor assay
			Registered Record Administrator
RPLC	reversed-phase liquid chromatography		right radial artery
			right renal artery
RPLND	retroperitoneal lymph node dissection	RRAM	rapid rhythmic alternating movements
RPN	renal papillary necrosis		
	resident's progress notes	RRC	cohort relative risk
R₂PN	second year resident's progress notes	RRCT, no(m)	regular rate, clear tones, no murmurs

R

RRD	rhegmatogenous retinal detachment	right side
		Ringer's solution
RRE	round, regular, and equal (pupils)	rumination syndrome
		R/S	reschedule
RRED®	Rapid Rare Event Detection	rest stress
		rupture spontaneous
RREF	resting radionuclide ejection fraction	R & S	restraint and seclusion
		R/S I	resuscitation status one (full resuscitative effort)
RRI	renal resistive index	
RR-IOL	remove and replace intraocular lens	
RRM	reduced renal mass	R/S II	resuscitation status two (no code, therapeutic measures only)
	right radial mastectomy	
RRMS	relapsing-remitting multiple sclerosis	R/S III	resuscitation status three (no code, comfort measures only)
RRNA	Resident Registered Nurse Anesthetist	
		RSA	right sacrum anterior
rRNA	ribosomal ribonucleic acid		right subclavian artery
RRND	right radical neck dissection	RSAPE	remitting seronegative arthritis with pitting edema
RROM	resistive range of motion	
R rot	right rotation	RSB	right sternal border
RRP	radical retropubic prostatectomy	RSC	right subclavian (artery) (vein)
RRR	recovery room routine	RScA	right scapuloanterior
	regular rhythm and rate	RSCL	Rotterdam Symptom Check List
	relative risk reduction	
RRRN	round, regular, and react normally	RScP	right scapuloposterior
		RSCS	respiratory system compliance score
RRRsM	regular rate and rhythm without murmur	rscu-PA	recombinant, single-chain, urokinase-type plasminogen activator
RRT	Registered Respiratory Therapist	
RRU	rapid reintegration unit	
RRVO	repair relaxed vaginal outlet	RSD	reflex sympathetic dystrophy
		RSDS	reflex-sympathetic dystrophy syndrome
RRVS	recovery room vital signs	
RRV-TV	rhesus rotavirus tetravalent (vaccine)	RSE	reactive subdural effusion
		refractory status epilepticus
RRW	rales, rhonchi or wheezes		right sternal edge
RS	Raynaud's syndrome	RSI	rapid sequence intubation
	rectal swab		repetitive strain (stress) injury
	recurrent seizures	
	Reed-Sternberg (cell)	R-SICU	respiratory-surgical intensive care unit
	Reiter's syndrome	
	reschedule	RSL	renal solute load
	restart	
	Reye's syndrome	RSLR	reverse straight leg raise
	rhythm strip	

RSM	remote study monitoring		renal tubular acidosis
RSNI	round spermatid nuclear injection		road traffic accident
		t-RA	tretinoin (*trans*-retinoic acid)
RSO	right salpingooophorectomy	RTAE	right atrial enlargement
	right superior oblique	RTAH	right anterior hemiblock
rS$_{O2}$	regional oxygen saturation	RTAT	right anterior thigh
RSOP	right superior oblique palsy	RTB	return to baseline
		RTC	Readiness to Change (questionnaire)
RSP	rapid straight pacing		return to clinic
	right sacroposterior		round the clock
RSR	regular sinus rhythm	RTCA	ribavirin
	relative survival rate	RTER	return to emergency room
	right superior rectus		
RSRI	renal:systemic renin index	rt.↑ext.	right upper extremity
RSS	reduced space symbologies	RTF	ready-to-feed
			return to flow
	representative sample sectioned	RTFS	return to flying status
		RTI	respiratory tract infection
RSSE	Russian spring-summer encephalitis		reverse transcriptase inhibitor
RST	rapid simple tests	RTK	rhabdoid tumor of the kidney
	right sacrum transverse		
RSTs	Rodney Smith tubes	RTL	reactive to light
RSV	respiratory syncytial virus	RTLF	respiratory-tract lining fluids
	right subclavian vein		
RSVC	right superior vena cava	RTM	regression to the mean
RSV$_{IGIV}$	respiratory syncytial virus immune globulin, intravenous		routine medical care
		RTMD	right mid-deltoid
		rTMS	repetitive transcranial magnetic stimulation
RSV$_{mab}$	respiratory syncytial virus monoclonal antibody, intramuscular (palivizumab; Synagis)	RTN	renal tubular necrosis
		RTNM	retreatment staging of cancer
RSW	right-sided weakness	RTO	return to office
RT	radiation therapy	RTOG	Radiation Therapy Oncology Group
	Radiologic Technologist		
	recreational therapy	RTP	renal transplant patient
	rectal temperature		return to pharmacy
	renal transplant	rtPA	alteplase (recombinant tissue-type plasminogen activator) (Activase)
	repetition time		
	Respiratory Therapist		
	reverse transcriptase	RT-PCR	reverse transcription polymerase chain reaction
	right		
	right thigh		
	room temperature	RTR	renal transplant recipient(s)
R/t	related to		
RTA	ready to administer		return to room

R

RT (R)	Radiologic Technologist (Registered)	RUQD	right upper quadrant defect
RTRR	return to recovery room	RURTI	recurrent upper respiratory tract infection
RTS	radial tunnel syndrome		
	raised toilet seat		
	real-time scan	RUSB	right upper scapular border
	Resolve Through Sharing		
	return to school		right upper sternal border
	return to sender	RUT	rapid urease test
	Revised Trauma Score	RUV	residual urine volume
	Rubinstein-Taybi syndrome	RUX	right upper extremity
		RV	rectovaginal
RTT	Respiratory Therapy Technician		residual volume
			respiratory volume
RT$_3$U	resin triiodothyronine uptake		retinal vasculitis
			return visit
RTUS	realtime ultrasound		right ventricle
RTV	ritonavir (Norvir)		rubella vaccine
	rotavirus vaccine, not otherwise specified	RVA	rabies vaccine, adsorbed
			right ventricular apex
RTV$_{rr}$	rotavirus vaccine, rhesus reassortant		right vertebral artery
		RVAD	right ventricular assist device
RTW	return to ward		
	return to work	RVCD	right ventricular conduction deficit
	Richard Turner Warwick (urethroplasty)		
		RVD	relative vertebral density
RTWD	return to work determination		renal vascular disease
		RVDP	right ventricular diastolic pressure
RTX	resiniferatoxin		
RTx	radiation therapy	RVE	right ventricular enlargement
	renal transplantation		
RU	residual urine	RVEDP	right ventricular end-diastolic pressure
	resin uptake		
	retrograde ureterogram	RVEDV	right ventricular end-diastolic volume
	right upper		
	routine urinalysis	RVEF	right ventricular ejection fraction
RU 486	mifepristone (Mifeprex)		
RUA	right upper arm	RVET	right ventricular ejection time
	routine urine analysis		
RUB	rubella virus vaccine	RVF	Rift Valley fever
RUE	right upper extremity		right ventricular function
RUG	resource utilization group		right visual field
		RVG	radionuclide ventriculography
	retrograde urethrogram		
RUL	right upper lid		Radio VisioGraphy
	right upper lobe		right ventrogluteal
RUOQ	right upper outer quadrant	RVH	renovascular hypertension
rupt.	ruptured		right ventricular hypertrophy
RUQ	right upper quadrant		

RVHT	renovascular hypertension	radiotherapy
RVI	right ventricle infarction	take
RVIDd	right ventricle internal	therapy
	dimension diastole	treatment
RVL	right vastus lateralis	RXN reaction
RVO	relaxed vaginal outlet	RXT radiation therapy
	retinal vein occlusion	right exotropia
	right ventricular outflow	
	right ventricular	
	overactivity	
RVOT	right ventricular outflow	
	tract	
RVOTH	right ventricular outflow	
	tract hypertrophy	
RVP	right ventricular pressure	
RVR	rapid ventricular response	
	renal vascular resistance	
	right ventricular rhythm	
RVSP	right ventricular systolic	
	pressure	
RVSW	right ventricular stroke	
	work	
RVSWI	right ventricular stroke	
	work index	
RVT	recurrent ventricular	
	tachycardia	
	renal vein thrombosis	
RV/TLC	residual volume to total	
	lung capacity ratio	
RVU	relative-value units	
RVV	rubella vaccine virus	
RVVT	Russell's viper venom	
	time	
RW	radiant warmer	
	ragweed	
	red welt	
	rolling walker	
R/W	return to work	
RWM	regional wall motion	
RWMA	regional wall motion	
	abnormalities	
RWP	ragweed pollen	
RWS	ragweed sensitivity	
RWT	relative wall thickness	
RXRs	retinoid X receptors	
Rx	drug	
	medication	
	pharmacy	
	prescription	

R

S

S	sacral		substance abuse
	second (s)		suicide alert
	sensitive		suicide attempt
	serum		surface area
	single		surgical assistant
	sister		sustained action
	son	S/A	same as
	South (as in the location		sugar and acetone
	2S would be second	S&A	sugar and acetone
	floor, South wing)	SAA	same as above
	sponge		serum amyloid A
	subjective findings		Stokes-Adams attacks
	suicide		synthetic amino acids
	suction	SAAG	serum-ascites albumin
	sulfur		gradient
	supervision	SAANDs	selective apoptotic
	susceptible		antineoplastic drugs
/S/	signature	SAARDs	slow-acting antirheumatic
s̄	without (this is a		drugs
	dangerous abbreviation)	SAB	serum albumin
S′	shoulder		sinoatrial block
S_1	first heart sound		Spanish-American Black
$S^{-1}...S^{-4}$	suicide risk classifications		spontaneous abortion
S_2	second heart sound		subarachnoid bleed
S_3	third heart sound		subarachnoid block
	(ventricular filling	SABR	screening auditory
	gallop)		brainstem response
S_4	fourth heart sound (atrial	SAC	segmental antigen
	gallop)		challenge
$S_1...S_5$	sacral vertebra or nerves		serum aminoglycoside
	1 through 5		concentration
SI..SIV	symbols for the first to		short arm cast
	fourth heart sounds		substance abuse counselor
SA	sacroanterior	SACC	short arm cylinder cast
	salicylic acid	SACD	subacute combined
	semen analysis		degeneration
	Sexoholics Anonymous	SACH	solid ankle, cushioned
	sinoatrial		heel
	sleep apnea	SACT	sinoatrial conduction time
	slow acetylator	SAD	seasonal affective disorder
	Spanish-American		Self-Assessment
	spinal anesthesia		Depression (scale)
	Staphylococcus aureus		social anxiety disorder
	subarachnoid		source-axis distance
			subacromial
			decompression
			subacute dialysis
			sugar, acetone, and
			diacetic acid

S

	sugar and acetone determination	SAL 12	sequential analysis of 12 chemistry constituents (see page 358)
	superior axis deviation		
SADD	Students Against Drunk Driving	SAM	methylprednisolone sodium succinate (Solu-Medrol), aminophylline, and metaproterenol (Metaprel)
SADL	simulated activities of daily living		
SADR	suspected adverse drug reaction		selective antimicrobial modulation
SADS	Schedule for Affective Disorders and Schizophrenia		self-administered medication
			short arc motion
			sleep apnea monitor
SADs	severe autoimmune diseases		Spanish-American male
			systolic anterior motion
SADS-C	Schedule for Affective Disorders And Schizophrenia – Change Version	SAMe	S-adenosylmethionine
		SAMHSA	Substance Abuse and Mental Health Services Administration
SAE	serious adverse event		
	short above elbow (cast)		
SAEG	signal averaging electrocardiogram	SAMPLE	symptoms/signs, allergies, medications, past medical history, last oral intake, and events prior to arrival (an EMT mnemonic used in initial patient questioning)
SAEKG	signaled average electrocardiogram		
SAESU	Substance Abuse valuating Screen Unit		
SAF	Self-Analysis Form		
	self-articulating femoral	SAN	side-arm nebulizer
	Spanish-American female		sinoatrial node
			slept all night
SAFHS	sonic accelerated fracture healing system	SANC	short arm navicular cast
		sang	sanguinous
SAG	sodium antimony gluconate	SANS	Schedule (Scale) for the Assessment of Negative Symptoms
Sag D	sagittal diameter		
SAGE	serial analysis of gene expression		sympathetic autonomic nervous system
SAH	subarachnoid hemorrhage	SAO	small airway obstruction
	systemic arterial hypertension	SaO_2	arterial oxygen percent saturation
SAHS	sleep apnea/hypopnea (hypersomnolence) syndrome	SAP	serum alkaline phosphate
			sporadic adenomatous polyps
SAI	Sodium Amytal® interview	SAPD	self-administration of psychotropic drugs
SAL	salicylate		
	Salmonella	SAPH	saphenous
	sensory acuity level		
	sterility assurance level		

S

SAPHO	synovitis, acne, pustulosis, hyperostosis, and osteomyelitis (syndrome)	SASH	saline, agent, saline, and heparin
SAPS	short arm plaster splint	SASP	sulfasalazine (salicylazo-sulfapyridine; Azulfidine)
	Simplified Acute Physiology Score	SASS	Social Adaptation Self-Evaluation Scale
SAPS II	Simplified Acute Physiology Score version II	SAT	methylprednisolone sodium succinate (Solu-Medrol), aminophylline, and terbutaline
SAQ	saquinavir (Invirase)		saturated
	Sexual Adjustment Questionnaire		saturation
	short-arc quadriceps		Saturday
SAR	seasonal allergic rhinitis		self-administered therapy
	Senior Assistant Resident		Senior Apperception Test
	sexual attitudes reassessment		speech awareness threshold
	structural activity relationships		subacute thyroiditis
SARA	sexually acquired reactive arthritis	SATC	substance abuse treatment clinic
	system for anesthetic and respiratory administration analysis	SATL	surgical Achilles tendon lengthening
		SATP	substance abuse treatment program
SARAN	senior admitting resident's admission note	SATS	refers to oxygen saturation levels
SARC	seasonal allergic rhinoconjunctivitis	SATU	substance abuse treatment unit
S Arrh	sinus arrhythmia	SAVD	spontaneous assisted vaginal delivery
SART	standard acid reflux test	SB	safety belt
SAS	saline, agent, and saline		sandbag
	scalenus anticus syndrome		scleral buckling
	see assessment sheet		seat belt
	Self-rating Anxiety Scale		seen by
	short arm splint		Sengstaken-Blakemore (tube)
	sleep apnea syndrome		sick boy
	Social Adjustment Scale		side bend
	Specific Activity Scale		side bending
	statistical applications software		sinus bradycardia
	subarachnoid space		slide board
	subaxial subluxation		small bowel
	sulfasalazine (Azulfidine)		spina bifida
	synthetic absorbable sutures		sponge bath
SASA	Sex Abuse Survivors Anonymous		stand-by
			Stanford-Binet (test)

	sternal border	SB-LM	Stanford-Binet Intelligence Test-Form LM
	stillbirth		
	stillborn		
	stone basketing	SBO	small bowel obstruction
Sb	antimony		specified bovine offals
SB+	wearing seat belt	SBOD	scleral buckle, right eye
SB−	not wearing seat belt	SBOE	surgical blood order equation
SBA	serum bactericidal activity		
	standby angioplasty	SBOH	State Board of Health
	standby assistant (assistance)	SBOM	soybean oil meal
		SBOS	scleral buckle, left eye
	Summary Basis of Approval	SBP	school breakfast program
			scleral buckling procedure
SBAC	small bowel adenocarcinoma		small bowel phytobezoars
			spontaneous bacterial peritonitis
SBB	stereotactic breast biopsy		
			systolic blood pressure
SBBO	small-bowel bacterial overgrowth	SBQC	small based quad cane
		SBR	sluggish blood return
SBC	sensory binocular cooperation		strict bed rest
		SBRN	sensory branch of the radial nerve
	single base cane		
	standard bicarbonate	SBS	serum blood sugar
	strict bed confinement		shaken baby syndrome
	superficial bladder cancer		short (small) bowel syndrome
SBD	straight bag drainage		sick-building syndrome
SBE	saturated base excess		side-by-side
	self-breast examination		small bowel series
	short below-elbow (cast)	SBT	serum bactericidal titers
	shortness of breath on exertion		special baby Travesol
		SBTB	sinus breakthrough beat
	subacute bacterial endocarditis	SBTT	small bowel transit time
		SBV	single binocular vision
SBFT	small bowel follow through	SBW	seat belts worn
		SBX	symphysis, buttocks, and xiphoid
SBG	stand-by guard		
SBGM	self blood-glucose monitoring	SC	schizophrenia
			self-care
SBH	State Board of Health		serum creatinine
SBI	silicone (gel-containing) breast implants		service connected
			sick call
	systemic bacterial infection		sickle cell
			small (blood pressure) cuff
SBJ	skin, bones, and joints		Snellen's chart
SBK	spinnbarkeit		spinal cord
SBL	sponge blood loss		sport cord
sBLA	supplemental Biologics License Application		sternoclavicular

S

	subclavian	SCCE	squamous cell carcinoma of the esophagus
	subclavian catheter		
	subcutaneous	SCCHN	squamous cell carcinoma of the head and neck
	succinylcholine		
	sulfur colloid	SCCI	subcutaneous continuous infusion
	surveillance cultures		
s̄c	without correction (without glasses)	SCD	sequential compression device
S&C	sclerae and conjunctivae		service connected disability
SCA	sickle cell anemia		sickle cell disease
	spinocerebellar ataxia		spinal cord disease
	subclavian artery		subacute combined degeneration
	subcutaneous abdominal (block)		
	superior cerebellar artery		sudden cardiac death
SCa	serum calcium	ScDA	scapulodextra anterior
SCAD	short chain acyl-coenzyme A dehydrogenase	SCDM	soybean-casein digest medium
SCAN	suspected child abuse and neglect	ScDP	scapulodextra posterior
		SCE	sister chromatid exchange
SCAP	scapula; scapulae; scapular		soft cooked egg
			specialized columnar epithelium
	stem cell apheresis		
SCARMD	severe childhood autosomal recessive muscular dystrophy	SCEMIA	self-contained enzymatic membrane immunoassay
SCAT	sheep cell agglutination titer	SCEP	somatosensory cortical evoked potential
	sickle cell anemia test	SCF	special care formula
SCB	strictly confined to bed		stem cell factor
SCBC	small cell bronchogenic carcinoma	SCFA	short-chain fatty acid
		SCFE	slipped capital femoral epiphysis
SCBE	single-contrast barium enema		
SCBF	spinal cord blood flow	SCFGT	Southern California Figure Ground Test
SCC	short course chemotherapy (for tuberculosis)	SCG	seismocardiography
			serum Chemogram
	sickle cell crisis		sodium cromoglycate
	small cell carcinoma	SCH	schistosomiasis (*Schistosoma* sp.) vaccine
	spinal cord compression		
	squamous cell carcinoma		
SCCA	semi-closed circle absorber	SCh	succinylcholine chloride
		SCHISTO	schistocytes
	squamous cell carcinoma antigen	SCHIZ	schizocytes
			schizophrenia
SCCa	squamous cell carcinoma	SCHLP	supracricord hemilaryngopharyngec-tomy
SCCB	small cell cancer of the bladder		

SCHNC	squamous cell head and neck cancer		special care nursery
SCI	specific COX-2 inhibitor		suprachiasmatic nucleus (nuclei)
	spinal cord injury	SCOB	Schedule-Controlled Operant Behavior
	subcoma insulin		
SCID	severe combined immunodeficiency disorders (disease)	SCOP	scopolamine
		SCOPE	arthroscopy
		SCP	secondary care provider
	structured clinical interview for DSM-III-R		sodium cellulose phosphate
			standardized care plan
SCII	Strong-Campbell Interest Inventory	SCPF	stem cell proliferation factor
SCIP	Screening and Crisis Intervention Program	S-CPK	serum creatine phosphokinase
SCIPP	sacrococcygeal to inferior pubic point	SCPP	spinal cord perfusion pressure
SCIU	spinal cord injury unit	SCR	special care room (seclusion room)
SCIV	subclavian intravenous		
SCI-WORA	spinal cord injury without radiographic abnormalities		spondylitic caudal radioculopathy
			stem cell rescue
SCL	skin conductance level	SCr	serum creatinine
	symptom checklist	sCR	soluble complement receptor
SCL-90	Symptoms Checklist—90 items	SCRIPT	prescription
ScLA	scapulolaeva anterior	SC/RP	scaling and root planing
SCLAX	subcostal long axis	SC-RNV	subcutaneous radionuclide venography
SCLC	small cell lung cancer		
SCLD	sickle cell lung disease	SCS	spinal cord stimulation
SCLE	subacute cutaneous lupus erythematosis		splatter control shield
			stem cell support
ScLP	scapulolaeva posterior		suspected catheter sepsis
SCLs	soft contact lenses		
	synthetic combinatorial libraries	SCSAX	subcostal short axis
SCM	scalene muscle	SCSIT	Southern California Sensory Integration Tests
	sensation, circulation, and motion		
		SCSVT	Southern California Space Visualization Test
	spondylitic caudal myelopathy		
	sternocleidomastoid	SCT	Sertoli cell tumor
	supraclavicular muscle		sex chromatin test
SCMD	senile choroidal macular degeneration		sickle cell trait
			stem cell transplant
SCMV	serogroup C meningococcal vaccine		sugar-coated tablet
		SCTX	static cervical traction
SCN	severe congenital neutropenia	SCU	self-care unit
			special care unit

S

295

SCUCP	small cell undifferentiated carcinoma of the prostate	SDAT	senile dementia of Alzheimer's type
SCUF	slow continuous ultrafiltration	SDB	Sabouraud dextrose broth self-destructive behavior sleep disordered breathing
SCUT	schizophrenia, chronic undifferentiated type	SDBP	seated diastolic blood pressure
SCV	subclavian vein subcutaneous vaginal (block)		standing diastolic blood pressure supine diastolic blood pressure
SCY	scytonemin	SDC	serum digoxin concentration
SD	scleroderma senile dementia sensory deficit severe deficit septal defect severely disabled shallow distance (aquatic therapy)		serum drug concentration Sleep Disorders Center sodium deoxycholate
		SD&C	suction, dilation, and curettage
		SDD	selective digestive (tract) decontamination sterile dry dressing subantimicrobial dose doxycycline (dental; Periostat)
	shoulder disarticulation single dose skin dose sleep deprived solvent-detergent somatic dysfunction spasmodic dysphonia speech discrimination	SDDT	selective decontamination of the digestive tract
		SDE	subdural empyema
	spontaneous delivery stable disease standard deviation standard diet step-down sterile dressing straight drainage streptozocin and doxorubicin sudden death surgical drain	SDES	symptomatic diffuse esophageal spasm
		SDF	sexual dysfunction stromal-cell-derived factor
		SDH	spinal detrusor hyperreflexia subdural hematoma
		SDI	Sandimmune (cyclosporine) State Disability Insurance
S & D	seen and discussed stomach and duodenum	SDII	sudden death in infancy
S/D	sharp/dull systolic-diastolic ratio	SDL	serum digoxin level serum drug level speech discrimination loss
SDA	sacrodextra anterior same day admission serotonin/dopamine antagonist Seventh-Day Adventist steroid-dependent asthmatic	SDLE	sex-difference in life expectancy somatic dysfunction lower extremity
		SDM	soft drusen maculopathy

	standard deviation of the mean		Starr-Edwards (valve, pacemaker)
S/D/M	systolic, diastolic, mean		status epilepticus
SD/N	signal-difference-to-noise ratio	Se	selenium
		S/E	suicidal and eloper
SDNN	standard deviation of normal-to-normal beats	S & E	seen and examined
		SEA	sheep erythrocyte agglutination (test)
SDO	surgical diagnostic oncology		Southeast Asia
			subdural electrode array
SDP	sacrodextra posterior		synaptic electronic activation
	single donor platelets		
	solvent-detergent plasma	SEAR	Southease Asia refugee
	stomach, duodenum, and pancreas	SEB	Staphylococcus enterotoxin B
SDPTG	second derivative of photoplethysmogram		surrogate end-point biomarker
SDR	selective dorsal rhizotomy	SEC	second
	short-duration response		secondary
SDS	same day surgery		secretary
	Self-Rating Depression Scale		size exclusion chromatography
	sodium dodecyl sulfate		steric exclusion chromatography
	somatropin deficiency syndrome	SECG	scalp electrocardiogram
	Speech Discrimination Score	SECL	seclusion
		SECPR	standard external cardiopulmonary resuscitation
	standard deviation score		
	sudden death syndrome	SE-CPT	single-electrode current perception threshold
	Symptom Distress Scale		
SDSO	same day surgery overnight	SED	sedimentation
			skin erythema dose
SDS-PAGE	sodium dodecyl sulfate – polyacrylamide gel electrophoresis		socially and emotionally disturbed
			spondyloepiphyseal dysplasia
SDT	sacrodextra transversa	SED-NET	severely emotional disturbed - network
	speech detection threshold		
SDU	step-down unit	sed rt	sedimentation rate
SDUE	somatic dysfunction upper extremity	SEER	Surveillance, Epidemiology, and End Results (program)
SE	saline enema (0.9% sodium chloride)		
	self-examination	SEG	segment
	side effect		sonoencephalogram
	soft exudates	segs	segmented neutrophils
	spin echo	SEH	spinal epidural hematomas
	staff escort		
	standard error		

S

	subependymal hemorrhage		standard electrolyte solution
SEI	subepithelial (comeal) infiltrate	SET	signal extraction technology
SELDI	surface enhanced laser desorption/ionization		social environmental therapy
SELFVD	sterile elective low forceps vaginal delivery	SEV	systolic ejection time sevoflurane (Ultane)
SEM	scanning electron microscopy	SEWHO	shoulder-elbow-wrist-hand orthosis
	semen	SF	salt-free
	slow eye movement		saturated fat
	standard error of mean		scarlet fever
	systolic ejection murmur		seizure frequency
SEMI	subendocardial myocardial infarction		seminal fluid skull fracture
SENS	sensitivity		soft feces
	sensorium		sound field
SEP	multiple sclerosis (French)		spinal fluid
	separate		starch-free
	serum electrophoresis		sugar-free
	somatosensory evoked potential		symptom-free synovial fluid
	syringe exchange program	S&F	soft and flat
	systolic ejection period	SF-6	sulfahexafluoride
SEQ	sequela	SF 36	36-item short form health survey
SER	scanning equalization radiography	SFA	saturated fatty acids superficial femoral artery
	sertraline (Zoloft)	SFB	single frequency bioimpedance
	side effects records		
	signal enhancement ratio	SFC	spinal fluid count
Serial 7's	a mental status examination (starting with a 100, count backward by 7's)		subarachnoid fluid collection
		SFD	scaphoid fossa depression small for dates
SER-IV	supination external rotation, type 4 fracture	SFE	supercritical fluid extraction
SERM	selective estrogen-receptor modulator	SFEMG	single-fiber electromyography
SERO-SANG	serosanguineous	SFH	schizophrenia family history
SERP-ACWA	Skin Exposure Reduction Paste Against Chemical Warfare Agents	SFP	simulated fluorescence process
			simultaneous foveal perception
SERs	somatosensory evoked responses		spinal fluid pressure
SES	sick euthyroid syndrome socioeconomic status	SFPT	standard fixation preference test

S

SFS	split function studies	SGTCS	secondarily generalized tonic-clonic seizures
SFTR	sagittal, frontal, transverse, rotation	SH	serum hepatitis
SFUP	surgical follow-up		sexual harassment
SFV	simian foamy viruses		short
	superficial femoral vein		shoulder
SFW	shell fragment wound		shower
SFWB	social/family well-being		social history
SFWD	symptom-free walking distance		sulfhydryl (group)
			surgical history
SG	salivary gland	S&H	speech and hearing
	scrotography		suicidal and homicidal
	serum glucose	S/H	suicidal/homicidal ideation
	side glide		
	skin graft	SH2	sarc homology region 2
	specific gravity	SHA	super-heated aerosol
	Swan-Ganz (catheter)	SHAL	standard hyperalimentation
S/G	swallow/gag	SHAS	supravalvular hypertrophic aortic stenosis
SGA	small for gestational age		
	subjective global assessment (dietary history and physical examination)	S Hb	sickle hemoglobin screen
		SHBG	sex hormone-binding globulin
	substantial gainful activity (employment)	sHBO₂T	systemic hyperbaric oxygen therapy
SGB	Swiss gym ball	SHC	subsequent hospital care
SGC	Swan-Ganz catheter		
SGCNB	stereotactic guided core-needle biopsy	SHEENT	skin, head, eyes, ears, nose, and throat
SGD	straight gravity drainage	SHG	shigellosis (*Shigella* sp.) vaccine
SGE	significant glandular enlargement		
		SHGT	somatic-cell human gene therapy
s̄ gl	without correction (without glasses)	SHI	standard heparin infusion
SGM	serum glucose monitoring	Shig	*Shigella*
		SHL	sudden hearing loss
SGOT	serum glutamic oxalo-acetic transaminase (same as AST)		supraglottic horizontal laryngectomy
		SHO	Senior House Officer
SGPT	serum glutamate pyruvate transaminase (same as ALT)	SHP	secondary hypertension, pulmonary
		SHR	scapulohumeral rhythm
SGRQ-A	St. George's Respiratory Questionnaire translated into American English	SHRC	shortened, held, resisted contraction
		SHS	student health service
SGS	second-generation sulfonylurea	SHV	short hepatic vein
	subglottic stenosis		sulfhydryl variant
sGS	surgical Gleason score		

S

299

SHx	social history	SICD	sudden infant crib death
SI	International System of Units	SICT	selective intracoronary thrombolysis
	sacroiliac	SICU	surgical intensive care unit
	sagittal index		
	sector iridectomy	SIDA	French and Spanish abbreviation for AIDS
	self-inflicted		
	sensory integration	SIDD	syndrome of isolated diastolic dysfunction
	seriously ill		
	sexual intercourse	SIDERO	siderocyte
	signal intensity	SIDFF	superimposed dorsiflexion of foot
	small intestine		
	strict isolation	SIDS	sudden infant death syndrome
	stress incontinence		
	stroke index	SIEP	serum immunoelectrophoresis
	suicidal ideation		
Si	silicon	SIG	let it be marked (appears on prescription before directions for patient)
S & I	suction and irrigation		
	support and interpretation		
SIA	small intestinal atresia		sigmoidoscopy
SIDAM	structured interview for the diagnosis of dementia of Alzheimer type	Signal 99	patient in cardiac or respiratory distress
		SIJ	sacroiliac joint
		SIJS	sacroiliac joint syndrome
SIDAM-A	structured interview for the diagnosis of dementia of the Alzheimer type, multi-infarct dementia, and dementias of other etiology according to ICD-10 and DSM-III-R	SIL	seriously ill list
			sister-in-law
			squamous intraepithelial lesion
		SILFVD	sterile indicated low forceps vaginal delivery
		SILV	simultaneous independent lung ventilation
SIADH	syndrome of inappropriate antidiuretic hormone secretion	SIM	selective ion monitoring
			Similac®
		SIMCU	surgical intermediate care unit
SIAT	supervised intermittent ambulatory treatment	Sim c̄ Fe	Similac with iron®
SIB	self-inflating bulb	SIMV	synchronized intermittent mandatory ventilation
	self-injurious behavior		
SIBC	serum iron-binding capacity	SIN	salpingitis isthmica nodose
sibs	siblings	SIP	Sickness Impact Profile
SIC	self-intermittent catheterization		stroke in progression
			sympathetically independent pain
	squamous intraepithelial cells	SIQ	sick in quarters
	Standard Industrial Classification	SIR	standardized incidence rate (ratio)

S

SIRS	systemic inflammatory response syndrome	SKU	stock keeping unit (related to product identification)
SIS	sister		
	Surgical Infection Stratification (system)	SKY	spectral karyotyping
		SL	scapholunate
SISI	Short Increment Sensitivity Index		secondary leukemia
			sensation level
SISS	severe invasion streptococcal syndrome		sentinel lymphadenectomy
			serious list
SIT	serum inhibitory titers		shortleg
	silicon-intensified target		side-lying
	Slossen Intelligence Test		slight
	specific immunotherapy (allergy)		sublingual
		S/L	slit lamp (examination)
	sperm immobilization test	SLA	sacrolaeva anterior
	supraspinatus, infraspinatus, teres (insertions)		sex and love addictions
			slide latex agglutination
			The Satisfaction with Life Areas
	surgical intensive therapy		
SITA	standard infertility treatment algorithm	SLAA	Sex and Love Addicts Anonymous
SIT BAL	sitting balance	SLAC	scapholunate advanced collapse
SIT TOL	sitting tolerance		
SIV	simian immunodeficiency virus	SLAM	Systemic Lupus Activity Measure
SIVP	slow intravenous push	SLAP	serum leucine amino-peptidase
SIW	self-inflicted wound		
SJC	swollen joint count		superior labral anteroposterior (shoulder lesion)
SJCRH	St. Jude Children's Research Hospital		
S-JRA	systemic juvenile rheumatoid arthritis	SLB	short leg brace
		SLC	short leg cast
SJS	Stevens-Johnson syndrome	SLCC	short leg cylinder cast
		SLCG	sulfolithocholyglycine
	Swyer-James syndrome	SLCT	Sertoli-Leydig cell tumor
S_{jv02}	jugular venous oxygen saturation	SLD	specific language disorder
			stealth liposomal doxorubicin
SK	seborrheic keratosis		
	senile keratosis	SLE	slit-lamp examination
	SmithKline		St. Louis encephalitis
	solar keratosis		systemic lupus erythematosus
	streptokinase		
S & K	single and keeping (baby)	SLEDAI	Systemic Lupus Erythematosus Disease Activity Index
SKAO	supracondylar knee-ankle orthosis		
SKB	SmithKline Beecham	SLEX	slit-lamp examination (biomicroscopy)
SKC	single knee to chest		
SK-SD	streptokinase streptodornase	SLFVD	sterile low forceps vaginal delivery

S

SLGXT	symptom-limited graded exercise test		single lung transplantation
SLK	superior limbic keratoconjunctivitis		swing light test
SLL	second-look laparotomy	SLT-I	Shiga-like toxin I
	small lymphocytic lymphoma	SLTA	standard language test for aphasia
SLMFVD	sterile low midforceps vaginal delivery	SLTEC	Shiga-like toxin-producing *Escherichia coli*
		sl. tr.	slight trace
SLMMS	slightly more marked since	SLUD	salivation, lacrimation, urination, and defecation
SLMP	since last menstrual period	SLUDGE	salivation, **l**acrimation, **u**rination, **d**iarrhea,
SLN	sentinel lymph node(s)		**g**astrointestinal upset,
	superior laryngeal nerve		and **e**mesis (signs and
SLND	sentinel lymph node detection		symptoms of cholinergic excess)
SLNM	sentinel lymph node mapping	SLV	since last visit
SLNTG	sublingual nitroglycerin	SLWB	severely low birth weight
SLNWBC	short leg nonweight-bearing cast	SLWC	short leg walking cast
SLNWC	short leg nonwalking cast	SM	sadomasochism
SLO	scanning laser ophthalmoscope		service mark (such as The Pause that
	second-look operation		Refreshes)
	shark liver oil		skim milk
	Smith-Lemli-Opitz (syndrome)		small
	streptolysin O		sports medicine
SLOA	short leave of absence		Stairmaster®
SLP	single-limb progression		streptomycin
	speech language pathology		systolic motion
			systolic murmur
		^{153}Sm	samarium 153
SLPI	secretory leukocyte protease inhibitor	SMA-6	simultaneous multichannel autoanalyzer (page 358)
SLPMS	short-leg posterior-molded splint	SMA-7	See page 358
		SMA-12	See page 358
SLR	straight-leg raising	SMA-18	See page 358
SLRT	straight-leg raising tenderness	SMA-23	See page 358
		SMAO	superior mesenteric artery occlusion
	straight-leg raising test	SMAR	self-medication administration record
SLS	second-look sonography		
	short leg splint		
	shrinking lungs syndrome	SMAS	superficial musculoaponeurotic
	single limb support		system (flap)
SLT	sacrolaeva transversa		superior mesenteric artery syndrome
	scanning laser tomography		

SMAST	Short Michigan Alcoholism Screening Test	SMO	Senior Medical Officer site management organization(s) slip made out
SMB	simulated moving bed (chromatography)		
SMBG	self-monitoring blood glucose	SMON	subacute myelo-opticoneuropathy
SMC	skeletal myxoid chondrosarcoma special mouth care	SMP	self-management program sympathetic maintained plan
SMCA	sorbitol MacConkey agar	SMPN	sensorimotor polyneuropathy
SMCD	senile macular chorioretinal degeneration	SMR	senior medical resident skeletal muscle relaxant standardized mortality ratio submucous resection
SMCs	smooth muscle cells		
SMD	senile macular degeneration		
SMDA	Safe Medical Defice Act		
SME	significant medical event	SMRR	submucous resection and rhinoplasty
SMF	streptozocin, mitomycin, and fluorouracil	SMS	scalded mouth syndrome senior medical student Smith-Magenis syndrome somatostatin (Zecnil) stiff-man syndrome
SMFA	sodium monofluoroacetate		
SMFVD	sterile midforceps vaginal delivery		
SMG	submandibular gland		
SMH	state mental hospital	SMSA	standard metropolitan statistical area
SMI	sensory motor integration (group) severely mentally impaired small volume infusion suggested minimum increment sustained maximal inspiration	SMT	smooth muscle tumors
		SMV	submentovertical superior mesenteric vein
		SMVT	sustained monomorphic ventricular tachycardia
		SMX-TMP	sulfamethoxazole and trimethoprim (SMZ-TMP)
SMIDS	suppertime mixed insulin and daytime sulfonylureas	SN	sciatic notch staff nurse student nurse suprasternal notch superior nasal
SMILE	safety, monitoring, intervention, length of stay and evaluation sustained maximal inspiratory lung exercises		
		Sn	tin
		S/N	signal to noise ratio
		SNA	specimen not available Student Nursing Assistant
SMIT	standard mycological identification techniques	SNa	serum sodium
		SNAP	scheduled nursing activities program Score for Neonatal Acute Physiology sensory nerve action potential
SMMVT	sustained monomorphic ventricular tachycardia		
SMN	second malignant neoplasia		

S

SNAP-PE	Score for Neonatal Acute Physiology-Perinatal Extension	SNOOP	Systematic Nursing Observation of Psychopathology
SNaRI	serotonin noradrenergic reuptake inhibitor	SNOs	S-nitrosothiols
SNAT	suspected nonaccidental trauma	SNP	simple neonatal procedure sodium nitroprusside
SNB	scalene node biopsy sentinel (lymph) node biopsy	SNP-LP	single nucleotide polymorphisms – linkage disequilibrium
SNC	skilled nursing care	SNPs	single nucleotide polymorphisms
SNc	substantia nigra compacta	SNR	signal-to-noise ratio
		SNr	substantia nigra reticularis
SNCV	sensory nerve conduction velocity	SNRI	serotonin norepinephrine reuptake inhibitor
SND	single needle device sinus node dysfunction	SNRT	sinus node recovery time
		SNS	sterile normal saline (0.9% sodium chloride, sterile)
SNDA	Supplemental New Drug Application		
SNE	subacute necrotizing encephalomyelopathy		sympathetic nervous system
SNEP	student nurse extern program	SNT	sinuses, nose, and throat suppan nail technique
SnET2	tin ethyl etiopurpurin	SNV	Sin Nombre virus
SNF	skilled nursing facility		skilled nursing visit
SnF₂	stannous fluoride		spleen necrosis virus
SNF/MR	skilled nursing facility for the mentally retarded	SO	second opinion sex offender
SNGFR	single nephron glomerular filtration rate		shoulder orthosis significant other
SNGP	supranuclear gaze palsy		special observation
SNHL	sensorineural hearing loss		sphincter of Oddi standing orders
SNIP	silver nitrate immunoperoxidase		suboccipital suggestive of
	strict no information in paper		superior oblique supraoptic
SNM	sentinel (lymph) node mapping		supraorbital sutures out
	student nurse midwife		sympathetic ophthalmia
SnMp	tin-mesoporphyrin	S/O	suggestive of
SNOMED	Systematized Nomenclature of Medicine	S-O	salpingo-oophorectomy
		S&O	salpingo-oophorectomy
		SO₃	sulfite
SNOMED-RT®	Systematized Nomenclature of Human and Veterinary Medicine—reference terminology	SO₄	sulfate
		SOA	serum opsonic activity shortness of air spinal opioid analgesia supraorbital artery

	swelling of ankles		space occupying lesion
SOAA	signed out against advice	SOL I	special observations level one (there are also SOL II and SOL III)
SOAM	sutures out in the morning		
SOAMA	signed out against medical advice		
SOAP	subjective, objective, assessment, and plans	SOM	secretory otitis media
			serous otitis media
			somatization
SOAPIE	subjective, objective, assessment, plan, implementation, (intervention), and evaluation	SOMI	sterno-occipital mandibular immobilizer
		Sono	sonogram
		SONP	solid organs not palpable
		SOOL	spontaneous onset of labor
SOB	see order book	SOP	standard operating procedure
	shortness of breath (this abbreviation has caused problems)		
		SOPM	sutures out in afternoon (or evening)
	side of bed	SOR	sign own release
SOBE	short of breath on exertion	SOS	if there is need
			may be repeated once if urgently required (Latin: *si opus sit*)
SOBOE	short of breath on exertion		
SOC	see old chart		self-obtained smear
	socialization		suicidal observation status
	standard of care	SOSOB	sit on side of bed
	start of care	SOT	solid organ transplant
	state of consciousness		something other than
	system organ class		stream of thought
S & OC	signed and on chart (e.g. permit)	SP	sacrum to pubis
			sequential pulse
SOD	sinovenous occlusive disease		serum protein
			shoulder press
	sphincter of Oddi dysfunction		silent period (related to electromyographic responses)
	superoxide dismutase		
	surgical officer of the day		spastic dysphonia
SODAS	spheriodal oral drug absorption system		speech
			Speech Pathologist
SOE	source of embolism		spinal
SOFA	sepsis-related organ failure assessment		spouse
			stand and pivot
SOG	suggestive of good		stand pivot
SOH	sexually oriented hallucinations		status post
			Streptococcus pneumoniae
SoHx	social history		systolic pressure
SOI	slipped on ice	sp	species
	surgical orthotopic implantation (implant)	S/P	status post
	syrup of ipecac		
SOL	solution		suprapubic

SP 1	suicide precautions number 1		serum protein electrophoresis
SP 2	suicide precautions number 2		solid-phase extraction
SPA	albumin human (formerly known as salt-poor albumin)		superficial punctate erosions
	serum prothrombin activity	SPEB	streptococcal pyrogenic exotoxins B
	single photon absorptiometry	SPEC	specimen
	Speech Pathology and Audiology	Spec Ed	streptococcal pyrogenic exotoxins C
	stimulation produced analgesia	SPECT	special education
			single-photon emission computed tomography
	student physician's assistant	SPEEP	spontaneous positive end-expiratory pressure
	subperiosteal abscess	SPEP	serum protein electrophoresis
	suprapubic aspiration	SPET	single-photon emission tomography
SpA	spondyloarthropathy		
SP-A	surfactant-specific protein A	SPF	semipermeable film
			split products of fibrin
SPAC	satisfactory postanesthesia course		sun protective factor
SPAG	small-particle aerosol generator	sp fl	spinal fluid
		SPG	scrotopenogram
SPAMM	spatial modulation of magnetization		sphenopalatine ganglion
		SpG	specific gravity
SPBE	saw palmetto berry extract	SPH	severely and profoundly handicapped
SPBI	serum protein bound iodine		sighs per hour
			spherocytes
SPBT	suprapubic bladder tap	SPHERO	spherocytes
SPC	saturated phosphatidylcholine	SPI	speech processor interface
	sclerosing pancreatocholangitis		surgical peripheral iridectomy
	statistical process control	SPIA	solid phase immunoabsorbent assay
	Summary of Product Characteristics		
	suprapubic catheter	SPIF	spontaneous peak inspiratory force
SPCT	simultaneous prism and cover test	SPIFE	serum protein and immunofixation electrophoresis (system)
SPD	subcorneal pustular dermatosis		
	Supply, Processing, and Distribution (department)	S-PIN	Steinmann pin
		SPK	single parent keeping (baby)
	suprapubic drainage		superficial punctate keratitis
SPE	saw palmetto extract		

SPL	sound pressure level	SPT	second primary tumors
SPL®	Staphylococcal Phage Lysate		skin prick test
			standing pivot transfer
SPLATTT	split anterior tibial tendon transfer		suprapubic tenderness
		SP TAP	spinal tap
SPM	scanning probe microscopy	SPTs	second primary tumors
	second primary malignancy	SP TUBE	suprapubic tube
		SPTX	static pelvic traction
SPMA	spinal progressive muscle atrophy	SPU	short procedure unit
		SPVR	systemic peripheral vascular resistance
SPME	solid-phase microextraction	SPX	smallpox vaccine, not otherwise specified
SPMSQ	Short Portable Mental Status Questionnaire	SPX_v	smallpox vaccine (vaccinia virus)
SPN	solitary pulmonary nodule	SQ	status quo
	student practical nurse		subcutaneous (this is a dangerous abbreviation, use subcut)
SPNK	single parent not keeping (baby)		
SPO	status postoperative	Sq CCa	squamous cell carcinoma
SpO_2	oxygen saturation by pulse oximeter	SQE	subcutaneous emphysema
		SQM	square meter(s)
spont	spontaneous	SQV	saquinavir (Fortovose; Invirase)
SponVe	spontaneous ventilation		
SPP	Sexuality Preference Profile	SR	screen
			sedimentation rate
	single presentation phenotype		see report
			senior resident
	species (specus)		service record
	super packed platelets		side rails
	suprapubic prostatectomy		sinus rhythm
SPR	surface plasmon resonance		slow release
			smooth-rough
SPRAS	Sheehan Patient Rated Anxiety Scale		social recreation
			stretch reflex
SP-RIA	solid-phase radioimmunoassay		superior rectus
			sustained release
SPROM	spontaneous premature rupture of membrane		suture removal
			system review
SPS	shoulder pain and stiffness	S/R	strong/regular (pulse)
	simple partial seizure	S&R	seclusion and restraint
	sodium polyethanol sulfonate		smooth and rough
		^{89}Sr	strontium 89
	sodium polystyrene sulfonate (Kayexalate; SPS®)	SRA	steroid-resistant asthma
		SRAN	surgical resident admission note
	status post surgery		
	systemic progressive sclerosis	SRBC	sheep red blood cells

S

	sickle red blood cells	SRR	surgical recovery room
SRBOW	spontaneous rupture of bag of waters	SRS	somatostatin receptor scintigraphy
SRCC	sarcomatoid renal cell carcinoma	s̄RS	without redness or swelling
SRD	service-related disability sodium-restricted diet	SRS-A	slow-reacting substance of anaphylaxis
SRE	skeletal related event	SRSV	small round structured viruses
SRF	somatotropin releasing factor	SRT	sedimentation rate test sleep-related tumescence
	subretinal fluid		speech reception threshold
SRF-A	slow-releasing factor of anaphylaxis		speech recognition threshold
SRGVHD	steroid-resistant graft-versus-host disease		surfactant replacement therapy
SRH	signs of recent hemorrhage		sustained release theophylline
SRI	serotonin reuptake inhibitor	SRU	side rails up
SRICU	surgical respiratory intensive care unit	SRUS	solitary rectal ulcer syndrome
SRIF	somatotropin-release inhibiting factor (somatostatin; Zecnil)	SR ↑ X2	both siderails up
		SS	half
SRMD	stress-related mucosal damage		sacral sulcus
			sacrosciatic
SRMS	sustained-release morphine sulfate		saline (sodium chloride 0.9%) soak
SRMs	specified risk materials		saline solution (0.9% sodium chloride)
SR/NE	sinus rhythm, no ectopy		saliva sample
SRNV	subretinal neovascularization		salt sensitivity (sensitive)
			salt substitute
SRNVM	subretinal neovascular membrane		serotonin syndrome
			serum sickness
SRO	sagittal ramus osteotomy		sickle cell
	single room occupancy		single-strength (as compared to double-strength)
	sustained-release oral		
SROA	sports-related osteoarthritis		Sjögren's syndrome
SROCPI	Self-Rating Obsessive-Compulsive Personality Inventory		sliding scale
			slip sent
			Social Security
SROM	spontaneous rupture of membrane		social service
			somatostatin (Zecnil)
SRP	scaling and root planing (dental)		stainless steel
			steady state
	septorhinoplasty		step stool
	stapes replacement prosthesis		subaortic stenosis
			susceptible

S

	suprasciatic (notch)		Social Security disability
	symmetrical strength		source to skin distance
S/S	Saturday and Sunday	SSDI	Social Security disability
SS#	Social Security number		income
S & S	shower and shampoo	SSE	saline solution enema
	signs and symptoms		(0.9% sodium chloride)
	sitting and supine		skin self-examination
	sling and swathe		soapsuds enema
	soft and smooth		subacute spongiform
	(prostate)		encephalopathy
	support and stimulation		systemic side effects
	swish and spit	SSEH	spontaneous spinal
	swish and swallow		epidural hematoma
SSA	sagittal split	SSEPs	somatosensory evoked
	advancement		potentials
	salicylsalicylic acid	SSF	subscapular skinfold
	(salsalate)	SSG	sodium stibogluconate
	Sjögren's syndrome		sublabial salivary gland
	antigen A	SSI	sliding scale insulin
	Social Security		Social Skills Inventory
	Administration		sub-shock insulin
	Subjective Symptoms		superior sector iridectomy
	Assessment (profile)		Supplemental Security
	sulfasalicylic acid (test)		Income
SSBP	sitting systolic blood		surgical site infection
	pressure	SSKI	saturated solution of
SSC	sign symptom complex		potassium iodide
	silver sulfadiazine and	SSL	second stage of labor
	chlorhexidine		subtotal supraglottic
	Similac® and special care		laryngectomy
	Special Services for	SSLR	seated straight leg raise
	Children	SSM	short stay medical
	stainless steel crown		skin surface microscopy
	standard straight cane		superficial spreading
SSc	systemic sclerosis		melanoma
SSCA	single shoulder contrast	SSN	severely subnormal
	arthrography		Social Security number
SSCP	single-stranded	SSO	second surgical opinion
	conformational		short stay observation
	polymorphism		(unit)
	substernal chest pain		Spanish speaking only
SSCr	stainless steel crown	SSOP	Second Surgical Opinion
SSCU	surgical special care unit		Program
SSCVD	sterile spontaneous	SSP	short stay procedure (unit)
	controlled vaginal		superior spermatic plexus
	delivery		supragingival scaling and
SSD	serosanguineous drainage		prophylaxis (dental)
	sickle cell disease	SSPE	subacute sclerosing
	silver sulfadiazine		panencephalitis

S

SSPG	steady-state plasma glucose	shock therapy
		sinus tachycardia
SSPL	saturation sound pressure level	skin tear
		skin test
SSPU	surgical short procedure unit	slight trace
		slow-twitch
SSQ	Staring Speel Questionnaire	smokeless tobacco
		sore throat
SSR	substernal retractions	speech therapist
	sympathetic skin response	speech therapy
		sphincter tone
SSRFC	surrounding subretinal fluid cuff	split thickness
		spondee threshold
SSRI	selective serotonin reuptake inhibitor	station (obstetrics)
		stomach
SSRP	subgingival scaling and root planing (dental)	straight
		stress testing
SSRs	simple sequence repeats	stretcher
SSS	layer upon layer	subtotal
	scalded skin syndrome	Surgical Technologist
	Scandinavian Stroke Scale	survival time
	Sepsis Severity Score	synapse time
	Severity Scoring System (Dart's Snakebite)	S & T	sulfamethoxazole and trimethoprim (SMZ-TMP or SMX-TMP)
	short stay service (unit)	
	sick sinus syndrome	STA	second trimester abortion
	skin and skin structures		staphylococcus vaccine, not otherwise specified
	sterile saline soak	
SSSB	sagittal split setback	
SSSDW	significant sharp, spike, or delta waves		superficial temporal artery
		STA$_{aur}$	*Staphylococcus aureus* vaccine
SSSE	self-sustained status epilepticus	
SSSIs	skin and skin structure infections	stab.	polymorphonuclear leukocytes (white blood cells, in nonmature form)
SSSS	staphylococcal scalded skin syndrome	
SSSs	small short spikes (encephalography)	STAI	State-Trait Anxiety Inventory
SST	sagittal sinus thrombosis	STAI-I	State-Trait-Anxiety Index—I
	somatostatin (Zecnil)	STA-MCA	superficial temporary artery-middle cerebral artery (anastomosis; bypass)
SSTI	skin and skin structure infections	
SSU	short stay unit	
SSX	sulfisoxazole acetyl	STAPES	stapedectomy
S/SX	signs/symptoms	staph	*Staphylococcus aureus*
ST	esotropic	STA$_{SPL}$	staphylococcus vaccine, bacteriophage lysate
	sacrum transverse	
	Schiotz's tonometry	STAT	immediately

S

	signal transducers and activators of transcription	STHB	said to have been
		STI	sexually transmitted infection
STATINS	HMG-CoA reductase inhibitors		soft tissue injury
STAXI	State-Trait Anger Expression Inventory		sum total impression
		STILLB	stillborn
STB	stillborn	STIR	short TI (tau) inversion recovery
STBAL	standing balance		
ST BY	stand by	STIs	sexually transmitted infections
STC	serum theophylline concentration		systolic time intervals
		STJ	scapulothoracic joint
	soft tissue calcification		subtalar joint
	special treatment center	STK	streptokinase
	stimulate to cry	STL	sent to laboratory
	stroke treatment center		serum theophylline level
	subtotal colectomy	STLE	St. Louis encephalitis
	sugar tongue cast	STLOM	swelling, tenderness, and limitation of motion
ST CLK	station clerk		
STD	sexually transmitted disease(s)	STLV	simian T-lymphotrophic viruses
	short-term disability	STM	scanning tunneling microscope
	skin test dose		
	skin to tumor distance		short-term memory
	sodium tetradecyl sulfate		soft tissue mobilization
STD TF	standard tube feeding		streptomycin
STE	ST-segment elevation	STMT	Seat Movement
STEAM	stimulated-echo acquisition mode	STN	subtalar neutral
			subthalamic nucleus
STEC	shiga toxin-producing *Escherichia coli*	STNI	subtotal nodal irradiation
		STNM	surgical evaluative staging of cancer
STEM	scanning transmission electron microscopic		
		STNR	symmetrical tonic neck reflex
Stereo	steropsis		
STET	single photon emission tomography	S to	sensitive to
		STOP	sensitive, timely, and organized programs (battered spouses)
	submaximal treadmill exercise test		
STETH	stethoscope	STORCH	syphilis, toxoplasmosis, other agents, rubella, cytomegalovirus, and herpes (maternal infections)
STF	special tube feeding		
	standard tube feeding		
STG	short-term goals		
	split-thickness graft	STP	short-term plans
	superior temporal gyri		sodium thiopental
STH	soft tissue hemorrhage		step training progression
	somatotrophic hormone		
	subtotal hysterectomy	STPD	standard temperature and pressure—dry
	supplemental thyroid hormone		

S

STPI	State-Trait Personality Inventory	STV inter	short-term variability-intermittent
STPS	Short-Term Performance Status	STX	stricture
		STZ	streptozocin (Zanosar)
STR	scotopic threshold response	SU	sensory urgency
	sister		Somogyi units
	small tandem repeat		stasis ulcer
	stretcher		stroke unit
Strab	strabismus		sulfonylurea
strep	streptococcus		supine
	streptomycin	S/U	shoulder/umbilicus
STRICU	shock/trauma/respiratory intensive care unit	S&U	supine and upright
		SUA	serum uric acid
Str Post MI	strictly posterior myocardial infarction		single umbilical artery
		SUB	Skene's urethra and Bartholin's glands
STS	serologic test for syphilis	Subcu	subcutaneous
	short-term survivors	SUBCUT	subcutaneous
	slide thin slab	Subepi M Inj	subepicardial myocardial injury
	sodium tetradecyl sulfate		
	sodium thiosulfate	SUBL	sublingual
	soft tissue sarcoma	SUB-MAND	submandibular
	soft tissue swelling		
	somatostatin (Zecnil)	sub q	subcutaneous (this is a dangerous abbreviation since the q is mistaken for every, when a number follows)
	staurosporine		
	Surgical Technology Student		
STSG	split thickness skin graft		
STSS	streptococcal-induced toxic shock syndrome	SUCC	succinylcholine
		SUCT	suction
STS-SPT	simple two-step swallowing provocation test	SUD	sudden unexpected death
		SuDBP	supine diastolic blood pressure
STT	scaphoid, trapezium trapezoid	SUDEP	sudden unexpected (unexplained) death in epilepsy
	serial thrombin time		
	skin temperature test	SUDS	Subjective Unit of Distress (Disturbance) (Discomfort) Scale
	soft tissue tumor		
STT#1	Schirmer tear test one		
STT#2	Schirmer tear test two		sudden unexplained death syndrome
STTb	basal Schirmer tear test		
STTOL	standing tolerance	SUF	symptomatic uterine fibroids
STU	shock trauma unit		
	surgical trauma unit	SUI	stress urinary incontinence
STV	short-term variability		
STV+	short-term variability-present		suicide
		SUID	sudden unexplained infant death
STV 0	short-term variability-absent		

SULF-PRIM	sulfamethoxazole and trimethoprim	SVC-RPA	superior vena cava and right pulmonary artery (shunt)
SUN	serum urea nitrogen		
SUNDS	sudden unexplained nocturnal death syndrome	SVCS	superior vena cava syndrome
SUO	syncope of unknown origin	SVD	single-vessel disease
			spontaneous vaginal delivery
SUP	stress ulcer prophylaxis	SVE	sterile vaginal examination
	superior		
	supination		*Streptococcus viridans* endocarditis
	supinator		
	symptomatic uterine prolapse		subcortical vascular encephalopathy
SUPAC	Scale-Up and Post Approval Change	SV&E	suicidal, violent, and eloper
supp	suppository	SVG	saphenous vein graft
SUR	suramin (Metaret)	SVI	seminal vesicle invasion
	surgery		stroke volume index
	surgical	S VISC	serum viscosity
Surgi	Surgigator	SVL	severe visual loss
SUUD	sudden unexpected, unexplained death	SVN	small volume nebulizer
SUV	standard uptake variable	SVO$_2$	mixed venous oxygen saturation
SUX	succinylcholine	SVP	spontaneous venous pulse
	suction		
SUZI	subzonal insertion	SVPB	supraventricular premature beat
SV	seminal vesical		
	severe	SVPC	supraventricular premature contraction
	sigmoid volvulus		
	single ventricle	SVR	supraventricular rhythm
	single vessel		systemic vascular resistance
	snake venom		
	stock volume	SVRI	systemic vascular resistance index
	subclavian vein		
Sv	sievert (radiation unit)	SVT	supraventricular tachycardia
SV40	simian virus 40		
SVA	small volume admixture	SVVD	spontaneous vertex vaginal delivery
SVB	saphenous vein bypass	SW	sandwich
SVBG	saphenous vein bypass graft		sea water
			seriously wounded
SVC	slow vital capacity		shallow walk (aquatic therapy)
	subclavian vein compression		short wave
			Social Worker
	superior vena cava		stab wound
SVCO	superior vena cava obstruction		sterile water
			swallowing reflex

S&W	soap and water	**T**
S/W	somewhat	
SWA	Social Work Associate	
SWD	short wave diathermy	
SWFI	sterile water for injection	
SWG	standard wire gauge	T — inverted T wave
SWI	sterile water for injection	tablespoon (15 mL)
	surgical wound infection	(this is a dangerous
S&WI	skin and wound isolation	abbreviation)
SWL	shock wave lithotripsy	temperature
SWMA	segmental wall-motion	tender
	abnormalities	tension
SWO	superficial white	testicles
	onychomycosis	testosterone
SWOG	Southwest Oncology	thoracic
	Group	thymine
SWOT	strengths, weaknesses,	trace
	opportunities, threats	t — teaspoon (5 mL) (this is
	(analysis)	a dangerous
SWP	small whirlpool	abbreviation)
SWR	surface wrinkling	T+ — increase intraocular
	retinopathy	tension
	surgical waiting room	T— — decreased intraocular
SWS	sheltered workshop	tension
	slow wave sleep	2,4,5-T — 2,4,5-
	social work service	trichlorophenoxyacetic
	student ward secretary	acid
	Sturge-Weber syndrome	T° — temperature
SWT	stab wound of the throat	$T_{1/2}$ — half-life
	shuttle-walk test	T_1 — tricuspid first sound
SWU	septic work-up	T_2 — tricuspid second sound
SWW	static wall walk (aquatic	T-2 — dactinomycin,
	therapy)	doxorubicin,
Sx	signs	vincristine, and
	surgery	cyclophosphamide
	symptom	T_3 — triiodothyronine
SXA	single-energy x-ray	(liothyronine)
	absorptiometry	T3 — transurethral thermo-
SXR	skull x-ray	ablation therapy
SYN	synovial	(Targis)
SYN Fl	synovial fluid	Tylenol with codeine 30
SYPH	syphilis	mg (this is a dangerous
SYR	syrup	abbreviation)
SYS BP	systolic blood pressure	$T_{3/4}$ind — triiodothyronine to
SZ	schizophrenic	thyroxine index
	seizure	T_4 — levothyroxine
	suction	thyroxine
SZN	streptozocin (Zanosar)	T4 — CD4 (helper-inducer cells)
		T-7 — free thyroxine factor

S

T-10	methotrexate, calcium leucovorin rescue, doxorubicin, cisplatin, bleomycin, cyclophosphamide, and dactinomycin	TACC	thoracic aortic cross-clamping
		TACE	transarterial chemoembolization
$T_1...T_{12}$	thoracic nerve 1 through 12	TACI	total anterior cerebral infarct
	thoracic vertebra 1 through 12	TAD	thoracic asphyxiant dystrophy
TA	Takayasu's arteritis		transverse abdominal diameter
	temperature axillary temporal arteritis	TADAC	therapeutic abortion, dilation, aspiration, and curettage
	tendon Achilles therapeutic abortion		
	tracheal aspirate	TAE	transcatheter arterial embolization
	traffic accident tricuspid atresia	TAF	tissue angiogenesis factor
	truncus arteriosus	TAG	tumor-associated glycoprotein
Ta	tonometry applanation	TA-GVHD	transfusion-associated graft-versus-host disease
T&A	tonsillectomy and adenoidectomy		
	tonsils and adenoids	TAH	total abdominal hysterectomy
T(A)	axillary temperature		total artificial heart
TA-55	stapling device	TAHBSO	total abdominal hysterectomy, bilateral salpingo-oophorectomy
TAA	Therapeutic Activities Aide		
	thoracic aortic aneurysm	TAHL	thick ascending limb of Henle's loop
	total ankle arthroplasty		
	transverse aortic arch	T Air	air puff tonometry
	triamcinolone acetonide	TAL	tendon Achilles lengthening
	tumor-associated antigen (antibodies)		total arm length
TAAA	thoracoabdominal aortic aneursym	T ALCON	Alcon® tonometry
		TALP	total alkaline phosphatase
TAB	tablet	TAML	therapy-related acute myelogenous leukemia
	therapeutic abortion		
	total androgen blockade	TAM	tamoxifen
	triple antibiotic (bacitracin, neomycin, and polymyxin—this is a dangerous abbreviation)		teenage mother
			total active motion
			tumor-associated macrophages
TAC	tetracaine, Adrenalin® and cocaine	TAN	Treatment Authorization Number
			tropical ataxic neuropathy
	tibial artery catheter	TANI	total axial (lymph) node irradiation
	total abdominal colectomy		
	total allergen content	TAO	thromboangitis obliterans
	triamcinolone cream		troleandomycin

TAP	tone and positioning		thrombin-antithrombin III
	tonometry by applanation		complex
	transabdominal		'til all taken
	preperitoneal		total adipose tissue
	(laparoscopic hernia		transactivator of
	repair)		transcription
	transesophageal atrial		transplant-associated
	paced		thrombocytopenia
	trypsinogen activation		turnaround time
	peptide	TAUC	target area under the curve
	tumor-activated prodrug		time-averaged urea
TAPP	transabdominal		concentration
	preperitoneal	TAX	cefotaxime (Claforan)
	polypropylene (mesh-	TB	Tapes for the Blind
	plasty)		terrible burning
T APPL	applanation tonometry		thought broadcasting
TAPVC	total anomalous		toothbrush
	pulmonary venous		total base
	connection		total bilirubin
TAPVD	total anomalous		total body
	pulmonary venous		tuberculosis
	drainage	TBA	to be absorbed
TAPVR	total anomalous		to be added
	pulmonary venous		to be administered
	return		to be admitted
TAR	thrombocytopenia with		to be announced
	absent radius		to be arranged
	total ankle replacement		to be assessed
	total anorectal		to be evaluated
	reconstruction		total body (surface) area
	treatment administration	TBAGA	term birth appropriate for
	record		gestational age
	treatment authorization	T-bar	tracheotomy bar (a device
	request		used in respiratory
TARA	total articular replacement		therapy)
	arthroplasty	TBARS	thiobarbituric acid
TART	tenderness, asymmetry,		reactive substances
	restricted motion, and	TBB	transbronchial biopsy
	tissue texture changes	TBC	to be cancelled
	tumorectomy and		total-blood cholesterol
	radiotherapy		total-body clearance
TAS	therapeutic activities		tuberculosis
	specialist	TBD	to be determined
	turning against self	TBE	tick-borne encephalitis
	typical absence seizures	TBE$_e$	tick-borne encephalitis,
TAT	tandem autotransplants		eastern subtype (Far
	tell a tale		eastern encephalitis,
	tetanus antitoxin		Russian spring-summer
	thematic apperception test		e., Taiga e.) vaccine

T

T-berg	Trendelenburg (position)		total-burn surface area
TBEV	tick-borne encephalitis virus	tbsp	tablespoon (15 mL)
TBE$_w$	tick-bone encephalitis, western subtype (Central European encephalitis) vaccine	TBT	tolbutamide test tracheal bronchial toilet transbronchoscopic balloon tipped
TBF	total-body fat	TBV	thiotepa, bleomycin, and vinblastine
TBG	thyroxine-binding globulin		total-blood volume transluminal balloon valvuloplasty
TBI	toothbrushing instruction total-body irradiation traumatic brain injury	TBW	total-body water
T bili	total bilirubin	TBZ	thiabendazole (Mintezol)
TBK	total-body potassium	TC	team conference
tbl	tablespoon (15 mL)		telephone call
TBLB	transbronchial lung biopsy		terminal cancer
TBLC	term birth, living child		testicular cancer
TBLF	term birth, living female		thioguanine and cytarabine
TBLI	term birth, living infant		thoracic circumference
TBLM	term birth, living male		throat culture
TBM	tracheobronchomalacia tuberculous meningitis tubule basement membrane		tissue culture tolonium chloride tonsillar coblation
TBMg	total-body magnesium		total cholesterol
TBN	total-body nitrogen		to (the) chest
TBNA	transbronchial needle aspiration		tracheal collar trauma center
	treated but not admitted		true conjugate
TBNa	total-body sodium		tubocurarine
TBOCS	Tale-Brown Obsessive-Compulsive Scale	Tc	technetium
		T/C	telephone call
TBP	thyroxine-binding protein toe blood pressure		ticarcillin-clavulanic acid (Timentin)
	total-body phosphorus		to consider
	total-body protein	3TC	lamivudine (Epivir)
	tuberculous peritonitis	TC7	Interceed®
TBPA	thyroxine-binding prealbumin	T&C	turn and cough type and crossmatch
TBR	total-bed rest	T&C#3	Tylenol with 30 mg codeine
TBS	tablespoon (15ml)(this is a dangerous abbreviation)	TCA	thioguanine and cytarabine
	The Bethesda System (reporting cervical and vagina cytology)		tissue concentrations of antibiotic(s) trichloroacetic acid
	total-serum bilirubin		tricuspid atresia
TBSA	total-body surface area		tricyclic antidepressant

T

	tumor chemosensitivity assay	TCL	tibial collateral ligament transverse carpal ligament
	tumor clonogenic assays	TCM	tissue culture media
TCABG	triple coronary artery bypass graft		traditional Chinese medicine
TCAD	transplant-related coronary-artery disease tricyclic antidepressant		transcutaneous (oxygen) monitor
TCAR	tiazofurin	^{99m}Tc-MAA	technetium Tc 99m albumin microaggregated
TCB	to call back tumor cell burden	TCMH	tumor-direct cell-mediated hypersensitivity
TCBS agar	thiosulfate-citrate-bile salt-sucrose agar	TCMS	transcranial cortical magnetic stimulation
TCC	transitional cell carcinoma	TCMZ	trichlormethiazide
TcCO$_2$	transcutaneous carbon dioxide	TCN	tetracycline triciribine phosphate (tricyclic nucleoside)
TCD	transcerebellar diameter transcranial Doppler (ultrasonography) transverse cardiac diameter	TCNS	transcutaneous nerve stimulator
		TCNU	tauromustine
TCCB	transitional cell carcinoma of bladder	TcO$_4$$^-$	pertechnetate
		TCOM	transcutaneous oxygen monitor
TC/CL	ticarcillin-clavulanate (Timentin)	T Con	temporary conservatorship
TCD	transcystic duct	TCP	thrombocytopenia transcutaneous pacing tranylcypromine (Parnate) tumor control probability
TCDB	turn, cough, and deep breath		
TCDD	tetrachlorodibenzo-p-dioxin (dioxin)	TcPCO$_2$	transcutaneous carbon dioxide
^{99m}Tc DTPA	technetium Tc 99m pentetate	TcPO$_2$	transcutaneous oxygen
		^{99m}TcPYP	technetium Tc 99m pyrophosphate
TCE	tetrachloroethylene total-colon examination transcatheter embolotherapy	TCR	T-cell receptor
		TCRE	transcervical resection of the endometrium
T cell	small lymphocyte	TCS	tonic-clonic seizure
^{99m}TcGHA	technetium Tc 99m gluceptate	^{99m}TcSC	technetium Tc 99m sulfur colloid
TCH	turn, cough, hyperventilate	TCT	thyrocalcitonin tincture triple combination tablet (abacavir, lamivudine, and zidovudine)
TCHRs	traditional Chinese herbal remedies		
TCI	target-control infusion to come in		
TCID	tissue culture infective dose	TCU	transitional care unit
TCIE	transient cerebral ischemic episode	TCVA	thromboembolic cerebral vascular accident

TD	Takayasu's disease	TDT	tentative discharge tomorrow
	tardive dyskinesia		transmission disequilibrium test
	temporary disability		Trieger Dot Test
	terminal device		tumor doubling time
	test dose	TdT	terminal deoxynucleotidyl transferase
	tetanus-diphtheria toxoids (pediatric use)	TDW	target dry weight
	tidal volume	TDWB	touch down weight bearing
	tolerance dose		
	tone decay	TDx®	fluorescence polarization immunoassay
	total disability		
	transverse diameter	TE	echo time
	travelers' diarrhea		tennis elbow
	treatment discontinued		terminal extension
Td	tetanus-diphtheria toxoids (adult type)		tooth extraction
			toxoplasmic encephalitis
TDAC	tumor-derived activated cell (cultures)		trace elements (chromium, copper, iodine, manganese, selenium, molybdenum and zinc)
TDD	telephone device for the deaf		
	thoracic duct drainage		tracheoesophageal
	total daily dose		transesophageal echocardiography
TDE	total daily energy (requirement)		transrectal electroejaculation
TDF	testis determining factor	tE	total expiratory time
	total-dietary fiber	T/E	testosterone to epitestosterone ratio
	tumor dose fractionation		
TDI	tolerable daily intake	T&E	testing and evaluation
	toluene diisocyanate		training and evaluation
TDK	tardive diskinesia		trial and error
TDL	thoracic duct lymph	TEA	thromboendarterectomy
TDLN	tumor-draining lymph nodes		total elbow arthroplasty
		TEB	thoracic electrical bioimpedance
TDM	therapeutic drug monitoring		
		TEBG	testosterone-estradiol binding globulin
TDMAC	tridodecylmethyl ammonium chloride		
		TeBG	testeosterone binding globulin
TDN	totally digestible nutrients		
	transdermal nitroglycerin	TeBIDA	technetium 99m trimethyl 1-bromo-imono diacetic acid
TDNTG	transdermal nitroglycerin		
TDNWB	touchdown non-weight-bearing	TEC	total eosinophil count
			toxic *Escherichia coli*
TdP	torsades de pointes		transient erythroblastopenia of childhood
TDPWB	touchdown partial weight-bearing		
TdR	thymidine		
TDS	three times a day (United Kingdom)		

T

	transluminal extraction-endarterectomy catheter	TEQ	tubal ectopic pregnancy
	triethyl citrate	TER	toxic equivalents
T&EC	trauma and emergency center		terlipressin
			total elbow replacement
TECA	titrated extract of *Centella asiatica*		total energy requirement
			transurethral electroresection
TED	thromboembolic disease	TERB	terbutaline
	thyroid eye disease	TERC	Test of Early Reading Comprehension
TEDS	thromboembolic disease stockings	TERM	full-term
TEE	total energy expended		terminal
	transnasal endoscopic ethmoidectomy	TERT	tertiary
			total end-range time
	transesophageal echocardiography	TES	therapeutic electrical stimulation
TEF	tracheoesophageal fistula		thoracic endometriosis syndrome
TEG	thromboelastogram (thromboelastography)		treatment emergent symptoms
TEI	total episode of illness	TESE	testicular sperm extraction
	transesophageal imaging		
TEL	telemetry	TESI	thoracic epidural steroid injection
	telephone	TESS	Treatment Emergent Symptom Scale
tele	telemetry		
TEM	temozolomide (Temodar)	TET	transcranial electrostimulation therapy
	transanal endoscopic microsurgery		
	transmission electron microscopy		treadmill exercise test
TEMI	transient episodes of myocardial ischemia	TETE	too early to evaluate
TEMP	temperature	TEU	token economy unit
	temporal	TEV	talipes equinovarus (deformity)
	temporary		
TEN	tension (intraocular pressure)	TEVAP	transurethral electrovaporization of the prostate
	toxic epidermal necrolysis		
TEN®	Total Enteral Nutrition	TF	tactile fremitus
TENS	transcutaneous electrical nerve stimulation		tail flick (reflex)
			tetralogy of Fallot
TEOAE	transient evoked otoacoustic emission (test)		to follow
			tube feeding
TEP	total endoprosthesis	TFA	topical fluoride application
	total extraperitoneal (laparoscopic hernia repair)		trans fatty acids
			trifluoroacetic acid
		TFB	trifascicular block
	tracheoesophageal puncture	TFBC	The Family Birthing Center

TFC	thoracic fluid content	TGGE	temperature-gradient gel electrophoresis
	time to following commands	TGR	tenderness, guarding, and rigidity
TFCC	transjugular fibrocartilage complex	TGS	tincture of green soap
TFF	tangential flow filtration	TGs	triglycerides
TF-Fe	transferrin-bound iron	TGT	thromboplastin generation test
TFL	tensor fasciae latae		
	trimetrexate, fluorouracil, and leucovorin	TGTL	total glottic transverse laryngectomy
TFM	transverse friction massage	TGV	thoracic gas volume
			transposition of great vessels
TFO	triplex-forming oligonucleotide	TGXT	thallium-graded exercise test
TFOs	triplex-forming oligonucleotides	TGZ	troglitazone (Rezulin)
TFPI	tissue factor pathway inhibitor	TH	thrill
			thyroid hormone
TFR	total fertility rate		total hysterectomy
TFT	thumb-finding test	T&H	type and hold
	trifluridine (trifluorothymidine)	THA	tacrine (tetrahydroacridine; Cognex)
TFTs	thyroid function tests		total hip arthroplasty
TG	total gym		transient hemispheric attack
	triglycerides		
Tg	thyroglobulin	THAA	thyroid hormone autoantibodies
6-TG	thioguanine		tubular hypoplasia aortic arch
TGA	Therapeutic Goods Administration (Australia)	THAL	thalassemia
	third-generation antidepressant	THBI	thyroid hormone binding index
	transient global amnesia	THBR	thyroid hormone-binding ratio
	transposition of the great arteries	THAM®	tromethamine
TGAR	total graft area rejected	THBO$_2$	topical hyperbaric oxygen
TGB	tiagabine (Gabatril)	THC	tetrahydrocannabinol (dronabinol)
TGCT	testicular germ cell tumor(s)		thigh circumference
TGD	thyroglossal duct		transhepatic cholangiogram
	tumor growth delay	THCT	triple-phase helical computer tomography
TGE	transmissible gastroenteritis	TH-CULT	throat culture
TGFA	triglyceride fatty acid	tHcy	total homocysteine
TGF	transforming growth factor	THE	total-head excursion
			transhepatic embolization
TGF-$_\beta$	transforming growth factor-beta	Ther Ex	therapeutic exercise

T

THF	thymic humoral factor		transplant intensive care unit
THI	transient hypogamma-globinemia of infancy		trauma intensive care unit
THKAFO	trunk-hip-knee-ankle-foot orthosis	*TID*	three times a day
THL	transvaginal hydrolaparoscopy	TIDM	three times daily with meals
THLAA	tubular hypoplasia left aortic arch	TIE	transient ischemic episode
		TIF	tracheal intubation fiberscope
THP	take home packs	TIG	tetanus immune globulin
	total hip prosthesis		
	transhepatic portography	TIH	tumor-inducing hypercalcemia
	trihexyphenidyl (Artane)		
THR	target heart rate	TIL	tumor-infiltrating lymphocytes
	thrombin receptor		
	total hip replacement	%tile	percentile
	training heart rate	TIMP	tissue inhibitor of metalloproteinase
THRL	total hip replacement, left		
		TIN	three times a night (this is a dangerous abbreviation)
THRR	total hip replacement, right		
			tubulointerstitial nephritis
THTV	therapeutic home trial visit		
		tinct	tincture
THV	therapeutic home visit	TIND	Treatment Investigational New Drug (application)
TI	terminal ileus		
	thought insertion	TINEM	there is no evidence of malignancy
	transischial		
	transverse diameter of inlet	TIP	toxic interstitial pneumonitis
			tubularized incised plate (urethroplasty)
	tricuspid incompetence		
	tricuspid insufficiency		
TIA	transient ischemic attack		
TIB	tibia	TIPS	transjugular intrahepatic portosystemic shunt (stent-shunt)
TIBC	total iron-binding capacity		
TIC	paclitaxel (Taxol), ifosfamide, and cisplain	TIPSS	transjugular intrahepatic portosystemic shunt (stent)
	trypsin-inhibitor capacity		
TICOSMO	**t**rauma, **i**nfection, **c**hemical/drug exposure, **o**rgan systems, **s**tress, **m**usculoskeletal, and **o**ther (prompts used during history taking for possible etiologies of problems)	TIRFM	total-internal reflection microscopy
		TIS	tumor *in situ*
		TISS	Therapeutic Intervention Scoring System
		TIT	*Treponema* (*pallidum*) immobilization test
			triiodothyronine (liothyronine)
TICS	diverticulosis		
TICU	thoracic intensive care unit	TIUP	term intrauterine pregnancy

T

TIVA	total intravenous anethesia		T-lymphocyte choriocarcinoma
TIVC	thoracic inferior vena cava		total lung capacity
+tive	positive		total lymphocyte count
TIW	three times a week (this is a dangerous abbreviation)	TLD	triple lumen catheter
			thermoluminescent dosimeter
TJ	tendon jerk	TLE	temporal lobe epilepsy
	triceps jerk	TLI	total lymphoid irradiation
TJA	total joint arthroplasty		translaryngeal intubation
TJC	tender joint count	TLK	thermal laser keratoplasty
TJN	tongue jaw neck (dissection)	TLM	torn lateral meniscus
		TLNB	term living newborn
	twin jet nebulizer	TLP	transitional living program
TJR	total joint replacement	TLR	target lesion reintervention
TK	thymidine kinase		tonic labyrinthine reflex
	toxicokinetics	TLS	tumor lysis syndrome
TKA	total knee arthroplasty	TLSO	thoracic lumbar sacral orthosis
	tyrosine kinase activity		
TKD	tokodynamometer	TLSSO	thoracolumbosacral spinal orthosis
TKE	terminal knee extension		
TKIC	true knot in cord	TLT	tonsillectomy
TKNO	to keep needle open	TLV	total lung volume
TKP	thermokeratoplasty	TM	temperature by mouth
	total knee prosthesis		thalassemia major
TKO	to keep open		Thayer-Martin (culture)
TKR	total knee replacement		trabecular meshwork
TKRL	total knee replacement, left		trademark (unregistered)
			transcendental meditation
TKRR	total knee replacement, right		treadmill
			tropical medicine
TKVO	to keep vein open		tumor
TL	team leader		tympanic membrane
	thoracolumbar	T & M	type and crossmatch
	total laryngectomy	TMA	thrombotic microangiopathy
	transverse line		
	trial leave		trained medication aid
	tubal ligation		transcription mediated amplification
T/L	terminal latency		
Tl	thallium		transmetatarsal amputation
TLA	translumbar arteriogram (aortogram)		trimethylamine
		T/MA	tracheostomy mask
TLAC	triple lumen Arrow catheter	TMAS	Taylor Manifest Anxiety Scale
TL BLT	tubal ligation, bilateral	TMA-uria	trimethylaminuria
TLC	tender loving care	T_{max}	temperature maximum
	thin layer chromatography	t_{max}	time of occurrence for maximum (peak) drug concentration
	titanium linear cutter		

T

TMB	tetramethylberizidine	TMR	trainable mentally retarded
	transient monocular blindness		transmyocardial revascularization
	trimethoxybenzoates		
TMC	transmural colitis	TMS	transcranial magnetic stimulation
	triamcinolone		
TMCA	trimethylcolchicinic acid	TMST	treadmill stress test
TMCN	triamcinolone	TMT	tarsometatarsal
TMD	temporomandibular dysfunction (disorder)		teratoma with malignant transformation
	treating physician		treadmill test
TME	thermolysin-like metalloendopeptidase		tympanic membrane thermometer
	total mesorectal excision	TMTC	too many to count
		TMTX	trimetrexate (Neutrexin)
TMET	treadmill exercise test	TMUGS	Tumor Marker Utility Grading Scale
TMEV	Theiler's murine encephalomyelitis virus	TMX	tamoxifen
TMH	trainable mentally handicapped	TMZ	temazepam (Restoril)
			temozolomide (Temodar)
TMI	threatened myocardial infarction	TN	normal intraocular tension
			team nursing
	transmandibular implant		temperature normal
	transmural infarct	T&N	tension and nervousness
T>MIC	time above minimum inhibitory concentration		tingling and numbness
		TNA	total nutrient admixture
TMJ	temporomandibular joint	TNAB	transthoracic needle biopsy
TMJD	temporomandibular joint dysfunction	TNB	term newborn
TMJS	temporomandibular joint syndrome		transnasal butorphanol
			transrectal needle biopsy (of the prostate)
TML	tongue midline		Tru-Cut® needle biopsy
	treadmill	TNBP	transurethral needle biopsy of prostate
TMLR	transmyocardial laser revascularization		
		TND	term, normal delivery
TMM	torn medial meniscus	TNDM	transient neonatal diabetes mellitus
	total muscle mass		
Tmm	McKay-Marg tension	TNF	tumor necrosis factor
TMNG	toxic multinodular goiter	TNF-bp	tumor necrosis factor binding protein
TMP	thallium myocardial perfusion		
		TNG	nitroglycerin
	transmembrane pressure	TNI	total nodal irradiation
	trimethoprim	TNKase®	tenecteplase
TMP/SMZ	trimethoprim and sulfamethoxazole (correct name is sulfamethoxazole and trimethoprin; SMZ-TMP)	TNM	primary tumor, regional lymph nodes, and distant metastasis (used with subscripts for the staging of cancer)

TNR	tonic neck reflex		trial of labor
TNS	transcutaneous nerve stimulation (stimulator)	TOLA	temporary leave of absence
	transient neurologic symptoms	TOLD	Test of Language Development
	Tullie-Niebörg syndrome	TOM	therapeutic outcomes monitoring
TNT	thiotepa, mitoxantrone (Novantrone), and paclitaxel (Taxol)		tomorrow
			transcutaneous oxygen monitor
	triamcinolone and nystatin	Tomo	tomography
TNTC	too numerous to count	TON	tonight
TNU	tobacco nonuser	TOP	termination of pregnancy
TNY	trichomonas and yeast		Topografov (virus)
TO	old tuberculin		topotecan (Hycamtin)
	telephone order	TOP-8	Treatment Outcome PTSD (post-traumatic stress disorder) (scale)
	time off		
	tincture of opium (warning: this is NOT paregoric)	TOPO	topotecan (Hycamtin)
		TOPO 1	topoisermerase
	total obstruction	TOPS	Take Off Pounds Sensibly
	transfer out	TOPV	trivalent oral polio vaccine
T(O)	oral temperature		
T/O	time out	TOR	toremifene (Faneston)
T&O	tubes and ovaries	TORC	Test of Reading Comprehension
TOA	time of arrival		
	tubo-ovarian abscess	TORCH	toxoplasmosis, others (other viruses known to attack the fetus), rubella, cytomegalovirus, and herpes simplex (maternal viral infections)
TOAA	to affected areas		
TOB	tobacco		
	tobramycin		
TOC	table of contents		
	total organic carbon		
TOCE	transcatheter oily chemoembolization		
TOCO	tocodynamometer	TORP	total ossicular replacement prosthesis
TOD	intraocular pressure of the right eye	TOS	intraocular pressure of the left eye
	time of death		thoracic outlet syndrome
	time of departure	TOT BILI	total bilirubin
	tubal occlusion device	TOTM	trioctyltrimellitate
TOF	tetralogy of Fallot	TOV	trial of void
	time of flight	TOWL	Test of Written Language
	total of four	TOXO	toxoplasmosis
	train-of-four	TP	temperature and pressure
TOFMS	time-of-flight mass spectrometry		temporoparietal
			tender point
TOGV	transposition of the great vessels		therapeutic pass
TOH	throughout hospitalization		thought process
TOL	tolerate		

	thrombophlebitis	TPF	trained participating father
	thymidine phosphorylase		
	time to progression	TPH	thromboembolic pulmonary hypertension
	Todd's paralysis		
	toe pressure		trained participating husband
	toilet paper		
	total protein	TPHA	*Treponema pallidum* hemagglutination
	"T" piece		
	treating physician	T PHOS	triple phosphate crystals
	trigger point	TPI	*Treponema pallidum* immobilization
T:P	trough-to-peak ratio		
T & P	temperature and pulse		triose phosphate isomerase
	turn and position		
TPA	alteplase, recombinant (tissue plasminogen activator) (Activase)	TPIT	trigger point injection therapy
		t_{pk}	time to peak
	temporary portacaval anastomosis	TPL	thromboplastin
		T plasty	tympanoplasty
	third-party administrator	TPLSM	two-photon laser-scanning microscope
	tissue polypeptide antigen		
	total parenteral alimentation	TPM	temporary pacemaker
			topiramate (Topamax)
TPAL	term infant(s), premature infant(s), abortion(s), living children	TPMT	thiopurine methyltransferase
		TPN	total parenteral nutrition
TPC	target plasma concentration	TPO	thrombopoietin
			thyroid peroxidase
	total patient care		trial prescription order
TPD	tropical pancreatic diabetes	TPP	thiamine pyrophosphate
		TpP	thrombus precursor protein
	typhoid vaccine, not otherwise specified	TP & P	time, place, and person
TPD$_a$	typhoid vaccine, attenuated live (oral Ty21a strain)	TPPN	total peripheral parenteral nutrition
		TPPS	Toddler-Preschooler Postoperative Pain Scale
TPD$_{AKD}$	typhoid vaccine, acetone-killed and dried (U.S. military)		
		TPPV	trans pars plana vitrectomy
TPD$_{HP}$	typhoid vaccine, heat and phenol inactivated, dried	TPR	temperature
			temperature, pulse, and respiration
TPD$_{VI}$	typhoid vaccine, *Vi* capsular polysaccharide		total peripheral resistance
TPE	therapeutic plasma exchange	TPRI	total peripheral resistance index
		T PROT	total protein
	total placental estrogens	TPS	typhus (*rickettsiae* sp.) vaccine
	total protective environment		
T-penia	thrombocytopenia	TPT	time to peak tension

	topotecan (Hycamtin)	TRAMP	transversus and rectus abdominis musculo-peritoneal (flap)
	transpyloric tube		
	treadmill performance test		
*t*PTEF	time to peak tidal expiratory flow	TRANCE	tumor necrosis factor–related activation-induced cytokine
TPU	tropical phagedenic ulcer		
T-putty	Theraputty	TRANS	transfers
TPVR	total peripheral vascular resistance	Trans D	transverse diameter
TPZ	tirapazamine	TRANS Rx	transfusion reaction
TQM	total quality management	TRAP	tartrate-resistant (leukocyte) acid phophatase
TR	therapeutic recreation		
	time to repeat		Telomeric Repeat Amplification Protocol
	tincture		
	to return		thrombospondin-related anonymous protein
	trace		
	transfusion reaction		total radical-trapping antioxidant parameter
	transplant recipients		
	treatment		trapezium
	tremor		trapezius muscle
	tricuspid regurgitation	TRAS	transplant renal artery stenosis
	tumor registry		
T(R)	rectal temperature		
T & R	tenderness and rebound	TRB	return to baseline
	treated and released	TRBC	total red blood cells
	turn and reposition	TRC	tanned red cells
TRA	therapeutic recreation associate	TRD	tongue-retaining device
	to run at		total-retinal detachment
	tumor regression antigen		traction retinal detachment
TRAb	thyrotropin-receptor antibody		treatment-related death
TRAC	traction		treatment-resistant depression
TRACH	tracheal	TRDN	transient respiratory distress of the newborn
	tracheostomy		
TRAFO	tone-reducing ankle/foot orthosis		
TRAIL	tumor-necrosis-factor-related apoptosis-inducing ligand	TREC	T-cell receptor-rearrangement excision circles
TRALI	transfusion-associated lung injury	Tren	Trendelenburg
TRAM	transverse rectus abdominis myocutaneous (flap)	TRH	protirelin (thyrotropin-releasing hormone) (Relefact TRH®; Thypinone®)
	transverse rectus abdominum muscle	TRI	transient radicular irritation
	Treatment Response Assessment Method		trimester
		T_3RIA	triiodothyronine level by radioimmunoassay

T

TRIC	trachoma inclusion conjunctivitis	TRUS	transrectal ultrasonography	
TRICH	*Trichomonas*	TRUSP	transrectal ultrasonography of the prostate	
TRICKS	time-resolved imaging contrast kinetics			
TRIG	triglycerides	TRUST	toluidine red unheated serum test	
TRISS	Trauma Related Injury Severity Score	TRZ	triazolam (Halcion)	
TR-LSC	time-resolved liquid scintillation counting	TS	Tay-Sachs (disease) telomerase	
TRM	transplant-related mortality		temperature sensitive test solution	
	treatment-related mortality		thoracic spine throat swab	
TRM-SMX	trimethoprim-sulfamethoxazole (correct name is sulfamethoxazole and trimethoprin; SMZ-TMP; SMX-TMP)		thymidylate synthase toe signs Tourette's syndrome transsexual Trauma Score tricuspid stenosis triple strength	
tRNA	transfer ribonucleic acid		tuberous sclerosis	
TRNBP	transrectal needle biopsy prostate		Turner's syndrome	
TRND	Trendelenburg (position)	T/S	trimethoprim/sulfamethoxazole (correct name is sulfamethoxazole and trimethoprin)	
TRNG	tetracycline-resistant *Neisseria gonorrhoeae*			
TRO	to return to office			
TROFO	trofosfamide			
TROM	torque range of motion	T&S	type and screen	
	total range of motion	Ts	Schiotz tension T suppressor cell	
TRP	tubular reabsorption of phosphate			
TrPs	trigger points	TSAb	thyroid stimulating antibodies	
TRPT	transplant			
TRS	Therapeutic Recreation Specialist	TSA	toluenesulfonic acid total shoulder arthroplasty tumor-specific antigen type-specific antibody tyramine signal amplification	
	the real symptom			
TRT	tangential radiation therapy thermoradiotherapy thoracic radiation therapy treatment-related toxicity			
		TSAR®	tape surrounded Appli-rulers	
TR/TE	time to repetition and time to echo in spin (echo sequence of magnetic resonance imaging)	TSAS	Total Severity Assessment Score	
		TSB	total serum bilirubin trypticase soy broth	
		TSBB	transtracheal selective bronchial brushing	
T_3RU	triiodothyronine resin uptake	TSC	technetium sulfur colloid	

	theophylline serum concentration	TSST	toxic shock syndrome toxin
	total symptom complex	TST	titmus stereocuity test
	tuberous sclerosis complex		trans-scrotal testosterone
T-score	number of standard deviations from the average bone mineral density (BMD) of a 25-30 year old woman		treadmill stress test tuberculin skin test(s)
		TSTA	tumor-specific transplantation antigens
		T&T	tobramycin and ticarcillin
TSD	target to skin distance		touch and tone
	Tay-Sachs disease	TT	Test Tape®
TSDP	tapered steroid dosing package		tetanus toxoid thiotepa (Thioplex)
TSE	targeted systemic exposure		thrombin time thrombolytic therapy
	testicular self-examination		thymol turbidity
	total skin examination		tilt table
	transmissible spongiform encephalopathy		tonometry total thyroidectomy
TSEBT	total skin electron beam therapy		transit time transtracheal
T set	tracheotomy set		tuberculin tested
TSF	tricep skin fold (thickness)		twitch tension tympanic temperature
		T-T	time-to-time
TSGs	tumor suppressor genes	T/T	trace of ____/ trace of ____
TSH	thyroid-stimulating hormone (thyrotropin)	T&T	tympantomy and tube (insertion)
TSH-RH	thyrotropin-releasing hormone	TT4	total thyroxine
TSI	thyroid stimulating immunoglobulin	TTA	total toe arthroplasty transtracheal aspiration
	tobramycin solution for inhalation (TOBI®)	TTAT	toe touch as tolerated
		TTC	transtracheal catheter
TSIs	thymidylate synthase inhibitors	TTD	tarsal tunnel decompression
T-SKULL	trauma skull		temporary total disability
tsp	teaspoon (5 mL)		total tumor dose
TSP	thrombospondin		transverse thoracic diameter
	total serum protein		
	tropical spastic paraparesis	TTDE	transthoracic color Doppler echocardiography
TSPA	thiotepa		
T-SPINE	thoracic spine	TTDM	thallim threadmill
TSR	total shoulder replacement	TTDP	time-to-disease progression
TSS	total serum solids	TTE	transthoracic echocardiography
	toxic shock syndrome		
	tumor score system	t test	Student's t-test

T

329

TTF	time-to-treatment failure		total tourniquet time
TTGE	timed-temperature gradient electrophoresis		turn-to-turn transfusion
		TTTS	twin-twin transfusion syndrome
TTI	Teflon tube insertion	TTUTD	tetanus toxoid up-to-date
	total time to intubate	TTV	transfusion-transmitted virus
	transfer to intermediate		
TTII	thyrotropin-binding inhibitory immunoglobulins	TTVP	temporary transvenous pacemaker
		TTWB	touch-toe weight bearing
TTJV	transtracheal jet ventilation	TTx	thrombolytic therapy
		TU	Todd units
TTM	total tumor mass		transrectal ultrasound
	transtelephonic monitoring		transurethral
	trichotillomania		tuberculin units
TTN	transient tachypnea of the newborn	1-TU	1 tuberculin unit
		5-TU	5 tuberculin units
		250-TU	250 tuberculin units
TTNA	transthoracic needle aspiration	TUB	tuberculosis vaccine, not BCG
TTNB	transient tachypnea of the newborn	TUE	transurethral extraction
		TUF	total ultrafiltration
TTND	time to nondetectable	TUG	total urinary gonadotropin
TTO	tea tree oil	TUIBN	transurethral incision of bladder neck
	time trade-off		
	to take out	TUIP	transurethral incision of the prostate
	transfer to open		
	transtracheal oxygen	TUL	tularemia (*Francisella tularensis*) vaccine
TTOD	tetanus toxoid outdated		
TTOT	transtracheal oxygen therapy	TULIP®	transurethral ultrasound-guided laser-induced prostatectomy (system)
TTP	tender to palpation		
	tender to pressure	TUMT	transurethral microwave thermotherapy
	thrombotic thrombocytopenic purpura		
		TUN	total urinary nitrogen
	time to pregnancy	TUNA	transurethral needle ablation
	time to tumor progression		
	time-to-progression	TUPR	transurethral prostatic resection
TTR	transthyretin		
	triceps tendon reflex	TUR	transurethral resection
TTS	tarsal tunnel syndrome	T₃UR	triiodothyronine uptake ratio
	temporary threshold shift		
	through the skin	TURB	transurethral resection of the bladder
	transdermal therapeutic system		
			turbidity
	transfusion therapy service	TURBN	transurethral resection bladder neck
TTT	tilt-table test		
	tolbutamide tolerance test	TURBT	transurethral resection bladder tumor

T

TURP	transurethral resection of prostate		tapwater
			test weight
			thought withdrawal
TURV	transurethral resection valves		*Trophermyma whippleii*
			T-wave
TURVN	transurethral resection of vesical neck	TW2	Tanner-Whitehouse mark 2 (bone-age assessment)
TUU	transureteroureterostomy		
TUV	transurethral valve	5TW	five times a week (this is a dangerous abbreviation)
TUVP	transurethral vaporization of the prostate		
TV	television	TWA	time-weighted average
	temporary visit		total wrist arthroplasty
	tidal volume		T-wave alternans
	transvenous	TWAR	*Chlamydia pneumoniae*
	trial visit	T wave	part of the electrocardiographic cycle, representing a portion of ventricular repolarization
	Trichomonas vaginalis		
	tricuspid value		
T/V	touch-verbal		
TVC	triple voiding cystogram		
	true vocal cord		
TVc	tricuspid valve closure	TWD	total white and differential count
TVD	triple vessel disease		
TVDALV	triple vessel disease with an abnormal left ventricle	TWE	tapwater enema
		TWETC	tapwater enema 'til clear
		TWG	total weight gain
TVF	tactile vocal fremitus	TWH	transitional wall hyperplasia
	true vocal fold		
TVH	total vaginal hysterectomy	TWHW ok	toe walking and heel walking all right
TVI	time velocity integral		
TVN	tonic vibration response	TWI	T-wave inversion
TVP	tensor veli palatini (muscle)	TWiST	time without symptoms of progression or toxicity
	transvenous pacemaker	TWR	total wrist replacement
	transvesicle prostatectomy	TWSTRS	Toronto Western Spasmodic Torticollis Rating Scale
TVR	tricuspid valve replacement		
TVRSS	total vasomotor rhinitis symptom score	T1WT	T1 weighted image
		TWWD	tap water wet dressing
TVS	transvaginal sonography	Tx	therapist
	transvenous system		therapy
	trigemino-vascular system		traction
TVSC	transvaginal sector scan		transcription
TVT	transvaginal tension-free		transfuse
TVU	total volume of urine		transplant
	transvaginal ultrasonography		transplantation
			treatment
TVUS	transvaginal ultrasonography		tympanostomy
TW	talked with	T & X	type and crossmatch
		TXA₂	thromboxane A_2

T

331

TXB$_2$	thromboxane B$_2$
TXE	Timoptic-XE®
TXL	paclitaxel (Taxol) (this is a dangerous abbreviation as it can be read as TXT)
TXM	type and crossmatch
TXS	type and screen
TXT	docetaxel (Taxotere) (this is a dangerous abbreviation as it can be read as TXL)
T & Y	trichomonas and yeast
TYCO #3	Tylenol with 30 mg of codeine (#1=7.5 mg, #2=15 mg and #4=60 mg of codeine present)
Tyl	Tylenol (acetaminophen)
	tyloma (callus)
TYMP	tympanogram
TYR	tyrosine
TZ	temozolomide (Temodar)
	transition zone
TZD	thiazolidinedione
TZDs	thiazolidinediones
TZM	temozolomide (Temodar)

U

U	Ultralente Insulin®
	units (this is the most dangerous abbreviation—spell out "unit")
	unknown
	upper
	urine
Ⓤ	Kosher
U/1	1 finger breadth below umbilicus
1/U	1 finger over umbilicus
U/	at umbilicus
24U	24 hour urine (collection)
U100	100 units per milliliters
UA	umbilical artery
	unauthorized absence
	uncertain about
	unstable angina
	upper airway
	upper arm
	uric acid
	urinalysis
UAC	umbilical artery catheter
	under active
	upper airway congestion
UA/C	uric acid to creatinine (ratio)
UAD	upper airway disease
UADT	upper aerodigestive tract
UAE	urinary albumin excretion
UAL	umbilical artery line
	up *ad lib*
UA&M	urinalysis and microscopy
UAO	upper airway obstruction
UAP	upper abdominal pain
UAPD	Union of American Physicians and Dentists
UAPF	upon arrival patient found
UAPs	unlicensed assistive personnel
U-ARM	upper arm
UARS	upper airway resistance syndrome

T

UAS	upstream activating sequence	UCHS	uncontrolled hemorrhagic shock
UASA	upper airway sleep apnea	UCI	urethral catheter in
UAT	up as tolerated		usual childhood illnesses
UAVC	univentricular atrioventricular connection	UCL	uncomfortable loudness level
UBC	University of British Columbia (brace)	UCLP	unilateral cleft lip and palate
UBD	universal blood donor	UCN-01	7-hydroxystaurosporin
UBE	upper body ergometer	UCO	urethral catheter out
UBF	unknown black female	UCP	umbilical cord prolapse
	uterine blood flow		urethral closure pressure
UBI	ultraviolet blood irradiation	UCPs	urine collection pads
		UCR	unconditioned reflex
UBM	unknown black male		unconditioned response
UBO	unidentified bright object		usual, customary, and reasonable (fees)
UBT	^{13}C-urea breath test	UCP-3	uncoupling protein −3
	uterine balloon therapy	UCRE	urine creatinine
UBW	usual body weight	UCRP	universal coagulation reference plasma
UC	ulcerative colitis		
	umbilical cord	UCS	unconscious
	unchanged	UC&S	urine culture and sensitivity
	unconscious		
	Unit clerk	UCTD	undifferentiated connective tissue disease
	United Church of Christ		
	urea clearance		
	urinary catheter	UCX	urine culture
	urine culture	UD	as directed
	usual care		ulnar deviation
	uterine contraction		urethral dilatation
U&C	urethral and cervical		urethral discharge
	usual and customary		urodynamics
UCAD	unstable coronary artery disease		uterine distension
		UDC	uninhibited detrusor (muscle) capacity
UCB	umbilical cord blood		
	unconjugated bilirubin (indirect)		usual diseases of childhood
	Unicorn Campbell Boy (orthotics)	UDCA	ursodeoxycholic acid
		UDN	updraft nebulizer
UCBT	unrelated cord-blood transplant	UDO	undetermined origin
		UDP	unassisted diastolic pressure
UCD	urine collection device		
	usual childhood diseases	UDPGT	uridinediphospho-glucuronyl transferase
UCE	urea cycle enzymopathy		
UCG	urinary chorionic gonadotropins	UDS	unconditioned stimulus
			urine drug screen
UCHD	usual childhood diseases	UDT	undescended testicle(s)
UCHI	usual childhood illnesses	UE	under elbow

U

	undetermined etiology upper extremity	UGIS	upper gastrointestinal series
U & E	urea and electrolytes (see page 358)	UGIT	upper gastrointestinal tract
UEC	uterine endometrial carcinoma	UGI w/SBFT	upper gastrointestinal (series) with small bowel follow through
UEDs	unilateral epileptiform discharges	UGK	urine, glucose, and ketones
UES	undifferentiated embryonal sarcoma upper esophageal sphincter	UGP	urinary gonadotropin peptide
UESEP	upper extremity somatosensory evoked potential	UGVA	ultrasound-guided vascular access
		UH	umbilical hernia unfavorable history
UESP	upper esophageal sphincter pressure		University Hospital
UF	ultrafiltration until finished	UHBI	upper hemibody irradiation
UFC	urinary free cortisol	UHDDS	Uniform Hospital Discharge Data Set
UFF	unusual facial features	UHP	University Health Plan
UFFI	urea formaldehyde foam insulation	UI	urinary incontinence
UFH	unfractionated heparin	UIB	Unemployment Insurance Benefits
UFN	until further notice		
UFO	unflagged order unidentified foreign object	UIBC	unbound iron binding capacity unsaturated iron binding capacity
UFOV	useful field of view	UID	once daily (this is a dangerous abbreviation, spell out "once daily")
UFR	ultrafiltration rate		
UFT	uracil and tegafur		
UFV	ultrafiltration volume	UIEP	urine (urinary) immunoelectrophoresis
UG	until gone urinary glucose urogenital	UIP	usual interstitial pneumonitis (pneumonia)
UGA	under general anesthesia urogenital atrophy	UIQ	upper inner quadrant
		UJ	universal joint (syndrome)
UGCR	ultrasound-guided compression repair	UK	United Kingdom unknown urine potassium urokinase
UGDP	University Group Diabetes Project		
UGH	uveitis, glaucoma, and hyphema (syndrome)	UK IC	urokinase intracoronary
UGI	upper gastrointestinal series	UKO	unknown origin
		UL	Unit Leader upper left upper lid upper limb upper lobe
UGIB	upper gastrointestinal bleeding		
UGIH	upper gastrointestinal (tract) hemorrhage		

U

U/L	upper and lower	UN/P	unpatched eye
U & L	upper and lower	UN/P OD	unpatched right eye
ULBW	ultra low birth weight (between 501 and 750 g)	UN/P OS	unpatched left eye
		UNS	unsatisfactory
		UNSAT	unsatisfactory
ULLE	upper lid, left eye	UO	under observation
ULN	upper limits of normal		undetermined origin
ULPA	ultra-low particulate air		ureteral orifice
ULQ	upper left quadrant		urinary output
ULRE	upper lid, right eye	UOP	urinary output
ULSB	upper left sternal border	UOQ	upper outer quadrant
ULTT1	upper limb tension test 1 (median nerve)	Uosm	urinary osmolality
		✓ up	check up
ULTT2a	upper limb tension test 2a (medial nerve)	UP	unipolar
			ureteropelvic
ULTT2b	upper limb tension test 2b (radial nerve)	U/P	urine to plasma (creatinine)
ULTT3	upper limb tension test 3 (ulnar nerve)	UPC	unknown primary carcinoma
ULYTES	electrolytes, urine	UPD	uniparental disomy
UM	unmarried	UPDRS	Unified Parkinson's Disease Rating Scale
Umb A Line	umbilical artery line		
		UPEP	urine protein electrophoresis
Umb V Line	umbilical venous line		
		UPG	uroporphyrinogen
umb ven	umbilical vein	UPIN	unique physician (provided) identification number
UMCD	uremic medullary cystic disease		
UMLS	Unified Medical Language System	UPJ	ureteropelvic junction
		UPLIF	unilateral posterior lumbar interbody fusion
UMN	upper motor neuron (disease)		
		UPN	unique patient number
UN	undernourished	UPO	metastatic carcinoma of unknown primary origin
	urinary nitrogen		
UNA	urinary nitrogen appearance		
		UPOR	usual place of residence
UNa	urine sodium	UPP	urethral pressure profile
unacc	unaccompanied	UPPP	uvulopalatopharyngo-plasty
UNC	uncrossed		
UNDEL	undelivered	U/P ratio	urine to plasma ratio
UNDP	United Nations Development Program	UPSC	uterine papillary serous carcinoma
UNG	ointment	UPT	uptake
UNHS	universal newborn hearing screening		urine pregnancy test
		UR	unrelated
UNK	unknown		upper respiratory
UNL	upper normal levels		upper right
UNOS	United Network for Organ Sharing		urinary retention

U

	utilization review	USED-CARP	**u**reterosigmoidostomy, **s**mall bowel fistula, **e**xtra chloride, **d**iarrhea, **c**arbonic anhydrase inhibitors, **a**drenal insufficiency, **r**enal tubular acidosis, and **p**ancreatic fistula (common causes of nonanion gap metabolic acidosis)
URA	unilateral renal agenesis		
URAC	Utilization Review Accreditation Commission		
UR AC	uric acid		
URAS	unilateral renal artery stenosis		
URD	undifferentiated respiratory disease		
URG	urgent	USG	ultrasonography
URI	upper respiratory infection	USH	United Services for Handicapped
URIC A	uric acid		usual state of health
url	unrelated	USI	urinary stress incontinence
UR&M	urinalysis, routine and microscopic	USM	ultrasonic mist
URO	urology	USMC	United States Marine Corps
UROD	ultra-rapid opiate detoxification [under anesthesia]	USN	ultrasonic nebulizer
			United States Navy
UROL	Urologist	USOGH	usual state of good health
	urology	USOH	usual state of health
UROB	urobilinogen	USP	unassisted systolic pressure
URQ	upper right quadrant		
URR	urea reduction ratio		United States Pharmacopeia
URS	ureterorenoscopy		
URSB	upper right sternal border	USPHS	United States Public Health Service
URT	uterine resting tone	USUCVD	unsterile uncontrolled vaginal delivery
URTI	upper respiratory tract infection	USVMD	urine specimen volume measuring device
US	ultrasonography		
	unit secretary	UT	upper thoracic
USA	unit services assistant	UTA	urinary tract anomaly
	United States Army	UTD	unable to determine
	unstable angina		up to date
USAF	United States Air Force	*ut dict*	as directed
USAN	United States Adopted Names	UTF	usual throat flora
		UTI	urinary tract infection
USAP	unstable angina pectoris	UTL	unable to locate
		UTM	urinary-tract malformations
USB	upper sternal border		
U-SCOPE	ureteroscopy	UTMDACC	University of Texas M.D. Anderson Cancer Center
USCVD	unsterile controlled vaginal delivery		
USDA	United States Department of Agriculture	UTO	unable to obtain
			upper tibial osteotomy

U

UTR	untranslated region	
UTS	ulnar tunnel syndrome	
	ultrasound	
U/U−	uterine fundus at umbilicus (usually modified as number of finger breadths below)	
U/U+	uterine fundus at umbilicus (usually modified as number of finger breadths above)	
UUD	uncontrolled unsterile delivery	
UUN	urinary urea nitrogen	
UUTI	uncomplicated urinary tract infections	
UV	ultraviolet	
	ureterovesical	
	urine volume	
UVA	ultraviolet A light	
	ureterovesical angle	
UVB	ultraviolet B light	
UVC	umbilical vein catheter	
	ultraviolet C light	
UVEB	unifocal ventricular ectopic beat	
UVH	univentricular heart	
UVJ	ureterovesical junction	
UVL	ultraviolet light	
	umbilical venous line	
UVR	ultraviolet radiation	
UVT	unsustained ventricular tachycardia	
U/WB	unit of whole blood	
UW	unilateral weakness	
UWF	unknown white female	
UWM	unknown white male	
	unwed mother	

V

V	five
	gas volume
	minute volume
	vaccinated
	vagina
	vein
	ventricular
	verb
	verbal
	vertebral
	very
	Viagra (sildenafil citrate) as in "vitamin V"
	viral
	vision
	vitamin
	vomiting
$\dot{V}$	ventilation (L/min)
+V	positive vertical divergence
V1	fifth cranial nerve, ophthalmic division
V2	fifth cranial nerve, maxillary division
V3	fifth cranial nerve, mandibular division
V_1 to V_6	precordial chest leads
VA	vacuum aspiration
	valproic acid
	ventriculoatrial
	vertebral artery
	Veterans Administration
	visual acuity
V_A	alveolar gas volume
V&A	vagotomy and antrectomy
VAAESS	Vaccine-Associated Adverse Events Surveillance System (Canada)
VAB	vinblastine, dactinomycin (actinomycin D), bleomycin
VABS	Vineland Adaptive Behavior Scales

V

337

VAC	vacuum-assisted closure (dressings)	VAHBE	ventricular atrial His bundle electrocardiogram
	ventriculoarterial conduction	VAHRA	ventricular atrial height right atrium
	vincristine, dactinomycin (actinomycin D), and cyclophosphamide	VAIN	vaginal intraepithelial neoplasia
	vincristine, doxorubicin (Adriamycin), and cyclophosphamide	VALE	visual acuity, left eye
		VAMC	Veterans Affairs Medical Center
VA cc	distance visual acuity with correction	VAMP®	venous-arterial management protection system
VA ccl	near visual acuity with correction	VAMS	Visual Analogue Mood Scale
VACE	*Vitex agnus-castus* extract (Chaste tree berry extract)	VANCO/P	vancomycin-peak
		VANCO/T	vancomycin-trough
		VAOD	visual acuity, right eye
VAC EXT	vacuum extractor	VAOS	visual acuity, left eye
VAC$_{ig}$	vaccinia immune globulin	VA OS LP with P	visual acuity, left eye, left perception with projection
VACO	Veterans Administration Central Office		
VACTERL	vertebral, anal, cardiac, tracheal, esophageal, renal, and limb anomalies	VAP	venous access port
			ventilator-associated pneumonia
			vincristine, asparaginase, and prednisone
VAD	vascular (venous) access device	VAPCS	ventricular atrial proximal coronary sinus
	ventricular assist device	VAPP	vaccine-associated paralytic poliomyelitis
	vertebral artery dissection	VAR	variant
	Veterans Administration Domiciliary		varicella (chickenpox) (*varicella zoster* virus) vaccine
	vincristine, doxorubicin (Adriamycin), and dexamethasone		
VaD	vascular dementia	VARE	visual acuity, right eye
VADCS	ventricular atrial distal coronary sinus	VAS	vasectomy
			vascular
VADRIAC	vincristine, doxorubicin (Adriamycin), and cyclophosphamide		Visual Analogue Scale (Score)
		VASC	Visual-Auditory Screen Test for Children
VAERS	Vaccine Adverse Events Reporting System	VA sc	distance visual acuity without correction
VAFD	vascular access flush device	VA scl	near visual acuity without correction
VAG	vagina	VASPI	Visual Analogue Self Assessment Scales For Pain Intensity
VAG HYST	vaginal hysterectomy		
VAH	Veterans Administration Hospital	VAS RAD	vascular radiology

VAT	ventilatory anaerobic threshold		videofluoroscopic barium swallow (evaluation)
	vertebral artery test	VC	color vision
	video-assist thoracoscopy		etoposide (VePesid) and carboplatin
	visceral adipose tissue		
VATER	vertebral, anal, tracheal, esophageal, and renal anomalies		pulmonary capillary blood volume
			vena cava
VATH	vinblastine, doxorubicin (Adriamycin), thiotepa, and fluoxymesterone (Halotestin)		verbal cues
			vincristine
			vital capacity
			vocal cords
VATS	video assisted thoracic surgery	V&C	vertical and centric (a bite)
VB	Van Buren (catheter)	VCA	vasoconstrictor assay
	venous blood	VCAM	vascular cell adhesion molecule
	vinblastine		
	vinblastine and bleomycin	VCAP	vincristine, cyclophospha-mide, doxorubicin (Adriamycin), and prednisone
VB_1	first voided bladder specimen		
VB_2	second midstream bladder specimen	Vcc	vision with correction
		VCCA	velocity common carotid artery
VB_3	third voided urine specimen		
		VCD	vocal cord dysfunction
VBAC	vaginal birth after cesarean	VCE	vaginal cervical endocervical (smear)
VBAI	vertebrobasilar artery insufficiency	VCF	Vaginal Contraception Film™
VBAP	vincristine, carmustine (BiCNU), doxorubicin (Adriamycin), and prednisone	VCG	vectorcardiography
			voiding cystogram
		vCJD	variant Creutzfeldt-Jakob disease
VBC	vinblastine, bleomycin, and cisplatin	VCO	ventilator CPAP oxyhood
		Vco_2	carbon dioxide output
VBG	venous blood gas	VCR	video cassette recorder
	vertical banded gastroplasty		vincristine sulfate
VBGP	vertical banded gastroplasty	VCT	venous clotting time
			voluntary counselling and testing
VBI	vertebrobasilar insufficiency	VCTS	vitreal corneal touch syndrome
VBL	vinblastine	VCU	voiding cystourethrogram
VBM	vinblastine, bleomycin, and methotrexate	VCUG	vesicoureterogram
			voiding cystourethrogram
VBP	vinblastine, bleomycin, and cisplatin	VCV	volume-control ventilation
		VD	venereal disease
VBR	ventricular brain ratio		viral diarrhea
VBS	vertebral-basilar system		voided

	volume of distribution	VE	vaginal examination
V_D	deadspace volume		vertex
V_d	volume of distribution		Vietnam era
V&D	vomiting and diarrhea		virtual endoscopy
VDA	venous digital angiogram		visual examination
	visual discriminatory acuity		vitamin E
			vocational evaluation
VDAC	vaginal delivery after cesarean	V_E	minute volume (expired)
		V/E	violence and eloper
VDC	vincristine, doxorubicin, and cyclophosphamide	VEA	ventricular ectopic activity
			viscoelastic agent
VDD	atrial synchronous ventricular inhibited pacing	VEB	ventricular ectopic beat
		VEC	vecuronium (Norcuron)
			velocity-encoded cine
VDDR I	vitamin D dependency rickets type I	VECG	vector electrocardiogram
		VED	vacuum erection device
VDDR II	vitamin D dependency rickets type II		vacuum extraction delivery
VDG	venereal disease–gon-orrhea		ventricular ectopic depolarization
Vdg	voiding	VEE	Venezuelan equine encephalitis
VDH	valvular disease of the heart	VEE_a	Venezuelan equine encephalitis vaccine, attenuated live
VDJ	variable diversity joining	VEE_I	Venezuelan equine encephalitis vaccine, inactivated
VDL	vasodepressor lipid		
	visual detection level	VEF	visually evoked field
VDO	varus derotational osteotomy	VEG	vegetation (bacterial)
		VEGF	vascular endothelial growth factor
VD or M	venous distention or masses	VeIP	vinblastine (Velban), ifosfamide, and cisplatin (Platinol AQ)
VDP	vinblastine, dacarbazine, and cisplatin (Platinol AQ)		
VDPCA	variable-dose patient-controlled analgesia	VENT	ventilation
			ventilator
VDRF	ventilator dependent respiratory failure		ventral
			ventricular
VDRL	Venereal Disease Research Laboratory (test for syphilis)	VEP	visual evoked potential
		VER	ventricular escape rhythm
			visual evoked responses
VDRR	vitamin D-resistant rickets	VERP	ventricular effective refractory period
VDRS	Verdun Depression Rating Scale	VERT	velocity-enhanced resistance training
VDS	vasodepressor syncope		
	venereal disease—syphilis	VES	ventricular extrasystoles
	vindesine		video-endoscopic surgery
VDT	video display terminal		
VD/VT	dead space to tidal volume ratio		

340

	vitamin E succinate		von Herrick (grading
VET	veteran		system)
	Veterinarian	VH I	very narrow anterior
	veterinary		chamber angles
VF	left leg (electrode)	VH II	moderately narrow
	ventricular fibrillation		anterior chamber angles
	vertical float (aquatic	VH III	moderately wide open
	therapy)		anterior chamber angles
	visual field	VH IV	wide open anterior
	vocal fremitus		chamber angles
VFC	Vaccines for Children	VHD	valvular heart disease
	(program)	VHL	von Hippel-Lindau
VFCB	vertical flow clean bench		disease (complex)
VFD	visual fields	VI	six
VFFC	visual fields full to		velocity index
	confrontation		volume index
VFI	visual fields intact	*via*	by way of
	Visual Functioning index	vib	vibration
V. Fib	ventricular fibrillation	VIBS	Victim's Information
VFL	vinflunine		Bureau Service
VFP	vertical float progression	VICA	velocity internal carotid
	(aquatic therapy)		artery
	vitreous fluorophotometry	VICP	Vaccine Injury
VFPN	Volu-feed premie nipple		Compensation Program
VFRN	Volu-feed regular nipple	VID	videodensitometry
VFT	venous filling time	VIG	vaccinia immune globulin
	ventricular fibrillation		vinblastine, ifosfamide,
	threshold		and gallium nitrate
VG	vein graft	VIH	Spanish and French
	ventricular gallop		abbreviation for human
	ventrogluteal		immunodeficiency
	very good		virus
V&G	vagotomy and	VIN	vulvar intraepithelial
	gastroenterotomy		neoplasm
VGAD	vein of Galen aneurysmal	VIP	etoposide (VePesid),
	dilatation		ifosfamide, and
VGAM	vein of Galen aneurysmal		cisplatin (Platinol AQ)
	malformation		vasoactive intestinal
VGB	vigabatrin (Sabril)		peptide
VGE	viral gastroenteritis		vasoactive intracorporeal
VGH	very good health		pharmacotherapy
VGM	vein graft myringoplasty		very important patient
VGPO	volume-guaranteed		vinblastine, ifosfamide,
	pressure option		and cisplatin (Platinol)
VH	vaginal hysterectomy		voluntary interruption of
	Veterans Hospital		pregnancy
	viral hepatitis	VIPomas	vasoactive intestinal
	visual hallucinations		peptide-secreting
	vitreous hemorrhage		tumors

V

VIQ	Verbal Intelligence Quotient (part of Wechsler tests)	VLH	ventrolateral nucleus of the hypothalamus
VIS	Vaccine Information Statement	VLM	visceral larva migrans
		VLP	virus-like particle
		VLR	vastus lateralis release
	Visual Impairment Service	VM	venous malformation
			ventilated mask
VISA	vancomycin-intermediate *Staphylococcus aureus*		ventimask
			Venturi mask
VISC	vitreous infusion suction cutter		vestibular membrane
		VM 26	teniposide (Vumon)
VISI	volar intercalated segmental instability	VMA	vanillylmandelic acid
		VMCP	vincristine, melphalan, cyclophosphamide, and prednisone
VISs	Vaccine Information Statements		
VIT	venom immunotherapy	VMD	Doctor of Veterinary Medicine (DVM)
	vital		
	vitamin		vertical maxillary deficiency
	vitreous		
VIT CAP	vital capacity	VME	vertical maxillary excess
VIU	visual internal urethrotomy	VMH	ventromedial hypothalamus
VIZ	namely	VMI	visual motor integration
V-J	ventriculo-jugular (shunt)	VMO	vastus medialis oblique
VKC	vernal keratoconjunctivitis	VMR	vasomotor rhinitis
VKDB	vitamin K deficiency bleeding	VMS	vanilla milkshake
		VN	visiting nurse
VKH	Vogt-Koyanagi-Harada's disease	VNA	Visiting Nurses' Association
VL	left arm (electrode)	VNB	vinorelbine (Navelbine)
	vial	VNC	vesicle neck contracture
VLA	very-late antigen	VNS	vagus nerve stimulation
VLAD	variable life-adjusted display	VNTR	variable number of tandem repeats
VLAP	vaporization laser ablation of the prostate	VO	verbal order
		VO$_2$	oxygen consumption
VLBW	very low birth weight (less than 1500 g)	VOCAB	vocabulary
		VOCOR	vaso-occlusive crisis
			void on-call to operating room
VLBWPN	very low birth weight preterm neonate		
VLCAD	very-long-chain acyl coenzyme A dehydrogenase	VOCs	volatile organic compounds
		VOCTOR	void on-call to operating room
VLCD	very low calorie diet		
VLCFA	very-long-chain fatty acids	VOD	veno-occlusive disease
			vision right eye
VLDL	very-low-density lipoprotein	VOE	vascular occlusive episode
VLE	vision left eye		

VO$_2$I	oxygen consumption index	VPR	virtual patient record
			volume pressure response
VOL	volume	VPS	valvular pulmonic
	voluntary		stenosis
VOM	vomited	VPT	vascularized patellar
VOO	continuous ventricular		tendon
	asynchronous pacing		vibration perception
VOR	vestibular ocular reflex		threshold
VOS	vision left eye	VQ	ventilation perfusion
VOSS	visual observation	VR	right arm (electrode)
	shivering score		valve replacement
VOT	Visual Organization Test		venous resistance
VOU	vision both eyes		ventricular rhythm
VP	etoposide (VePesid) and		verbal reprimand
	cisplatin (Platinol AQ)		vocational rehabilitation
	variegate porphyria	V$_3$R··V$_6$R	right sided precordial
	venipuncture		leads
	venous pressure	VRA	visual reinforcement
	ventriculo-peritoneal		audiometry
	visual perception		visual response
	voiding pressure		audiometry
V & P	vagotomy and	VRB	vinorelbine (Navelbine)
	pyloroplasty	VRC	vocational rehabilitation
	ventilation and perfusion		counselor
VP-16	etoposide	VRE	vancomycin-resistant
VPA	valproic acid		enterococci
	ventricular premature		vision right eye
	activation	VREF	vancomycin-resistant
V-Pad	sanitary napkin		*Enterococcus faecium*
VPB	ventricular premature beat	VRI	viral respiratory infection
VPC	ventricular premature	VRL	ventral root, lumbar
	contractions		vinorelbine (Navelbine)
VPD	ventricular premature	VRP	vocational rehabilitation
	depolarization		program
VPDC	ventricular premature	VRS	viral rhinosinusitis
	depolarization	VRSA	vancomycin-resistant
	contraction		*Staphylococcus aureus*
VPDF	vegetable protein diet plus	VRT	variance of resident time
	fiber		ventral root, thoracic
VPDs	ventricular premature		vertical radiation
	depolarizations		topography
VPI	velopharyngeal		Visual Retention Test
	incompetence		vocational rehabilitation
	velopharyngeal		therapy
	insufficiency	VRTA	Vocational Rehabilitation
VPL	ventro-posterolateral		Therapy Assistant
VPLS	ventilation-perfusion lung	VRU	ventilator rehabilitation
	scan		unit
VPM	venous pressure module	VS	vagal stimulation

V

	vegetative state	VTS	Volunteer Transport Service
	versus *(vs)*		
	very sensitive	VT-S	ventricular tachycardia sustained
	visit		
	visited	VTSRS	Verdun Target Symptom Rating Scale
	vital signs (temperature, pulse, and respiration)	VT/VF	ventricular tachycardia/fibrillation
VSADP	vocational skills assessment and development program	VTX	vertex
		VU	vesicoureteral (reflux)
VSBE	very short below elbow (cast)	V/U	verbalize understanding
		VUJ	vesico ureteral junction
VSD	ventricular septal defect	VUR	vesicoureteric reflux
VSI	visual motor integration	VV	vaccina virus
VSMC	vascular smooth muscle cell		varicose veins
		V-V	ventriculovenous (shunt)
VSN	vital signs normal	V&V	vulva and vagina
VSO	vertical subcondylar oblique	V/V	volume to volume ratio
		VVB	venovenous bypass
VSOK	vital signs normal	VVC	vulvovaginal candidiasis
VSP	vertical stabilization program	VVD	vaginal vertex delivery
		VVETP	Vietnam Veterans Evaluation and Treatment Program
VSQOL	Vital Signs Quality of Life		
VSR	venous stasis retinopathy	VVFR	vesicovaginal fistula repair
VSS	vital signs stable		
V_{SS}	apparent volume of distribution	V/VI	grade 5 on a 6 grade basis
VSSAF	vital signs stable, afebrile	VVI	ventricular demand pacing
VST	visual search task	VVIR	ventricular demand inhibited pacemaker (V = chamber paced-ventricle, V = chamber sensed-ventricle, I = response to sensing-inhibited, R = programmability–rate modulation)
VSV	vesicular stomatitis virus		
VT	validation therapy		
	ventricular tachycardia		
V_t	tidal volume		
VTA	ventral tegmentum area		
VTBI	volume to be infused		
v. tach.	ventricular tachycardia		
VTE	venous thromboembolism	VVL	varicose veins ligation
			verruca vulgaris of the larynx
VTEC	verotoxin-producing *Escherichia coli*		
		VVOR	visual-vestibulo-ocular-reflex
VTED	venous thromboembolic disease		
		VVR	ventricular response rate
VT-NS	ventricular tachycardia non-sustained	VVT	ventricular synchronous pacing
VTOP	voluntary termination of pregnancy	VW	vessel wall
		VWD	ventral wall defect
VTP	voluntary termination of pregnancy	vWD	von Willebrand disease

V

vWF	von Willebrand factor		
VWM	ventricular wall motion		
V_x	vitrectomy		
V-XT	V-pattern exotropia		
VY	surgical replacement flap		
VZ	varicella zoster		
VZIG	varicella zoster immune globulin		
VZV	varicella zoster virus		

W

W	wash
	watts
	wearing glasses
	week
	weight
	well
	West (as in the location e.g. 2W, is second floor, West wing)
	white
	widowed
	wife
	with
	work
W-1	insignificant (allergies)
W-3	minimal (allergies)
W-5	moderate (allergies)
W-7	moderate-severe (allergies)
W-9	severe (allergies)
WA	when awake
	while awake
	White American
	wide awake
	with assistance
W-A	Wyeth-Ayerst Laboratories
W & A	weakness and atrophy
W or A	weakness or atrophy
WACH	wedge adjustable cushioned heel
WAF	weakness, atrophy, and fasciculation
	white adult female
WAGR	Wilms' tumor, aniridia, genitourinary malformations, and mental retardation (syndrome)
WAIS	Wechsler Adult Intelligence Scale
WAIS-R	Wechsler Adult Intelligence Scale-Revised

W

WALK	weight-activated locking knee (prosthesis)	WBRT	whole-brain radiotherapy
WAM	white adult male	WBS	weeks by size (for gestational age)
WAP	wandering atrial pacemaker		whole body scan
WARI	wheezing associated respiratory infection	WBTF	Waring Blender tube feeding
WAS	whiplash-associated disorders	WBTT	weight bearing to tolerance
	Wiskott-Aldrich syndrome	WBUS	weeks by ultrasound
WASO	wakefulness after sleep onset	WBV	whole blood volume
		WC	ward clerk
WASP	Wiskott-Aldrich syndrome protein		ward confinement
			warm compress
WASS	Wasserman test		wet compresses
WAT	word association test		wheelchair
WB	waist belt		when called
	weight bearing		white count
	well baby		whooping cough
	Western blot		will call
	whole blood		workers' compensation
WBACT	whole-blood activated clotting time	WCA	work capacity assessment
		WCC	well-child care
WBAT	weight bearing as tolerated		white cell count
		WCE	white coat effect
WBC	weight bearing with crutches		work capacity evaluation
		WCH	white coat hypertension
	well baby clinic	WC/LC	warm compresses and lid scrubs
	white blood cell (count)		
WBCT	whole-blood clotting time	WCM	whole cow's milk
		WCS	work capacity specialist
WBD	weeks by dates (for gestational age)	WD	ward
			well developed
WBE	weeks by examination (for gestational age)		well differentiated
			wet dressing
WBH	weight-based heparin (dosing)		Wilson's disease
			word
			working distance
	whole-body hyperthermia		wound
WBI	whole-bowel irrigation	W/D	warm and dry
W Bld	whole blood		withdrawal
WBN	wellborn nursery	W → D	wet to dry
WBNAA	whole-brain *N*-acetylaspartate	W4D	Worth four-dot (test for fusion)
WBOS	wide base of support	WDCC	well-developed collateral circulation
WBPTT	whole-blood partial thromboplastin time	WDF	white divorced female
		WDHA	watery diarrhea, hypokalemia, and achlorhydria
WBQC	wide-base quad cane		
WBR	whole-body radiation		

W

WDHH	watery diarrhea, hypokalemia, and hypochlorhydria		WFL	within full limits within functional limits
WDL	within defined limits		WFLC	white female living child
WDLL	well-differentiated lymphocytic lymphoma		WF-O	will follow in office
			WFR	wheel-and-flare reaction
WDM	white divorced male		WG	Wegener's granulomatosis
WDS	word discrimination score		WGA	wheat germ agglutinin
			WH	walking heel (cast) well healed well hydrated
WDWN-AAF	well-developed, well-nourished African-American female			
			WHA	warmed humidified air
			WHIS	War Head-Injury Score
WDWN-BM	well-developed, well-nourished black male		WHNR	well-healed, no residuals
			WHNS	well-healed, no sequelae well-healed, nonsymptomatic well-healed, no sequelae
WDWN-WF	well-developed, well-nourished white female			
			WHO	World Health Organization wrist-hand orthosis
WDXRF	wavelength-dispersive x-ray fluorescence			
WE	weekend		WHOART	World Health Organization Adverse Reaction Terms (Terminology)
W/E	weekend			
WEBINO	wall-eyed bilateral internuclear ophthalmoplegia			
			WHOQOL-100	World Health Organization Quality of Life 100-Item (instrument)
WE-D	withdrawal-emergent dyskinesia			
WEE	Western equine encephalitis		WHP	whirlpool
			WHPB	whirlpool bath
WEMINO	wall-eyed monocular internuclear ophthalmoplegia		WHR	ratio of waist to hip circumference
			WHV	woodchuck hepatitis virus
WEP	weekend pass		WHVP	wedged hepatic venous pressure
WESR	Westergren erythrocyte sedimentation rate Wintrobe erythrocyte sedimentation rate			
			WHZ	wheezes
			WI	ventricular demand pacing walk-in
WEUP	willful exposure to unwanted pregnancy		W/I	within
			W+I	work and interest
WF	well flexed wet film white female		WIA	wounded in action
			WIC	Women, Infants, and Children (program)
W/F	weakness and fatigue		WID	widow widower
WFE	Williams flexion exercises		WIED	walk-in emergency department
W FEEDS	with feedings		WIP	work in progess
WFH	white-faced hornet		WIS	Ward Incapacity Scale
WFI	water for injection			

W

WISC	Wechsler Intelligence Scale for Children	WNL x 4	upper and lower extremities within normal limits
WISC-R	Wechsler Intelligence Scale for Children-Revised	WNM	well-nourished male
		WNLS	weighted nonlinear least squares
WIT	water-induced thermotherapy	WNR	within normal range
WK	week	WNt^{50}	Wagner-Nelson time 50 hours
	work	WO	weeks old
WKI	Wakefield Inventory		wide open
WKS	Wernicke-Korsakoff Syndrome		written order
WL	waiting list	W/O	water in oil
	wave length		without
	weight loss	WOB	work of breathing
WLE	wide local excision	WOCN	Wound, Ostomy and Continence Nurses (Society)-formerly known as the International Association for Enterostomal Therapy (IEAT)
WLM	working level months		
WLS	wet lung syndrome		
WLT	waterload test		
WM	wall motion		
	warm, moist		
	wet mount		
	white male		
	white matter	WOMAC	Western Ontario and McMaster Universities Osteoarthritis Index
	whole milk		
WMA	wall motion abnormality	WOP	without pain
WMD	warm moist dressings (sterile)	W or A	weakness or atrophy
		WORD	Wechsler objective reading dimensions
WMF	white married female		
WMI	wall motion index	WORLD/ DLROW	a test used in mental status examinations (patient is asked to spell WORLD backwards)
	weighted mean index		
WML	white matter lesions (cerebral)		
WMLC	white male living child	WP	whirlpool
WMM	white married male	WPBT	whirlpool, body temperature
WMP	warm moist packs (unsterile)		
		WPCs	washed packed cells
	weight management program	WPFM	Wright peak flow meter
WMS	Wechsler Memory Scale	WPOA	wearing patch on arrival
	Wilson-Mikity syndrome		
WMX	whirlpool, massage, and exercise	WPP	Wechsler Preschool and Primary Scale of Intelligence
WN	well nourished		
WND	wound	WPPSI	Wechsler Preschool and Primary Scale of Intelligence
WNE	West Nile encephalitis		
WNF	well-nourished female	WPPSI-R	WPPSI revised
	West Nile fever	WPV	within-person variability
WNL	within normal limits		

W

WPW	Wolff-Parkinson-White (syndrome)		wisdom teeth
		0WT	zero work tolerance
WR	Wassermann reaction	W-T-D	wet to dry
	wrist	WTP	willingness to pay
WRA	with-the-rule astigmatism	WTS	whole tomography slice
WRAIR	Walter Reed Army Institute of Research	W/U	work-up
		WV	whispered voice
WRAMC	Walter Reed Army Medical Center	W/V	weight-to-volume ratio
		WW	Weight Watchers
WRARU	Walter Reed AFRIMS (Armed Forces Research Institute of Medical Sciences) Research Unit		wheeled walker
		WWI	World War One
		WWII	World War Two
		W/W	weight-to-weight ratio
		W → W	wet to wet
WRAT	Wide Range Achievement Test	WWAC	walk with aid of cane
		WW Brd	whole wheat bread
WRAT-R	The Wide Range Achievement Test, Revised	WWidF	white widowed female
		WWidM	white widowed male
		WWW	World Wide Web
WRBC	washed red blood cells	WYOU	women years of usage
WRC	washed red (blood) cells		
WRIOT	Wide Range Interest-Opinion Test (for career planning)		
WRT	weekly radiation therapy		
WRUED	work-related upper-extremity disorder		
WS	walking speed		
	ward secretary		
	watt seconds		
	Williams syndrome		
	work simplification		
	work simulation		
	work status		
W&S	wound and skin		
WSEP	Williams syndrome, early puberty		
WSepF	white separated female		
WSepM	white separated male		
WSF	white single female		
WSLP	Williams syndrome, late puberty		
WSM	white single male		
WSP	wearable speech processor		
WT	walking tank		
	walking training		
	weight (wt)		
	wild type		
	Wilms' tumor		

W

X

X	break	XL	extended release (once a day oral solid dosage form)
	cross		extra large
	crossmatch		forty
	exophoria for distance	XLA	X-linked infantile agammaglobulinemia
	extra		
	female sex chromosome	X-leg	cross leg
	start of anesthesia	XLFDP	cross-linked fibrin degradation products
	ten		
	times	XLH	X-linked hypophos-phatemia
	xylocaine		
$\bar{x}$	except	XLJR	X-linked juvenile retinoschisis
X′	exophoria at 33 cm		
X^2	chi-square	XLMR	X-linked mental retardation
X+#	xyphoid plus number of fingerbreadths	XM	crossmatch
x	mean	X-mat.	crossmatch
X3	orientation as to time, place and person	XML	extensible markup language
XBT	xylose breath test	XMM	xeromammography
XC	excretory cystogram	XNA	xenoreactive natural antibodies
XCF	aortic cross clamp off		
XCO	aortic cross clamp on	XOM	extraocular movements
XD	times daily	XOP	x-ray out of plaster
X&D	examination and diagnosis	XP	xeroderma pigmentosum
		XR	x-ray
X2d	times two days	XRF	x-ray fluorescence
XDP	xeroderma pigmentosum	XRT	radiation therapy
Xe	xenon	XS	excessive
^{133}Xe	xenon, isotope of mass 133	X-SCID	X-linked severe combined immunodeficiency disease
XeCT	xenon-enhanced computed tomography		
		XS-LIM	exceeds limits of procedure
X-ed	crossed	XT	exotropia
XEM	xonics electron mammography		extract
			extracted
XES	x-ray energy spectrometer	X(T')	intermittent exotropia at 33 cm
XFER	transfer	X(T)	intermittent exotropia
XGP	xanthogranulomatous pyelonephritis	XTLE	extratemporal-lobe epilepsy
		XU	excretory urogram
XI	eleven	XULN	times upper limit of normal
XII	twelve		
XIP	x-ray in plaster	XV	fifteen
XKO	not knocked out	3X/WK	three times a week

XX	normal female sex chromosome type
	twenty
XX/XY	sex karyotypes
XXX	thirty
XY	normal male sex chromosome type
XYL	Xylocaine®
	xylose
XYLO	Xylocaine®

Y

Y	male sex chromosome
	year
	yellow
YAC	yeast artificial chromosome
YACs	yeast artificial chromosomes
YACP	young adult chronic patient
YAG	yttrium aluminum garnet (laser)
YAS	youth action section (police)
Yb	ytterbium
YBOCS	Yale-Brown Obsessive-Compulsive Scale
Yel	yellow
YF	yellow fever
YFH	yellow-faced hornet
YFI	yellow fever immunization
YHL	years of healthy life
YJV	yellow jacket venom
Y2K	year 2,000
YLC	youngest living child
YLD	years of life with disability
YLL	years of life lost
YMC	young male Caucasian
YMRS	Young Mania Rating Scale
Y/N	yes/no
YO	years old
YOB	year of birth
YOD	year of death
YORA	younger-onset rheumatoid arthritis
YPC	YAG (yttrium aluminum garnet) posterior capsulotomy
YPLL	years of potential life lost before age 65
yr	year

YSC	yolk sac carcinoma
YTD	year to date
YTDY	yesterday

Z	impedance
ZAP	zoster-associated pain
ZDV	zidovudine (Retrovir)
Z-E	Zollinger-Ellison (syndrome)
ZEEP	zero end-expiratory pressure
ZES	Zollinger-Ellison syndrome
Z-ESR	zeta erythrocyte sedimentation rate
ZIFT	zygote intrafallopian (tube) transfer
ZIG	zoster serum immune globulin
ZIP	zoster immune plasma
ZMC	zygomatic zygomatic maxillary compound (complex)
Zn	zinc
ZnO	zinc oxide
ZnOE	zinc oxide and eugenol
ZnPc	zinc phthalocyanine
ZnPP	zinc protoporphyrin
ZNS	zonisamide (Zonegran)
ZOOM	Guarana
ZOT	zonula occludens toxin
ZPC	zero point of charge zopiclone
z-Plasty	surgical relaxation of contracture
ZPO	zinc peroxide
ZPP	zinc protoporphyrin
ZPT	zinc pyrithione
ZSB	zero stools since birth
ZSR	zeta sedimentation rate
ZSRDS	Zung Self-Rating Depression Scale

Y

Chapter 4

Symbols and Numbers

Symbols

↑	above	↔	same as
	alive		stable
	elevated		to and from
	greater than		unchanging
	high		
	improved	↓↓	flexor
	increase		plantar response
	rising		(Babinski)
	up		testes descended
	upper		
		↑↑	extensor
↑g	increasing		extensor response
			(positive Babinsky)
↓	dead		testes undescended
	decrease		
	depressed	‖	parallel
	diminished		parallel bars
	down	√	check
	falling		flexion
	lower		
	lowered	√'d	checked
	normal plantar reflex		
	restricted	√'ing	checking
↓g	decreasing	#	fracture
			number
→	causes to		pound
	greater than		weight
	progressing		
	results in	∴	therefore
	showed	∵	because
	to the right	Δ scan	delta scan (computed
	transfer to		tomography scan)
←	less than	+	plus
	resulted from		positive
	to the left		present

Symbol	Meaning
−	absent minus negative
/	slash mark signifying per, and, or with (this is a dangerous symbol as it is mistaken for a one)
±	either positive or negative no definite cause plus or minus very slight trace
└	right lower quadrant
┌	right upper quadrant
┐	left upper quadrant
┘	left lower quadrant
>	greater than left ear-bone conduction threshold
≥	greater than or equal to
<	caused by less than right ear-bone conduction threshold
≤	less than or equal to
≮	not less than
≯	not more than
∧	above diastolic blood pressure increased
∨	below systolic blood pressure
≠	not equal to
≅	approximately equal to
=	equal equal to
′	feet minutes (as in 30′)
″	inches seconds
~	about approximately difference
≈	approximately equal to
≡	identical
×	left ear-air conduction threshold ten
]	left ear-masked bone conduction threshold
△	right ear-masked air conduction threshold change
[	right ear-masked bone conduction threshold
▽	reversible
?	questionable not tested
Ø	no none without
⊙	start of an operation
⊗	end of anesthesia
@	at
ῑ	one
ΤΤ	two
♂	male
♀	female
♂	gay
♀	lesbian
■	deceased male
●	deceased female
□	living male left ear-masked air conduction threshold

○	living female	777	Ortho Novum 777®
	respiration		(a triphasic oral
	right ear-air conduction		contraceptive)
	threshold		

Symbol	Meaning
○	living female respiration right ear-air conduction threshold
◇	sex unknown
(□)	adopted living male
*	birth
†	dead death
♀	standing
O—<	recumbent position
♀	sitting position
♥	heart

Numbers (Arabic and Roman)

1/2 and 1/2	half Dakin's solution and half glycerin
1°	first degree primary
1:1	one-to-one (individual session with staff)
2°	second degree secondary
2×2	gauze dressing folded 2″×2″
3°	tertiary third degree
3×	three times
4×4	gauze dressing folded 4″×4″
5+2	cytarabine and daunorubicin
Serial 7's	a mental status examination (starting with 100, count backward by 7's)
24°	twenty-four hours (24 hr is safer as the ° is seen as a zero)

777	Ortho Novum 777® (a triphasic oral contraceptive)
1500	Health Insurance Claim Form HCFA 1500
1,000	one thousand (1×10^3)
10,000	ten thousand (1×10^4)
100,000	one hundred thousand (1×10^5)
1,000,000	one million (1×10^6)
10,000,000	ten million (1×10^7)
100,000,000	one hundred million (1×10^8)
1,000,000,000	one billion (1×10^9)
i	one (Roman numerals are dangerous expressions and should not be used)
ii	two
iii	three
iiii	four
iv	four (this is a dangerous abbreviation as it is read as intravenous, use 4)
v	five
vi	six
vii	seven
viii	eight
ix	nine
x	ten
xi	eleven
xii	twelve
XL	forty extended release dosage form

Greek Letters

A α	alpha
β B	beta
Γ γ	gamma

Δ δ	anion gap	O o	omicron
	change	Π π	pi
	delta	P ρ	rho
	delta gap	Σ σ	sigma
	prism diopter		sum of
	temperature		summary
	trimester		
		T τ	tau
E ε	epsilon	Υ υ	upsilon
Z ζ	zeta	Φ φ	phenyl
H η	eta		phi
Θ θ	negative		thyroid
	theta	X χ	chi
		Ψ ψ	psi
I ι	iota		psychiatric
K κ	kappa	Ω ω	omega
Λ λ	lambda		
M μ	micro		
	mu		
N ν	nu		
Ξ ξ	xi		

Miscellaneous

L M
K — O — T   liver, kidneys, and spleen
S   negative, no masses, or tenderness

Chapter 5
Tables and Lists

Numbers and letters for teeth

Two adult numbering systems and a deciduous system are shown. The adult systems are shown as numbers, whereas deciduous teeth are lettered. The system commonly used in the U.S. is 1 to 32 (shown in bold face type).

1 (18)	upper right 3rd molar	
2 (17) (A)	upper right 2nd molar	
3 (16) (B)	upper right 1st molar	
4 (15)	upper right 2nd bicuspid	
5 (14)	upper right 1st bicuspid	
6 (13) (C)	upper right canine (eyetooth)	
7 (12) (D)	upper right lateral incisor	
8 (11) (E)	upper right central incisor	
9 (21) (F)	upper left central incisor	
10 (22) (G)	upper left lateral incisor	
11 (23) (H)	upper left canine	
12 (24)	upper left 1st bicuspid	
13 (25)	upper left 2nd bicuspid	
14 (26) (I)	upper left 1st molar	
15 (27) (J)	upper left 2nd molar	
16 (28)	upper left 3rd molar	
17 (38)	lower left 3rd molar	
18 (37) (K)	lower left 2nd molar	
19 (36) (L)	lower left 1st molar	
20 (35)	lower left 2nd bicuspid	
21 (34)	lower left 1st bicuspid	
22 (33) (M)	lower left canine	
23 (32) (N)	lower left lateral incisor	
24 (31) (O)	lower left central incisor	
25 (41) (P)	lower right central incisor	
26 (42) (Q)	lower right lateral incisor	
27 (43) (R)	lower right canine	
28 (44)	lower right 1st bicuspid	
29 (45)	lower right 2nd bicuspid	
30 (46) (S)	lower right 1st molar	
31 (47) (T)	lower right 2nd molar	
32 (48)	lower right 3rd molar	

UPPER   UPPER

1	**2**	**3**	**4**	**5**	**6**	**7**	**8**	**9**	**10**	**11**	**12**	**13**	**14**	**15**	**16**
18	17	16	15	14	13	12	11	21	22	23	24	25	26	27	28
A	B				C	D	E	F	G	H			I	J	
T	S				R	Q	P	O	N	M			L	K	
48	47	46	45	44	43	42	41	31	32	33	34	35	36	37	38
32	**31**	**30**	**29**	**28**	**27**	**26**	**25**	**24**	**23**	**22**	**21**	**20**	**19**	**18**	**17**

Right   **Left**

LOWER   LOWER

Laboratory Test Panels*

	Cl CO$_2$ K Na	BUN Ca Creat Gluc	Alb Alk P AAST(SGOT) ALT(SGPT) T Bili TP	ANA ESR RF Ur Ac	Calc LDL HDL T Chol Trig VLDL	Alb Phos	HAAb, IgM Ab HbcAb, IgM Ab HbsAG HCAb
Lytes (electrolyte panel)	X						
BMP (basic metabolic panel) or MBP, MPB	X	X					
CMP (comprehensive metabolic panel)	X	X	X				
HFP (hepatitis function panel)			X plus D Bili				
AP (arthritis panel)				X			
LP (lipid Panel)					X		
RFP (renal function panel)	X	X				X	
AHP (acute hepatitis panel)							X

*These can vary from institution to institution and from year to year

Abbreviation Key
Ab–antibody
Alb–albumin
Alk P–alkaline phosphate
ALT (SGPT)–alanine transaminase (serum glutamate pyruvate)
ANA–antinuclear antibody
AST (SGOT)–aspartate-transaminase (serum glutamate oxaloacetic transaminase)
BUN–blood urea nitrogen
Ca–calcium
Calc LDL–calculated low-density lipoprotein
LDL–low density lipoprotein
Cl–chloride
CO$_2$–carbon dioxide
Creat–creatinine
D Bili–direct bilirubin
ESR–erythrocyte sedimentation rate
Gluc–glucose
HAAb–hepatitis A antibody
HBcAb–hepatitis B core antibody
HBsAg–hepatitis B surface antigen
HCAb–hepatitis C antibody
HDL–high-density lipoprotein
IgM–immunoglobulin M
K–potassium
Na–sodium
Phos–phosphate
RF–rheumatoid factor
T Bili–total bilirubin
T Chol–total cholesterol
TP–total protein
Trig–triglycerides
Ur Ac–uric acid
VLDI–very low-density lipoprotein

358

See text for meaning of the abbreviations shown

Complete Blood Count

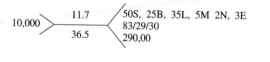

$10,000$ ⟩ $\dfrac{11.7}{36.5}$ ⟨ 50S, 25B, 35L, 5M 2N, 3E
83/29/30
290,00

WBC ⟩ $\dfrac{HgB}{HCT}$ ⟨ Segs/Bands/Lymphs/Monos/Basos/Eos
MCV-MCH-MCHC
platelet count

Electrolyte Panel

142	99	sodium		chloride
4.7	25	potassium		carbon dioxide

Blood Gases

$7.4/80/48/98/25$ pH/PO_2/PCO_2/% O_2 saturation/bicarbonate

Obstetrical shorthand

$\dfrac{2\ cm|80\%}{-2\ Vtx}$ 2 cm = dilation of cervix

80% = degree of cer-   Vtx = vertex; presen-
    vix effacement   tation of fetus,
                                (breech = Br)

−2 = station; distance
    above (−) or
    below (+) the
    spine of the ischium measured in cm

Reflexes

Reflexes are usually graded on a 0 to 4+ scale

4+ may indicate disease
    often associated with clonus
    very brisk, hyperactive (or ++++)
3+ brisker than average
    possibly but not necessarily indicative of disease
        (or +++)
2+ average
    normal (or ++)

1+ low normal
    somewhat diminished (or +)
0   may indicate neuropathy
    no response

Muscle strength[1]
0—No muscular contraction detected
1—A barely detectable flicker or trace of contraction
2—Active movement of the body part with gravity eliminated
3—Active movement against gravity
4—Active movement against gravity and some resistance
5—Active movement against full resistance without evident fatigue. This is
     normal muscle strength

Pulse[1]
0   completely absent
+1 markedly impaired (or 1+, or +)
+2 modererely impaired (or 2+, or ++)
+3 slightly impaired (or 3+, or +++)
+4 normal (or 4+, or ++++)

Gradation of intensity of heart murmurs[1]
1/6 or I/VI   may not be heard in all positions
                very faint, heard only after the listener has
                   "tuned in"
2/6 or II/VI   quiet, but heard immediately upon placing
                   the stethoscope on the chest
3/6 or III/VI   moderately loud
4/6 or IV/VI   loud
5/6 or V/VI   very loud, may be heard with a stethoscope
                   partly off the chest (thrills are associated)
6/6 or VI/VI   may be heard with the stethoscope entirely
                   off the chest (thrills are associated)

Tonsil Size
0   no tonsils
1   less than normal
2   normal
3   greater than normal
4   touching

Metric Prefixes and Symbols
Prefix	Symbol	
tera-	T	1,000,000,000,000 or (10^{12}) one trillion
giga-	G	1,000,000,000 or (10^{9}) one billion
mega-	M	1,000,000 or (10^{6}) one million
kilo-	k	1,000 or (10^{3}) one thousand
hecto-	h	100 or (10^{2}) one hundred
deka-	da	10 or (10^{1}) ten

deci-	d	0.1 or (10^{-1}) one-tenth
centi-	c	0.01 or (10^{-2}) one-hundredth
milli-	m	0.001 or (10^{-3}) one-thousandth
micro-	μ	0.000,001 or (10^{-6}) one-millionth
nano-	n	0.000,000,001 or (10^{-9}) one-billionth
pico-	p	0.000,000,000,000,001 or (10^{-12}) one-trillionth
femto-	f	0.000,000,000,000,001 or (10^{-15}) one-quadrillionth
atto-	a	0.000,000,000,000,000,001 or (10^{-18}) one-quintillionth

Apothecary symbols (Should never be used)

The symbols presented below are for informational use. The apothecary system should *not* be used. Only the metric system should be used. The methods of expressing the symbols, the meanings, and the equivalence are not the classic ones, nor are they accurate, but reflect the usual intended meanings when used by some older physicians in writing prescription directions.

ℨ or ℨ ɨ	dram, teaspoonful, (5 mL)	℥ or ℥ ɨ	ounce, (30 mL)
		gr	grain (approximately 60 mg)
ℨ ɨɨ	two drams, 2 tea-spoonfuls, (10 mL)		
		ɱ	minim (approximately 0.06 mL)
℥ss	half ounce, table-spoonful, (15 mL)	gtt	drop

Reference

1. Bates B. A guide to physical examinations and history taking, 6th ed. Philadelphia: J.B. Lippincott; 1999.

Chapter 6

Cross-Referenced List of Drug Generic and Brand Names

Listed below is a cross-referenced index of generic and brand drug names. Generic names begin with a lower case letter while brand names begin with a capital letter. This partial list consists of frequently prescribed and new drugs.

The meanings of abbreviated and coded drug names can be found in Chapter 3 (Lettered Abbreviations and Acronyms).

Complete indices of United States drug names can be found in current editions of Drug Facts and Comparisons[1], the American Drug Index[2], and Physicians GenRx[3]. A complete list of world-wide names may be found in Martindales.[4] These and other references should be used to determine the equivalence of products, strengths, and dosage forms. Although several products may be listed under one generic name they may differ in strength, dosage form, or concentration available, as is the case with estradiol transdermal (Climara, Estraderm, and Vivelle).

Some products are marketed without a brand name, as in the case of thioguanine. In such cases only the generic name is listed. When a product is often prescribed and/or labeled generically, the generic name is shown in italics.

The following abbreviations are used in this listing:

EC	enteric coated	SR	sustained release tablets or capsules
HCl	hydrochloride		(and other forms of extended
IM	intramuscular		release)
IV	intravenous	susp	suspension
inj	injection	(W)	withdrawn or discontinued from
oint	ointment		US market
ophth	ophthalmic	(WA)	withdrawn or discontinued from
soln	solution		US market but available under
			different name from another
			manufacturer

A

abacavir sulfate	Ziagen
Abbokinase	urokinase
abciximab	ReoPro
Abelcet	amphotericin B lipid complex
acarbose	Precose
Accolate	zafirlukast
Accupril	quinapril HCl
Accuretic	quinapril; hydrochlorothiazide
Accutane	isotretinoin
Accuzyme	papain; urea oint
acebutolol HCl	Sectral
Acel-Imune	diphtheria & tetanus toxoids & acellular pertussis vaccine
Aceon	perindopril erbumine
acetaminophen	paracetamol Tylenol
acetaminophen 300 mg with Codeine Phosphate (15, 30, and 60 mg)	Phenaphen with Codeine (#2, 3, and 4) Tylenol with Codeine (#2, 3, and 4)
acetazolamide	Diamox
acetohexamide	Dymelor
acetohydroxamic acid	Lithostat
acetylcholine ophth	Miochol E
acetylcysteine	Mucomyst
Achromycin (WA)	tetracycline HCl
Aciphex	rabeprazole sodium
acitretin	Soriatane
argatroban	argatroban
Acthar	corticotropin
ActHIB/Tripedia	*Haemophilus b* conjugate vaccine reconstituted with diphtheria and tetanus toxoids and acellular pertussis vaccine adsorbed
Acthrel	corticorellin ovine triflutate
Actifed	triprolidine HCl; pseudoephedrine HCl
Actigall	ursodiol
Actimmune	interferon gamma 1-b
Actiq	fentanyl oral transmucosal
Activase	alteplase, recombinant
Activella	norethindrone acetate; estradiol
Actonel	risedronate sodium
Actos	pioglitazone HCl
Acular	ketorolac tromethamine ophth
acyclovir	Zovirax
Adalat	nifedipine
Adalat CC	nifedipine SR
adapalene	Differin
Adapin	doxepin HCl
Adderall	amphetamine; dextroamphetamine mixed salts
adefovir dipivoxil	Preveon
Adenocard	adenosine
adenosine	Adenocard
Adrenalin	epinephrine

Adriamycin	doxorubicin HCl	Aldactone	spironolactone
Advair Diskus	fluticasone propionate; salmeterol inhalation powder	Aldara	imiquimod cream
		aldesleukin	Proleukin
		Aldomet	methyldopa
		Aldoril	methyldopa; hydrochloro-thiazide
Advil	ibuprofen		
AeroBid	flunisolide	alendronate sodium	Fosamax
Afrin nasal spray	oxymetazoline HCl		
		Alesse	levonorgestrel; ethinyl estradiol
Agenerase	amprenavir		
Aggrastat	tirofiban HCl	Alfenta	alfentanil HCl
Aggrenox	aspirin; extended-release dipyridamole	alfentanil HCl	Alfenta
		alglucerase	Ceredase
Agrylin	anagrelide HCl	alitretinoin	Panretin
Akineton	biperiden	Allegra	fexofenadine HCl
Alamast	pemirolast potassium ophth soln		
		Alkeran	melphalan
		allopurinol	Zyloprim
alatrovafloxacin mesylate IV	Trovan inj	Alocril	nedocromil ophth soln
albendazole	Albenza		
Albenza	albendazole	Alomide	lodoxamide tromethamine ophth soln
albumin human	Albuminar Albutein Buminate Plasbumin		
		alosetron (W)	Lotronex (W)
		Alphagan	brimonidine tartrate ophth
albumin (human), sonicated	Albunex		
Albuminar	albumin human	alpha₁-proteinase inhibitor (human)	Prolastin
Albunex	albumin (human), sonicated		
		alprazolam	Xanax
Albutein	albumin human	alprostadil	Caverject Edex Prostin VR
albuterol	Proventil salbutamol Ventolin		
		alprostadil urethral suppository	Muse
albuterol SR	Proventil Repetabs Volmax		
		Alrex	loteprednol etabonate ophth susp
albuterol sulfate inhalation aerosol	Proventil HFA		
		Altace	ramipril
		alteplase, recombinant	Activase
Aldactazide	spironolactone; hydrochloro-thiazide	altretamine	Hexalen
		aluminum acetate	Domeboro

aluminum carbonate	Basaljel
aluminum hydroxide	Amphojel
aluminum hydroxide; magnesium hydroxide	Maalox
Alupent	metaproterenol sulfate
amantadine HCl	Symmetrel
Amaryl	glimepiride
Ambien	zolpidem tartrate
AmBisome	liposomal amphotericin B
amcinonide	Cyclocort
Amerge	naratriptan HCl
Amicar	aminocaproic acid
Amidate	etomidate
amifostine	Ethyol
amikacin sulfate	Amikin
Amikin	amikacin sulfate
amiloride HCl	Midamor
amiloride; hydrochlorothiazide	Moduretic
amino acid inj	Aminosyn / Travasol / TrophAmine
amino acid with electrolytes in dextrose with calcium inj (various concentrations)	Clinimix E
aminocaproic acid	Amicar
aminocaproic acid gel	Caprogel
aminoglutethimide	Cytadren
aminolevulinic acid HCl topical soln	Levulan Kerastick
aminophylline	aminophylline
Aminosyn	amino acid inj
amiodarone HCl	Cordarone
amitriptyline HCl	Elavil / Endep
AmLactin	ammonium lactate lotion
amlexanox oral paste	Aphthasol
amlodipine besylate	Norvasc
amlodipine besylate; benazepril HCl	Lotrel
ammonium lactate lotion	AmLactin
amobarbital sodium	Amytal
amoxapine	Asendin
amoxicillin	Amoxil / Trimox / Wymox
amoxicillin; clavulanic acid	Augmentin
Amoxil	amoxicillin
amphetamine resins (W)	Biphetamine (W)
amphetamine; dextroamphetamine mixed salts	Adderall
Amphojel	aluminum hydroxide
Amphotec	amphotericin B cholesteryl sulfate
amphotericin B	Fungizone
amphotericin B cholesteryl sulfate	Amphotec
amphotericin B lipid complex	Abelcet
ampicillin	Principen
ampicillin sodium; sulbactam sodium	Unasyn
amprenavir	Agenerase

amrinone (former name)	inamrinone (new name)	antithymocyte globulin, (rabbit),	Thymoglobulin
amsacrine	Amsidyl	Antivert	meclizine
Amsidyl	amsacrine	Antizol	fomepizole
Amvisc	sodium hyaluronate	Anturane	sulfinpyrazone
		Anzemet	dolasetron mesylate
Amytal	amobarbital sodium	Aphthasol	amlexanox oral paste
Anadrol-50	oxymetholone		
Anafranil	clomipramine HCl	A.P.L.	chorionic gonadotropin
anagrelide HCl	Agrylin	apligraf	Graftskin
Anaprox	naproxen sodium	Aplisol	tuberculin skin test
anastrozole	Arimidex	apomorphine HCl	Uprima
Anbesol	benzocaine	Apresazide	hydralazine HCl; hydrochloro-thiazide
Ancef	cefazolin sodium		
Ancobon	flucytosine		
Androderm	testosterone transdermal system	Apresoline	hydralazine HCl
		aprotinin	Trasylol
		AquaMEPHY-TON	phytonadione
AndroGel	testosterone gel		
Androgel-DHT	dihydro-testosterone transdermal	Aralen	chloroquine phosphate
		Aramine	metaraminol bitartrate
Anectine	succinylcholine chloride	Arava	leflunomide
		arbutamine HCl	GenEsa
Anexsia	hydrocodone bitartrate; acetamino-phen	arcitumomab	CEA-Scan
		ardeparin sodium	Normiflo
		Arduan	pipecuronium bromide
Ansaid	flurbiprofen	Aredia	pamidronate disodium
Antabuse	disulfiram		
Antagon	ganirelix acetate	Arfonad	trimethaphan camsylate
antihemophilic factor (recombinant)	ReFacto		
		argatroban	argatroban
		arginine HCl	R-Gene
antihemophilic factor (recombinant), formulated with sucrose	Kogenate	Aricept	donepezil HCl
		Arimidex	anastrozole
		Aristocort	triamcinolone acetonide
		Aromasin	exemestane
Antilirium	physostigmine salicylate	arsenic trioxide	Trisenox
		Artane	trihexyphenidyl HCl
antipyrine otic	Auralgan		
antithrombin III (human)	Thrombate III	Arthrotec	diclofenac; misoprostol

Asacol	mesalamine
Asendin	amoxapine
asparaginase	Elspar
aspirin 325 mg with codeine phosphate (30 and 60 mg)	Empirin with codeine #3 and #4
aspirin buffered	Bufferin
aspirin EC	Ecotrin
Astelin	azelastine HCl nasal spray
astemizole (W)	Hismanal (W)
Atacand	candesartan cilexetil
Atarax	hydroxyzine HCl
atenolol	Tenormin
atenolol; chlorthalidone	Tenoretic
Atgam	lymphocyte immune globulin
articaine; epinephrine	Septocaine
aspirin; extended-release dipyridamole	Aggrenox
Atacand HCT	candesartan cilexetil; hydrochloro-thiazide
Ativan	lorazepam
atorvastatin calcium	Lipitor
atovaquone	Mepron
atovaquone; proguanil HCl	Malarone
atracurium besylate	Tracrium
Atridox	doxycycline hyclate gel
Atromid-S	clofibrate
atropine sulfate tablets	Sal-Tropine
Atrovent	ipratropium bromide
Augmentin	amoxicillin; clavulanic acid
Auralgan	antipyrine otic
auranofin	Ridaura
Aurolate	gold sodium thiomalate
aurothioglucose	Solganal
Avalide	irbesartan; hydrochloro-thiazide
Avandia	Rosiglitazone maleate
Avanir	docosanol cream
Avapro	irbesartan
Avelox	moxifloxacin HCl
Aventyl	nortriptyline HCl
Avita	tretinoin cream 0.025%
Avitene	collagen hemostat
Avonex	interferon beta-la
Axid	nizatidine
Azactam	aztreonam
azatadine maleate	Optimine
azathioprine	Imuran
azelaic acid cream	Azelex
azelastine HCl nasal spray	Astelin
azelastine HCl ophth soln	Optivar
Azelex	azelaic acid cream
azithromycin	Zithromax
Azmacort	triamcinolone acetonide aerosol
Azopt	brinzolamide ophth susp
aztreonam	Azactam
Azulfidine	sulfasalazine

B

Baciguent	bacitracin ointment
bacitracin ointment	Baciguent

baclofen	Lioresal		Hurricaine
Bactrim	sulfamethoxa-zole; trimeth-oprim		Orabase
			Orajel
		benzocaine; tetracaine HCl	Cetacaine
Bactroban	mupirocin nasal ointment	benztropine mesylate	Cogentin
BAL in Oil	dimercaprol	bepridil	Vascor
Basaljel	aluminum carbonate	beractant	Survanta
		Berroca	vitamin B complex; folic acid; vitamin C
balsalazide disodium	Colazal		
basiliximab	Simulect	Betadine	povidone iodine
Baycol	cerivastatin sodium	17β-estradiol; norgestimate	Ortho-Prefest
BCG intravesical	Pacis TheraCys TICE BCG	Betagan	levobunolol HCl
		betaine anhydrous	Cystadane
becaplermin gel	Regranex		
beclomethasone dipropionate	Beclovent Beconase AQ Nasal	betamethasone	Celestone
		betamethasone dipropionate	Diprosone
	Qvar Vancenase	betamethasone; clotrimazole cream	Lotrisone
	Vancenase AQ Nasal		
	Vanceril	betamethasone valerate (foam)	Luxiq
Beclovent	beclomethasone dipropionate	Betapace	sotalol
		Betaseron	interferon beta-1b
Beconase AQ Nasal	beclomethasone dipropionate	betaxolol	Kerlone
		betaxolol HCl ophth soln	Betoptic
belladonna alkaloids; phenobarbital	Donnatal		
		betaxolol HCl ophth susp	Betoptic S
Bellergal-S	phenobarbital; ergotamine; belladonna	betaxolol HCl; pilocarpine HCl ophth soln	Betoptic Pilo
Benadryl	diphenhydramine HCl		
		bethanechol chloride	Urecholine
benazepril HCl	Lotensin	Betoptic	betaxolol HCl ophth soln
BeneFix	factor IX, (recombinant)		
Benemid	probenecid	Betoptic Pilo	betaxolol HCl; pilocarpine HCl, ophth soln
bentoquatam	IvyBlock		
Bentyl	dicyclomine HCl		
Benzamycin	erythromycin; benzoyl peroxide topical gel	bexarotene gel	Targretin
		Betoptic S	betaxolol HCl ophth suspension
benzocaine	Anbesol		

Biaxin	clarithromycin	bretylium tosylate	Bretylol
Biaxin XL	clarithromycin SR		
bicalutamide	Casodex	Bretylol	bretylium tosylate
Bicillin C-R	penicillin G benzathine; penicillin G procaine (for IM use only)	Brevibloc	esmolol HCl
		Brevital Sodium	methohexital sodium
		Bricanyl	terbutaline sulfate tablets and inj
Bicillin L-A	penicillin G benzathine (for IM use only)		
		brimonidine tartrate ophth	Alphagan
Bicitra	sodium citrate; citric acid	brinzolamide ophth suspension	Azopt
BiCNU	carmustine		
Bilopaque	tyropanoate sodium	bromocriptine mesylate	Parlodel
biperiden	Akineton	brompheniramine maleate	Dimetane
Biphetamine (W)	amphetamine resins (W)	brompheniramine maleate; phenylpropan- olamime	Dimetapp Extentabs
bisacodyl	Dulcolax		
bismuth subsalicylate; metronidazole; tetracycline HCl	Helidac		
		Bronkometer	isoetharine HCl aerosol
		Bronkosol	isoetharine HCl soln
bisoprolol fumarate; hydrochlorothi- azide	Ziac	Bucladin-S	buclizine HCl
		buclizine HCl	Bucladin-S
		budesonide inhalation powder	Pulmicort Turbuhaler
bitolterol mesylate	Tornalate		
		budesonide nasal inhaler	Rhinocort
Blenoxane	bleomycin sulfate		
		Bufferin	aspirin buffered
bleomycin sulfate	Blenoxane	bumetanide	Bumex
Blocadren	timolol maleate	Bumex	bumetanide
B & O Supprettes	opium; belladonna suppositories	Buminate	albumin human
		Buphenyl	phenylbutyrate sodium
Botox	botulinum toxin type A		
		bupivacaine HCl	Marcaine HCl
botulinum toxin type A	Botox	bupropion HCl	Wellbutrin
		bupropion HCl SR	Wellbutrin SR Zyban
Brethaire	terbutaline sulfate aerosol		
		BuSpar	buspirone HCl
		buspirone HCl	BuSpar
Brethine	terbutaline sulfate tablets and inj	busulfan	Myleran
		busulfan inj	Busulfex
		Busulfex	busulfan inj

butabarbital sodium	Butisol
butalbital; acetaminophen; caffeine	Fioricet
butalbital; aspirin; caffeine	Fiorinal
butenafine HCl	Mentax
Butisol	butabarbital sodium
butoconazole nitrate vaginal cream	Gynazole
butorphanol tartrate inj	Stadol
butorphanol tartrate nasal spray	Stadol NS

C

cabergoline	Dostinex
Cafergot	ergotaminetartrate; caffeine
Cafcit	caffeine citrate inj
caffeine citrate inj	Cafcit
Calan SR	verapamil HCl SR
Calciferol	ergocalciferol
Calcimar	calcitonin
calcipotriene cream	Dovonex
calcitonin	Calcimar
calcitonin-salmon	Miacalcin
calcitriol	Rocaltrol
calcium carbonate	Os-Cal 500 Tums Viactiv
calcium carbonate; vitamin D and K chewable	

calfactant intratracheal susp	Infasurf
camphorated tincture of opium	paregoric
Camptosar	irinotecan HCl
candesartan cilexetil	Atacand
candesartan cilexetil; hydrochlorothi-azide	Atacand HCT
Capastat Sulfate	capreomycin sulfate
capecitabine	Xeloda
Capital w/ Codeine Suspension	codeine phosphate; acetaminophen suspension
Capitrol	chloroxine
Capoten	captopril
capreomycin sulfate	Capastat Sulfate
Caprogel	aminocaproic acid gel
capromab pendetide	ProstaScint
captopril	Capoten
Carafate	sucralfate
carbachol	Isopto Carbachol
carbamazepine	Tegretol
carbamazepine SR	Carbatrol Tegretol-XR
carbamide peroxide otic	Debrox
Carbatrol	carbamazepine SR
carbenicillin	Geocillin
Carbex	selegiline
Carbocaine	mepivacaine HCl
carboplatin	Paraplatin
Cardene	nicardipine HCl
Cardiolite	technetium Tc99m sestamibi

Cardiotec	technetium Tc-99m teboroxime kit	cefpodoxime proxetil	Vantin
Cardizem	diltiazem HCl	cefprozil	Cefzil
Cardizem CD	diltiazem HCl SR	ceftazidime	Ceptaz
			Fortaz
Cardura	doxazosin mesylate		Tazicef
			Tazidime
carisoprodol	Soma	ceftibuten	Cedax
carmustine	BiCNU	Ceftin	cefuroxime axetil
carmustine implantable wafer	Gliadel	ceftizoxime sodium	Cefizox
Carnitor	levocarnitine	ceftriaxone sodium	Rocephin
Cartia XR	diltiazem HCl SR	cefuroxime axetil	Ceftin
carvedilol	Coreg	cefuroxime sodium	Kefurox
Casodex	bicalutamide		Zinacef
Cataflam	diclofenac potassium	Cefzil	cefprozil
		Celebrex	celecoxib
Catapres	clonidine HCl	celecoxib	Celebrex
Caverject	alprostadil	Celestone	betamethasone
CEA-SCAN	arcitumomab	Celexa	citalopram hydrobromide
Ceclor	cefaclor		
Cedax	ceftibuten	CellCept	mycophenolate mofetil
CeeNu	lomustine		
cefaclor	Ceclor	Cenestin	synthetic conjugated estrogens, A
cefadroxil	Duricef		
Cefadyl	cephapirin sodium		
		Centrum	vitamins; minerals
cefamandole nafate	Mandol		
cefazolin sodium	Ancef	cephalexin	Keflex
	Kefzol	cephalexin HCl	Keftab
cefdinir	Omnicef	cephalothin sodium (W)	Keflin (W)
cefepime HCl	Maxipime		
cefixime	Suprax	cephapirin sodium	Cefadyl
Cefizox	ceftizoxime sodium		
		cephradine	Velosef
Cefobid	cefoperazone sodium	Cephulac	lactulose
		Ceptaz	ceftazidime
cefonicid sodium	Monocid	Cerebyx	fosphenytoin sodium
cefoperazone sodium	Cefobid		
		Ceredase	alglucerase
Cefotan	cefotetan	Cerezyme	imiglucerase
cefotaxime sodium	Claforan	cerivastatin sodium	Baycol
cefotetan	Cefotan		
cefoxitin sodium	Mefoxin	Cernevit-12	multivitamins for infusion

Cerubidine	daunorubicin HCl	chlorzoxazone 250 mg	Paraflex
Cervidil	dinoprostone vaginal insert	chlorzoxazone 500 mg	Parafon Forte DSC
Cetacaine	benzocaine; tetracaine HCl	Cholebrine	iocetamic acid
		Choledyl	oxtriphylline
cetirizine HCl	Zyrtec	cholestyramine	Questran
cetrorelix	Cetrotide	choline chloride inj	Intrachol
Cetrotide	cetrorelix		
cevimeline HCl	Evoxac	choline magnesium trisalicylate	Trilisate
Chirocaine	levobupivacaine		
chloral hydrate	chloral hydrate	Choloxin	dextrothyroxine sodium
chlorambucil	Leukeran		
chloramphenicol	Chloromycetin	chorionic gonadotropin	A.P.L.
chloramphenicol ophth	Chloroptic ophth	choriogona-dotropin alfa	Ovidrel
chlordiazepoxide HCl	Librium	Chronulac	lactulose
		Chymodiactin	chymopapain
chlordiazepoxide HCl; amitriptyline HCl	Limbitrol	chymopapain	Chymodiactin
		Cibalith-S	lithium citrate
		ciclopirox cream and lotion	Loprox
chlorhexidine gluconate	Hibiclens PerioChip	ciclopirox soln	Penlac Nail Lacquer
chlorhexidine gluconate mouth rinse	Peridex	cidofovir	Vistide
		cilostazol	Pletal
Chloromycetin	chloramphenicol	Ciloxan	ciprofloxacin ophth soln
chloroprocaine HCl	Nesacaine		
Chloroptic ophth	chloramphenicol ophth	cimetidine HCl	Tagamet
		Cipro	ciprofloxacin HCl
chloroquine phosphate	Aralen	ciprofloxacin HCl	Cipro
chlorothiazide	Diuril	ciprofloxacin; hydrocortisone otic	Cipro HC Otic
chloroxine	Capitrol		
chlorpheniramine maleate	Chlor-Trimeton	ciprofloxacin ophth soln	Ciloxan
chlorpheniramine maleate SR	Teldrin	Cipro HC Otic	ciprofloxacin; hydrocortisone otic
chlorpromazine	Thorazine		
chlorpropamide	Diabinese	cisapride (W)	Propulsid (W)
chlorthalidone	Hygroton	cisatracurium besylate	Nimbex
chlorthalidone; reserpine	Regroton	cisplatin	Platinol AQ
		citalopram hydrobromide	Celexa
Chlor-Trimeton	chlorpheniramine maleate	cladribine	Leustatin

C
R

Claforan	cefotaxime sodium	clotrimazole	Gyne-Lotrimin Lotrimin Mycelex
clarithromycin	Biaxin		
clarithromycin SR	Biaxin XL	clozapine	Clozaril
Claritin	loratadine	Clozaril	clozapine
Claritin D	loratadine; pseudoephedrine sulfate	coagulation factor IX (recombinant)	BeneFix
clemastine fumarate	Tavist	coagulation factor VII a (recombinant)	NovoSeven
Cleocin	clindamycin HCl		
clidinium bromide	Quarzan	coal tar product codeine	Zetar Capital w/
clidinium; chlordiazepoxide	Librax	phosphate; acetaminophen suspension	Codeine Suspension
Climara	estradiol transdermal	coenzyme Q10 Cogentin	UbiQGel benztropine
clindamycin HCl	Cleocin		mesylate
clindamycin phosphate pledgets	Clindets	Cognex Colace	tacrine HCl docusate sodium
Clindets	clindamycin phosphate pledgets	Colazol	balsalazide disodium
Clinimix E	amino acid with electrolytes in dextrose with calcium inj (various concentrations)	ColBENEMID (W) colchicine colesevelam HCl Colestid colestipol HCl	probenecid; colchicine (W) colchicine Welchol colestipol HCl Colestid
Clinoril	sulindac	colistimethate s odium	Coly-Mycin M
clioquinol	Vioform	colistin sulfate;	Coly-Mycin S
clobetasol foam	Olux	hydrocortisone,	
clofibrate	Atromid-S	and neomycin	
Clomid	clomiphene citrate	otic soln	
clomiphene citrate	Clomid	collagen hemostat	Avitene
clomipramine HCl	Anafranil	collagenase Collyrium	Santyl tetrahydrozoline
clonazepam	Klonopin		HCl ophth
clonidine HCl	Catapres	Colomed	short chain fatty
clonidine HCl inj	Duraclon		acids enema
clopidogrel bisulfate	Plavix	Coly-Mycin M	colistimethate sodium
clorazepate dipotassium	Tranxene	Coly-Mycin S	colistin sulfate; hydrocortisone,
Clorpactin WCS-90	oxychlorosene sodium		and neomycin otic soln

CoLyte	polyethylene glycol-electrolyte soln
CombiPatch	norethindrone acetate; estradiol transdermal
Combivent	ipratropium bromide; albuterol sulfate
Combivir	lamivudine; zidovudine
Compazine	prochlorperazine
Comtan	entacapone
Comvax	*Haemophilus b* conjugate; Hepatitis B vaccine
Concerta	methylphenidate HCl SR
Condylox	podofilox gel
Copaxone	glatiramer acetate
Cordarone	amiodarone HCl
Coreg	carvedilol
Corgard	nadolol
Corlopam	fenoldopam mesylate
Cortef	hydrocortisone
corticorellin ovine triflutate	Acthrel
corticotropin	Acthar
cortisone acetate	Cortone Acetate
Cortone Acetate	cortisone acetate
Cortrosyn	cosyntropin
Corvert	ibutilide fumarate
Cosmegen	dactinomycin
Cosopt	dorzolamide HCl; timolol maleate ophth soln
cosyntropin	Cortrosyn
Cotazym	pancrelipase
Cotazym-S	pancrelipase EC
Cotrim	sulfamethoxazole; trimethoprim

co-trimoxazole	Bactrim Cotrim Septra sulfamethoxazole; trimethoprim
Coumadin	warfarin sodium
Covera HS	verapamil HCl SR bedtime formulation
Cozaar	losartan potassium
Crinone	progesterone gel
Crixivan	indinavir
cromolyn sodium	Gastrocrom Nasalcrom Opticrom
crotamiton	Eurax
Crystodigin	digitoxin
Cuprimine	penicillamine
Curosurf	poractant alpha intratracheal susp
Cutivate	fluticasone propionate cream & ointment
cyanocobalamin nasal gel	Nascobal
cyclobenzaprine HCl	Flexeril
Cyclocort	amcinonide
Cyclogyl	cyclopentolate HCl
cyclopentolate HCl	Cyclogyl
cyclophosphamide	Cytoxan Neosar
cycloserine	Seromycin
cyclosporine	Sandimmune
cyclosporine capsules (modified) and oral soln	Neoral
cyclosporine capsules, (modified)	Gengraf
cyclosporine ophth emulsion	Restasis

Cycrin	medroxyproges- terone acetate	Darvon Compound 65	propoxyphene HCl; aspirin; caffeine
Cylert	pemoline		
cyproheptadine HCl	Periactin	daunorubicin citrate liposomal	DaunoXome
Cystadane	betaine anhydrous	daunorubicin HCl	Cerubidine
Cystospaz-M	hyoscyamine sulfate SR	DaunoXome	daunorubicin citrate liposomal
Cytadren	aminogluteth- imide		
cytarabine	Cytosar-U	Daypro	oxaprozin
cytarabine, liposomal inj	DepoCyt	DDAVP	desmopressin acetate
Cytomel	liothyronine sodium	Debrox	carbamide peroxide otic
Cytosar-U	cytarabine	Decadron	dexamethasone
Cytotec	misoprostol	Deca-Durabolin	nandrolone decanoate
Cytovene	ganciclovir		
Cytoxan	cyclophosphamide	Declomycin	demeclocycline HCl
		deferoxamine mesylate	Desferal

D

		delavirdine mesylate	Rescriptor
		Delestrogen	estradiol valerate
dacarbazine	DTIC-Dome	Deltasone	prednisone
daclizumab	Zenapax	Demadex	torsemide
dactinomycin	Cosmegen	demecarium bromide	Humorsol
Dalmane	flurazepam HCl		
dalteparin sodium	Fragmin	demeclocycline HCl	Declomycin
danaparoid sodium	Orgaran	Demerol	meperidine HCl
		Demser	metyrosine
danazol	Danocrine	Demulen	ethynodiol diacetate; ethinyl estradiol
Danocrine	danazol		
Dantrium	dantrolene sodium		
dantrolene sodium	Dantrium	Denavir	penciclovir cream
		denileukin diftitox	Ontak
dapsone	dapsone		
Daranide	dichlorphena- mide	Depacon	valproate sodium inj
Daraprim	pyrimethamine	Depakene	valproic acid
Darvocet-N 100	propoxyphene napsylate; acetaminophen	Depakote	divalproex sodium
Darvon	propoxyphene HCl	Depakote ER	divalproex sodium SR

DepoCyt	cytarabine, liposomal inj	dextrothyroxine sodium	Choloxin
Depo-Medrol	methylprednisolone acetate SR	D.H.E. 45	dihydroergotamine mesylate inj
Depo-Provera	medroxyprogesterone acetate SR	DiaBeta	glyburide
		Diabinese	chlorpropamide
Depo-Testosterone	testosterone cypionate SR	Diamox	acetazolamide
		Diapid	lypressin
Desferal	deferoxamine mesylate	Diastat	diazepam rectal gel
desflurane	Suprane	diazepam	Valium
desipramine HCl	Norpramin	diazepam emulsified inj	Dizac
desmopressin acetate	DDAVP		
Desogen	desogestrel; ethinyl estradiol	diazepam rectal gel	Diastat
		diazoxide	Hyperstat
desogestrel; ethinyl estradiol	Desogen Ortho-Cept	Dibenzyline	phenoxybenzamine HCl
		dibucaine	Nupercainal
desogestrel and ethinyl estradiol; ethinyl estradiol	Mircette	dichlorphenamide	Daranide
		diclofenac potassium	Cataflam
		diclofenac sodium	Voltaren
desonide	Tridesilon	diclofenac sodium; misoprostol	Arthrotec
desoximetasone	Topicort		
Desoxyn	methamphetamine HCl	diclofenac sodium SR	Voltaren-XR
Desyrel	trazodone HCl	dicloxacillin sodium	Dynapen
Detrol	tolterodine tartrate		
dexamethasone	Decadron Hexadrol	dicyclomine HCl	Bentyl
		didanosine	Videx
dexchlorpheniramine maleate SR	Polaramine Repetabs	Didronel	etidronate disodium
Dexedrine	dextroamphetamine sulfate	diethylcarbamazine citrate	Hetrazan
		diethylpropion HCl	Tenuate
dexfenfluramine HCl (W)	Redux (W)	diethylstilbestrol diphosphate	Stilphostrol
Dexferrum	iron dextran inj		
dexmedetomidine HCl inj	Precedex	Differin	adapalene
		diflorasone diacetate	Florone
dexrazoxane	Zinecard		
dextroamphetamine sulfate	Dexedrine	Diflucan	fluconazole
		diflunisal	Dolobid

D
Rx

Digibind	digoxin immune fab	diphtheria and tetanus toxoids and pertussis vaccine, adsorbed	DTwP Tri-Immunol
digitoxin	Crystodigin		
digoxin	Lanoxin		
digoxin capsules	Lanoxicaps		
digoxin immune fab	Digibind	diphtheria and tetanus toxoids; pertussis vaccine, adsorbed and haemophilus b conjugate vaccine	Tetramune
dihydroergota-mine mesylate inj	D.H.E. 45		
dihydroergota-mine mesylate nasal spray	Migranol		
dihydrotestoster-one transdermal	Androgel-DHT	dipivefrin	Propine
		Diprivan	propofol
Dilacor XR	diltiazem HCl SR	Diprosone	betamethasone dipropionate
Dilantin	phenytoin		
Dilaudid	hydromorphone HCl	dipyridamole	Persantine
		dirithromycin	Dynabac
diltiazem HCl	Cardizem	Disalcid	salsalate
diltiazem HCl SR	Cardizem CD Cartia XR Dilacor XR Tiazac	disopyramide phosphate	Norpace
		disulfiram	Antabuse
		Ditropan	oxybutynin chloride
diltiazem maleate SR	Tiamate		
		Diulo	metolazone
dimenhydrinate	Dramamine	Diuril	chlorothiazide
dimercaprol	BAL in Oil	divalproex sodium	Depakote
Dimetane	brompheniramine maleate		
		divalproex sodium SR	Depakote ER
dinoprostone gel	Prepidil		
dinoprostone vaginal insert	Cervidil	Dizac	diazepam emulsified inj
dinoprostone vaginal suppositories	Prostin E2		
		dobutamine HCl	Dobutrex
Diovan	valsartan	Dobutrex	dobutamine HCl
Dipentum	olsalazine sodium	docetaxel	Taxotere
diphenhydramine HCl	Benadryl	docosanol cream	Avanir
		docusate calcium	Surfak
diphenoxylate HCl; atropine sulfate	Lomotil	docusate calcium; phenolphthalein	Doxidan
		docusate sodium	Colace
diphtheria and tetanus toxoids and acellular pertussis vaccine	Acel-Imune Tripedia	docusate sodium; casanthranol	Peri-Colace
		dofetilide	Tikosyn
		dolasetron mesylate	Anzemet

Drug	Equivalent
Dolobid	diflunisal
Dolophine	methadone HCl
Domeboro	aluminum acetate
donepezil HCl	Aricept
Donnatal	belladonna alkaloids; phenobarbital
dopamine HCl	Intropin
Dopar	levodopa
Dopram	doxapram HCl
dornase alpha	Pulmozyme
dorzolamide HCl	Trusopt
dorzolamide HCl; timolol maleate ophth soln	Cosopt
Dostinex	cabergoline
Dovonex	calcipotriene cream
doxacurium chloride	Nuromax
doxapram HCl	Dopram
doxazosin mesylate	Cardura
doxepin HCl	Adapin Sinequan
doxepin HCl cream	Prudoxin
doxercalciferol	Hectorol
Doxidan	docusate calcium; phenolphthalein
Doxil	doxorubicin, liposomal
doxorubicin HCl	Adriamycin Rubex
doxorubicin, liposomal	Doxil
doxycycline hyclate	Vibramycin
doxycycline hyclate gel	Atridox
Dramamine	dimenhydrinate
Drisdol	ergocalciferol
Dristan Long Lasting	oxymetazoline HCl
Drixoral Syrup	pseudoephedrine HCl; bromphiramine maleate
dronabinol	Marinol
droperidol	Inapsine
Droxia	hydroxyurea
DTIC-Dome	dacarbazine
Dulcolax	bisacodyl
Durabolin	nandrolone phenpropionate
Duraclon	clonidine HCl inj
Duragesic	fentanyl transdermal
Duramorph	morphine sulfate inj
Duranest	etidocaine HCl
Duricef	cefadroxil
Dyazide	triamterene 37.5 mg; hydrochlorothiazide 25 mg
Dymelor	acetohexamide
Dynabac	dirithromycin
DynaCirc	isradipine
Dynapen	dicloxacillin sodium
dyphylline	Lufyllin
Dyrenium	triamterene

D R

E

Drug	Equivalent
EchoGen	perflenapent emulsion
echothiophate iodide	Phospholine Iodide
Ecotrin	aspirin EC
Edecrin	ethacrynic acid
edetate disodium	Endrate
Edex	alprostadil inj
edrophonium chloride	Tensilon
E.E.S. 400	erythromycin ethylsuccinate
efavirenz	Sustiva

Effexor	venlafaxine HCl	Endep	amitriptyline HCl
Effexor XR	venlafaxine HCl SR	Endocet	oxycodone HCl; acetaminophen
eflornithine HCl cream	Vaniqa	Endrate	edetate disodium
		Enduron	methyclothiazide
Elavil	amitriptyline HCl	enflurane	Ethrane
Eldepryl	selegiline HCl	Engerix-B	hepatitis B vaccine
Eldisine	vindesine sulfate		
Elixophyllin	theophylline	Enkaid	encainide HCl
Ellence	epirubicin HCl		
Elmiron	pentosan polysulfate sodium	enoxaparin sodium	Lovenox
		entacapone	Comtan
Elocon	mometasone furoate topical	Entex LA	phenylpropanol- amine HCl; guaifenesin SR
Elspar	asparaginase	epinephrine	Adrenalin
Emadine	emedastine difumarate opthth soln	epinephrine racemic	Vaponefrin
		epirubicin HCl	Ellence
Emcyt	estramustine phosphate sodium	Epivir	lamivudine
		Epivir HBV	lamivudine
		epoetin alfa	Epogen
emedastine difumarate opthth soln	Emadine		Procrit
		Epogen	epoetin alfa
EMLA Cream	lidocaine; prilocaine cream	epoprostenol sodium	Flolan
		eprosartan mesylate	Teveten
Empirin with codeine #3 and #4	aspirin 325 mg with codeine phosphate (30 and 60 mg)	eptifibatide	Integrilin
		Equanil	meprobamate
		Ergamisol	levamisole HCl
E-Mycin	erythromycin	ergocalciferol	Calciferol
enalapril maleate	Vasotec		Drisdol
enalapril maleate; diltiazem malate	Teczem	ergoloid mesylates	Hydergine
		ergotamine tartrate; caffeine	Cafergot
enalapril maleate; felodipine SR	Lexxel	ergotamine tartrate	Ergostat
		Ergotrate	ergonovine maleate
enalapril maleate; hydrochlorothi- azide	Vaseretic	Ery-Tab	erythromycin EC
Enbrel	etanercept	Erythrocin Stearate	erythromycin stearate
encainide HCl	Enkaid		

E
Rx

erythromycin	E-Mycin	estramustine	Emcyt
erythromycin base coated particles	PCE Dispertab	phosphate sodium	
		Estratest	estrogens, esterified; methyltestos-terone
erythromycin; benzoyl peroxide topical gel	Benzamycin		
		Estratest H.S.	estrogens, esterified; methyltestos-terone, half strength
erythromycin EC	Ery-Tab		
erythromycin estolate	Ilosone		
erythromycin ethylsuccinate	E.E.S. 400	Estring	estradiol vaginal ring
erythromycin ethylsuccinate; sulfisoxazole	Pediazole	estrogens, conjugated	Premarin
		estrogens conjugate, A synthetic	Cenestin
erythromycin stearate	Erythrocin Stearate	estrogens, conjugated; medroxyproges-terone acetate	Premphase Prempro
Esclim	estradiol transdermal		
Eserine Sulfate	physostigmine ophth ointment		
Esidrix	hydrochlorothi-azide	estrogens, esterified; methyltestoster-one	Estratest
Esimil	guanethidine monosulfate; hydrochloro-thiazide		
		estrogens, esterified methyltestost-erone, half strength	Estratest H.S.
Eskalith	lithium carbonate		
esmolol HCl	Brevibloc		
estazolam	ProSom	estropipate	Ogen
Estinyl	ethinyl estradiol	Estrostep	norethindrone acetate; ethinyl estradiol
Estrace	estradiol		
Estraderm	estradiol transdermal		
estradiol	Estrace	etanercept	Enbrel
estradiol hemihydrate vaginal tab	Vagifem	ethacrynic acid	Edecrin
		ethambutol HCl	Myambutol
		ethchlorvynol	Placidyl
estradiol transdermal	Climara Esclim Estraderm FemPatch Vivelle	Ethezyme	papain; urea oint
		ethinyl estradiol	Estinyl
		ethionamide	Trecator-SC
		Ethmozine	moricizine
		ethopropazine HCl	Parsidol
estradiol vaginal ring	Estring		
estradiol valerate	Delestrogen	ethosuximide	Zarontin
		Ethrane	enflurane

ethyl chloride	ethyl chloride	Fareston	toremifene citrate
ethynodiol diacetate; ethinyl estradiol	Demulen	Fastin	phentermine HCl
		fat emulsion	Intralipid Liposyn II and III
Ethyol	amifostine		
etidocaine HCl	Duranest	felbamate	Felbatol
etidronate disodium	Didronel	Felbatol	felbamate
		Feldene	piroxicam
etodolac	Lodine	felodipine	Plendil
etodolac SR	Lodine XL	Femara	Ietrozole
etomidate	Amidate	Femhrt	norethindrone acetate; ethinyl estradiol
Etopophos	etoposide phosphate diethanolate		
		FemPatch	estradiol transdermal
etoposide	VePesid		
etoposide phosphate diethanolate	Etopophos	fenfluramine HCl (W)	Pondimin (W)
		fenofibrate	Tricor
Etrafon	perphenazine; amitriptyline HCl	fenoldopam mesylate	Corlopam
		fenoprofen calcium	Nalfon
Eulexin	flutamide	fentanyl citrate	Sublimaze
Eurax	crotamiton	fentanyl citrate; droperidol	Innovar
Euthroid (WA)	liotrix		
Eutonyl	pargyline HCl	Fentanyl Oralet	fentanyl transmucosal
Evista	raloxifene HCl		
Evoxac	cevimeline HCl	fentanyl transdermal	Duragesic
Exelon	rivastigmine tartrate	fentanyl transmucosal	Actiq Fentanyl Oralet
exemestane	Aromasin		
Ex-Lax	sennosides	Feosol	ferrous sulfate
		Fer-In-Sol	ferrous sulfate
		Fergon	ferrous gluconate
F		Feridex	ferumoxide HCl
		Ferrlecit	sodium ferric gluconate complex in sucrose inj
factor IX, concentrate	BeneFix		
		ferrous gluconate	Fergon
Factrel	gonadorelin HCl	*ferrous sulfate*	Feosol
famciclovir	Famvir		Fer-In-Sol
famotidine	Pepcid		
famotidine, oral disintegrating tablet	Pepcid RPD	ferrous sulfate SR	SlowFe
		Fertinex	urofollitropin for inj
Famvir	famciclovir		
Fansidar	sulfadoxine; pyrimethamine	ferumoxetil oral suspension	Gastromark

E
R

ferumoxide HCl	Feridex	Flumadine	rimantadine
fexofenadine HCl	Allegra	flumazenil	Romazicon
		flunisolide	Aero Bid
filgrastim	Neupogen	fluocinolone acetonide	Synalar
finasteride	Propecia 1 mg tablet		
		fluocinonide	Lidex
	Proscar 5 mg tablet	Fluor-I-Strip	fluorescein sodium strips
Fioricet	butalbital; acetamino-phen; caffeine	fluorescein sodium soln	Fluorescite
Fiorinal	butalbital; aspirin; caffeine	fluorescein sodium strips	Fluor-I-Strip
Flagyl	metronidazole	Fluorescite	fluorescein sodium soln
Flagyl ER	metronidazole SR	fluorometholone	FML
flavoxate HCl	Urispas	Fluothane	halothane
Flaxedil	gallamine triethiodide	fluoxetine HCl	Prozac
			Sarafem
flecainide acetate	Tambocor	fluoxymesterone	Halotestin
Flexeril	cyclobenzaprine HCl	fluphenazine HCl	Permitil
			Prolixin
Flolan	epoprostenol sodium	flurazepam HCl	Dalmane
		flurbiprofen	Ansaid
Flomax	tamsulosin HCl	flutamide	Eulexin
Flonase	fluticasone propionate spray	fluticasone propionate spray	Flonase
			Flovent
Florinef	fludrocortisone acetate	fluticasone propionate cream & ointment	Cutivate
Florone	diflorasone diacetate		
Floropryl	isoflurophate	fluticasone propionate; salmeterol inhalation powder	Advair Diskus
Flovent	fluticasone propionate spray		
		fluvastatin sodium	Lescol
Floxin	ofloxacin		
Floxin Otic	ofloxacin otic soln	fluvoxamine maleate	Luvox
floxuridine	FUDR	FML	fluorometholone
fluconazole	Diflucan	Folex PFS	methotrexate inj
flucytosine	Ancobon	folic acid	Folvite
Fludara	fludarabine phosphate	Follistim	follitropin beta
		follitropin alfa	Gonal-F
fludarabine phosphate	Fludara	follitropin beta	Follistim
fludrocortisone acetate	Florinef	Folvite	folic acid
		fomepizole	Antizol

F
R/

fomivirsen sodium inj	Vitravene	ganciclovir ophthalmic implant	Vitrasert
Forane	isoflurane	ganirelix acetate	Antagon
Fortaz	ceftazidime	Ganite	gallium nitrate
Fortovase	saquinavir soft gel capsule	Gantanol	sulfamethoxazole
Fosamax	alendronate sodium	Garamycin	*gentamicin sulfate*
foscarnet	Foscavir	Gastrocrom	cromolyn sodium
Foscavir	foscarnet		
fosfomycin tromethamine	Monurol	Gastromark	ferumoxetil oral suspension
fosinopril sodium	Monopril	gatifloxacin	Tequin
fosphenytoin sodium	Cerebyx	gemcitabine HCl	Gemzar
Fragmin	dalteparin sodium	gemfibrozil	Lopid
		gemtuzumab ozogamicin	Mylotarg
FUDR	floxuridine	Gemzar	gemcitabine HCl
Fulvicin P/G	griseofulvin	GenEsa	arbutamine HCl
Fungizone	amphotericin B	Gengraf	cyclosporine capsules, (modified)
Furacin	nitrofurazone		
furosemide	Lasix	Genora	norethindrone; mestranol
		Genotropin	somatropin for inj
# G		*gentamicin sulfate*	Garamycin
gabapentin	Neurontin	Geocillin	carbenicillin
Gabitril	tiagabine HCl	Geref	sermorelin acetate
gadoteridol	ProHance	glatiramer acetate	Copaxone
gadoversetamide	OptiMark	Gliadel	carmustine implantable wafer
galanthamine HBr	Reminyl		
gallamine triethiodide	Flaxedil	glimepiride	Amaryl
gallium nitrate	Ganite	glipizide	Glucotrol
Galzin	zinc acetate	glipizide SR	Glucotrol XL
Gamimune N	immune globulin intravenous	GlucaGen	glucagon (rDNA origin)
gamma hydroxybutyrate	Xyrem	glucagon	glucagon
Gammagard S/D	immune globulin intravenous	glucagon (rDNA origin)	GlucaGen
Gammar-P IV	immune globulin intravenous	Glucophage	metformin HCl
ganciclovir	Cytovene	Glucotrol	glipizide

Glucotrol XL	glipizide SR	guanfacine HCl	Tenex
Glucovance	glyburide; metformin HCl	Gynazole	butoconazole nitrate vaginal cream
glyburide	DiaBeta Micronase	Gyne-Lotrimin	clotrimazole
glyburide; metformin HCl	Glucovance		
glyburide micronized	Glynase		

H

glycerin ophth soln	Ophthalgan		
glycopyrrolate	Robinul		
Glynase	glyburide micronized	Habitrol	nicotine transdermal system
Glyset	miglitol	*Haemophilus b* conjugate vaccine reconstituted with diphtheria and tetanus toxoids and acellular pertussis vaccine adsorbed	ActHIB/Tripedia
gold sodium thiomalate	Aurolate		
GoLYTELY	polyethylene glycol-electrolyte soln		
gonadorelin HCl	Factrel		
Gonal-F	follitropin alfa		
goserelin acetate implant	Zoladex		
graftskin	Apligraf		
granisetron HCl	Kytril	*Haemophilus b* conjugate; Hepatitis B vaccine	Comvax
grepafloxacin HCl (W)	Raxar (W)		
Grifulvin V	griseofulvin	haemophilus b vaccine	Hib-Immune HibTITER PedvaxHIB ProHIBiT
griseofulvin	Fulvicin P/G Grifulvin V		
guaifenesin	Organidin NR Robitussin		
guaifenesin; codeine phosphate	Robitussin A-C Tussi-Organidin NR	halcinonide	Halog
		Halcion	triazolam
		Haldol	haloperidol
guaifenesin; dextromethor-phan	Robitussin-DM	Halfan	halofantrine HCl
		halofantrine HCl	Halfan
guanabenz acetate	Wytensin	Halog	halcinonide
		haloperidol	Haldol
guanadrel sulfate	Hylorel	haloprogin	Halotex
guanethidine monosulfate	Ismelin	Halotestin	fluoxymesterone
		Halotex	haloprogin
guanethidine monosulfate; hydrochlorothi-azide	Esimil	halothane	Fluothane
		Havrix	hepatitis A vaccine, inactivated

G Rx

385

R

Healon	sodium hyaluronate
Hectorol	doxercalciferol
Helidac	bismuth subsalicylate; metronidazole; tetracycline HCl
heparin sodium	*heparin sodium*
hepatitis A vaccine, inactivated	Havrix / Vaqta
hepatitis B immune globulin (human)	NABI-HB
hepatitis B vaccine	Engerix-B / Recombivax HB
Herceptin	trastuzumab
Herplex	idoxuridine
Hespan	hetastarch
hetastarch	Hespan
hetastarch in lactated electrolyte inj	Hextend
Hetrazan	diethylcarbamazine citrate
Hexadrol	dexamethasone
Hexalen	altretamine
Hextend	hetastarch in lactated electrolyte inj
Hib-Immune	haemophilus b vaccine
Hibiclens	chlorhexidine gluconate
HibTITER	haemophilus b vaccine
Hiprex	methenamine hippurate
Hismanal (W)	astemizole (W)
Hivid	zalcitabine
homatropine hydrobromide ophth	Isopto Homatropine
Humalog	insulin, lispro (human)
Humalog Mix75/25	insulin lispro protamine susp 75%; insulin lispro inj 25% [rDNA origin]
Humatin	paromomycin sulfate
Humatrope	somatropin
Humorsol	demecarium bromide
Humulin 70/30	isophane insulin suspension 70%, insulin inj 30% (human)
Humulin L	insulin zinc suspension (Lente) (human)
Humulin N	isophane insulin suspension (NPH) (human)
Humulin R	insulin inj (human)
Humulin U Ultralente	insulin zinc suspension, extended, (human)
Hurricane	benzocaine
Hyalgan	sodium hyaluronate
hyaluronidase	Wydase
Hycamtin	topotecan HCl
Hydergine	ergoloid mesylates
hydralazine HCl	Apresoline
hydralazine HCl; hydrochlorothiazide	Apresazide
hydralazine; hydrochlorothiazide; reserpine	Ser-Ap-Es
Hydrea	hydroxyurea
hydrochlorothiazide	Esidrix / HydroDIURIL / Microzide / Oretic

hydrocodone bitartrate; acetaminophen	Anexsia 5/500 Anexsia 7.5/650 Lorcet 10/650 Lorcet-HD (5/500) Lorcet plus (7.5/650) Lortab 2.5/500; 5/500; 7.5/500; 10/500 Norco Vicodin Vicodin ES Zydone 5/400, 7.5/400, 10/400	Hygroton hylan G-F 20 Hylorel hyoscyamine sulfate SR Hyperab Hyperstat Hyper-Tet Hytrin Hyzaar	chlorthalidone Synvisc guanadrel sulfate Cystospaz-M Levbid rabies immune globulin, human diazoxide tetanus immune globulin (human) terazosin HCl losartan potassium; hydrochlorothi- azide
hydrocodone bitartrate 7.5 mg; ibuprofen 200 mg	Vicoprofen		

hydrocodone polistirex; chlorphenira- mine	Tussionex	**I-J**	
hydrocortisone hydrocortisone buteprate cream	Cortef Hydrocortone Pandel	*ibuprofen* ibutilide fumarate	Advil Motrin Nuprin Corvert
hydrocortisone sodium succinate	Solu-Cortef	Idamycin idarubicin idoxuridine	idarubicin Idamycin Herplex
Hydrocortone HydroDIURIL	hydrocortisone hydrochlorothia- zide	IFEX ifosfamide Ilosone	ifosfamide IFEX erythromycin estolate
hydroflumethia- zide	Saluron	Imagent GI imciromab pentetate	perflubron Myoscint
hydromorphone HCl hydromorphone HCl SR	Dilaudid Palladone XL	Imdur	isosorbide mononitrate SR
Hydromox hydroxychloro- quine sulfate	quinethazone Plaquenil	imiglucerase imipenem- cilastatin sodium	Cerezyme Primaxin
hydroxyurea hydroxyzine HCl	Droxia Hydrea Atarax	imipramine HCl imiquimod cream	Tofranil Aldara
hydroxyzine pamoate	Vistaril		

Imitrex	sumatriptan	insulin zinc	Humulin L
immune globulin	Gamimune N	suspension	Novolin L
intravenous	Gammagard S/D	(Lente)	
	Gammar-P IV	(human)	
	Sandoglobulin	insulin zinc	Ultralente U
Imodium	loperamide HCl	suspension,	
Imogam	rabies immune	extended	
	globulin,	(beef)	
	human	insulin zinc	Humulin U
Imuran	azathioprine	suspension,	Ultralente
inamrinone	Inocor	extended,	
Inapsine	droperidol	(human)	
indapamide	Lozol	Integrilin	eptifibatide
Inderal	propranolol HCl	interferon alfa-2a	Roferon-A
Inderide	propranolol HCl;	interferon alfa-2b	Intron A
	hydrochlorothi-	interferon alfa-n[1]	Wellferon
	azide	lymphoblastoid	
indinavir	Crixivan	interferon	Infergen
indium In-111	OctreoScan	alfacon-1	
pentetreotide		interferon beta-la	Avonex
Indocin	indomethacin	interferon beta-	Betaseron
indomethacin	Indocin	1b	
Infasurf	calfactant	interferon gamma	Actimmune
	intratracheal	1-b	
	susp	Intrachol	choline chloride
INFeD	iron dextran inj		inj
Infergen	interferon	Intralipid	fat emulsion
	alfacon-1	Intron A	interferon alfa-2b
infliximab	Remicade	Intropin	dopamine HCl
Innohep	tinzaparin sodium	Inversine	mecamylamine
Innovar	fentanyl citrate;		HCl
	droperidol	Invirase	saquinavir
Inocor	inamrinone		mesylate
INOmax	nitric oxide for	iocetamic acid	Cholebrine
	inhalation	iodamide	Renovue 65
insulin aspart	NovoLog	meglumine	
(rDNA origin)		iodixanol	Visipaque
insulin glargine	Lantus	iohexol	Omnipaque
(rDNA origin)		Ionamin	phentermine
insulin inj	Humulin R		resin
(human)	Novolin R	iopamidol	Isovue
	Velosulin Human	iopanoic acid	Telepaque
insulin lispro	Humalog	iopromide	Ultravist
(human)		iotrolan	Osmovist
insulin lispro	Humalog	ioversol	Optiray
protamine susp	Mix75/25	ioxilan	Oxilan
75%; insulin		Ipol	poliovirus
lispro inj 25%			vaccine
[rDNA origin]			inactivated

ipratropium bromide	Atrovent	isosorbide dinitrate	Isordil
ipratropium bromide; albuterol sulfate	Combivent	isosorbide mononitrate	ISMO
irbesartan	Avapro	isosorbide mononitrate SR	Imdur
irbesartan; hydrochlorothi-azide	Avalide	isotretinoin	Accutane
irinotecan HCl	Camptosar	Isovue	iopamidol
iron dextran inj	INFeD Dexferrum	isoxsuprine HCl	Vasodilan
		isradipine	DynaCirc
Ismelin	guanethidine monosulfate	Isuprel	isoproterenol HCl
ISMO	isosorbide mononitrate	itraconazole	Sporanox
		ivermectin	Stromectol
isocarboxazid	Marplan	IvyBlock	bentoquatam
isoetharine HCl aerosol	Bronkometer		
isoetharine HCl soln	Bronkosol		

K

isoflurane	Forane		
isoflurophate	Floropry l	Kadian	morphine sulfate SR
isoniazid	Nydrazid	kanamycin sulfate	Kantrex
isoniazid; rifampin	Rifamate	Kantrex	kanamycin sulfate
isophane insulin suspension (NPH) (human)	Humulin N Novolin N	Kaon	potassium gluconate
isophane insulin suspension (NPH) 70%, insulin inj 30% (human)	Humulin 70/30 Novolin 70/30	Kaon-Cl	potassium chloride SR
		Kayexalate	polystyrene sulfonate sodium
isoproterenol HCl	Isuprel	K-Dur	potassium chloride SR
Isoptin	verapamil HCl	Keflex	cephalexin
Isopto Carbachol	carbachol ophth	Keflin (W)	cephalothin sodium (W)
Isopto Carpine	pilocarpine HCl ophth	Keftab	cephalexin HCl
Isopto Homatropine	homatropine hydrobromide ophth	Kefurox	cefuroxime sodium
		Kefzol	cefazolin sodium
		Kemadrin	procyclidine HCl
Isopto Hyoscine	scopolamine hydrobromide ophth	Kenalog	triamcinolone acetonide
		Keppra	levetiracetam
Isordil	isosorbide dinitrate	Kerlone	betaxolol

Ketalar	ketamine HCl	Lac-Hydrin	lactic acid; ammonium lactate lotion
ketamine HCl	Ketalar		
ketoconazole	Nizoral	lactic acid; ammonium lactate lotion	Lac-Hydrin
ketoprofen	Orudis		
ketoprofen SR	Oruvail		
ketorolac tromethamine	Toradol	lactulose	Cephulac Chronulac
ketorolac tromethamine ophth	Acular	Lamictal	lamotrigine
		Lamisil	terbinafine HCl
ketotifen fumarate ophth soln	Zaditor	lamivudine	Epivir Epivir HBV
		lamivudine; zidovudine	Combivir
Klaron	sodium sulfacetamide lotion	lamotrigine	Lamictal
		Lanoxicaps	digoxin capsules
Klonopin	clonazepam	Lanoxin	digoxin
Klor-Con 10	potassium chloride SR	lansoprazole	Prevacid
K-Lyte	potassium bicarbonate; potassium citrate effervescent	lansoprazole; amoxicillin; clarithromycin	Prevpac
		Lantus	insulin glargine (rDNA origin)
K-Lyte/Cl	potassium chloride potassium bicarbonate effervescent	Lariam	mefloquine HCl
		Larodopa	levodopa
		Lasix	furosemide
		latanoprost	Xalatan
		leflunomide	Arava
		lepirudin	Refludan
Kogenate	antihemophilic factor (recombinant), formulated with sucrose	Lescol	fluvastatin sodium
		letrozole	Femara
		leucovorin calcium	Wellcovorin
Kolyum	potassium chloride; potassium gluconate	Leukeran	chlorambucil
		Leukine	sargramostim
		leuprolide acetate	Lupron
Konsyl-D	psyllium	leuprolide acetate implant	Viadur
Kwell (WA)	lindane		
Kytril	granisetron HCl	Leustatin	cladribine
		levalbuterol HCl inhalation soln	Xopenex
L		levamisole HCl	Ergamisol
		Levaquin	levofloxacin
		Levbid	hyoscyamine sulfate SR
labetalol HCl	Normodyne Trandate	levetiracetam	Keppra

Levlite	levonorgestrel; ethinyl estradiol	Librax	clidinium; chlordiaz-epoxide
levobupivacaine	Chirocaine	Librium	chlordiazepoxide HCl
levocabastine HCl ophth susp	Livostin		
		Lidex	fluocinonide
Levo-Dromoran	levorphanol tartrate	lidocaine HCl	Xylocaine HCl
		lidocaine patch	Lidoderm
levobunolol HCl	Betagan	lidocaine; prilocaine cream	EMLA Cream
levocarnitine	Carnitor		
levodopa	Dopar Larodopa	Lidoderm	lidocaine patch
		Limbitrol	chlordiazepoxide HCl; amitrip-tyline HCl
levodopa; carbidopa	Sinemet		
levodopa; carbidopa SR	Sinemet CR	Lincocin	lincomycin HCl
		lincomycin HCl	Lincocin
		lindane	Kwell (WA) lindane
levofloxacin	Levaquin	linezolid	Zyvox
levofloxacin ophth soln	Quixin	Lioresal	baclofen
		liothyronine sodium	Cytomel
levomethadyl acetate HCl	Orlaam		
		liothyronine sodium inj	Triostat
levonorgestrel	Plan B		
levonorgestrel implant	Norplant	liotrix	Thyrolar
		Lipitor	atorvastatin calcium
levonorgestrel; ethinyl estradiol	Alesse Levlite Nordette Preven Emergency Contraceptive Kit Tri-Levlen Triphasil		
		liposomal amphotericin B	AmBisome
		Liposyn II and III	fat emulsion
		lisinopril	Prinivil Zestril
Levophed	norepinephrine bitartrate	lisinopril; hydrochloro-thiazide	Zestoretic
levorphanol tartrate	Levo-Dromoran	*lithium carbonate*	Eskalith Lithobid
levothyroxine sodium	Levoxyl Synthroid	lithium citrate	Cibalith-S
		Lithobid	lithium carbonate
Levoxyl	levothyroxine sodium	Lithostat	acetohydroxamic acid
Levulan Kerastick	aminolevulinic acid HCl topical soln	Livostin	levocabastine HCl ophth susp
Lexxel	enalapril maleate; felodipine SR	Lodine	etodolac
		Lodine XL	etodolac SR

Iodoxamide tromethamine ophth soln	Alomide	Lotrel	amlodipine besylate; benazepril HCl
Loestrin	norethindrone acetate; ethinyl estradiol	Lotrimin	clotrimazole
		Lotrisone	betamethasone; clotrimazole cream
lomefloxacin	Maxaquin	Lotronex (W)	alosetron (W)
Lomotil	diphenoxylate HCl; atropine sulfate	lovastatin	Mevacor
		Lovenox	enoxaparin sodium
lomustine	CeeNu	loxapine succinate	Loxitane
Loniten	minoxidil tablets		
Lo/Ovral	norgestrel; ethinyl estradiol	Loxitane	loxapine succinate
		Lozol	indapamide
loperamide HCl	Imodium	Ludiomil	maprotiline HCl
Lopid	gemfibrozil	Lufyllin	dyphylline
Lopressor	metoprolol tartrate	LumenHance	manganese chloride
Loprox	ciclopirox cream and lotion	Lunelle	medroxy-progesterone acetate; estradiol cypionate inj
Lorabid	loracarbef		
loracarbef	Lorabid		
loratadine	Claritin	Lupron	leuprolide acetate
loratadine; pseudoephedrine sulfate	Claritin D	Luride	sodium fluoride
		Luvox	fluvoxamine maleate
lorazepam	Ativan	Luxiq	betamethasone valerate (foam)
Lorcet (various combinations)	hydrocodone bitartrate; acetaminophen	Lyme disease vaccine	LYMErix
Lortab (various combinations)	hydrocodone bitartrate; acetaminophen	LYMErix	Lyme disease vaccine
losartan potassium	Cozaar	lymphocyte immune globulin	Atgam
losartan potassium; hydrochlorothiazide	Hyzaar	lypressin	Diapid
		Lysodren	mitotane
Lotemax	loteprednol etabonate ophth susp		

M

Lotensin	benazepril HCl	Maalox	aluminum hydroxide; magnesium hydroxide
loteprednol etabonate ophth susp	Alrex Lotemax		

Macrobid	nitrofurantoin macrocrystals and mono-hydrate
Macrodantin	nitrofurantoin macrocrystals
magaldrate	Riopan
manganese chloride	LumenHance
magnesium chloride SR	Slow-Mag
magnesium sulfate	magnesium sulfate
Malarone	atovaquone; proguanil HCl
Mandol	cefamandole nafate
mangofodipir trisodium	Teslascan
maprotiline HCl	Ludiomil
Marcaine HCl	bupivacaine HCl
Marinol	dronabinol
Marplan	isocarboxazid
Matulane	procarbazine HCl
Mavik	trandolapril
Maxalt	rizatriptan benzoate
Maxalt-MLT	rizatriptan oral disintegrating tablet
Maxaquin	lomefloxacin
Maxipime	cefepime HCl
Maxzide	triamterene 75 mg; hydrochlorothiazide 50 mg
Maxzide-25MG	triamterene 37.5 mg; hydrochlorothiazide 25 mg
mazindol	Sanorex
measles, mumps, rubella vaccines, combined	M-M-R II
Mebaral	mephobarbital
mebendazole	Vermox
mecamylamine HCl	Inversine
mechlorethamine HCl	Mustargen
Meclan	meclocycline sulfosalicylate
meclizine	Antivert
meclocycline sulfosalicylate	Meclan
meclofenamate sodium	Meclomen
Meclomen	meclofenamate sodium
Medrol	methylprednisolone
medroxyprogesterone acetate	Cycrin Provera
medroxyprogesterone acetate; estradiol cypionate inj	Lunelle
medroxyprogesterone acetate SR	Depo-Provera
mefenamic acid	Ponstel
mefloquine HCl	Lariam
Mefoxin	cefoxitin sodium
Megace	megestrol acetate
megestrol acetate	Megace
Mellaril	thioridazine HCl
meloxicam	Mobic
melphalan	Alkeran
menadiol sodium diphosphate	Synkayvite
menotropins	Pergonal Repronex
Mentax	butenafine HCl
meperidine HCl	Demerol
mephentermine sulfate	Wyamine
mephenytoin	Mesantoin
mephobarbital	Mebaral
mepivacaine HCl	Carbocaine
meprobamate	Equanil Miltown
Mepron	atovaquone
mercaptopurine	Purinethol

M
Rx

Meridia	sibutramine HCl monohydrate
meropenem	Merrem
Merrem	meropenem
Meruvax II	rubella virus vaccine live attenuated
mesalamine	Asacol
	Rowasa
Mesantoin	mephenytoin
mesna	Mesnex
Mesnex	mesna
mesoridazine	Serentil
Mestinon	pyridostigmine bromide
Metadate ER	methylphenidate HCl SR
Metamucil	psyllium
Metaprel	metaproterenol sulfate
metaproterenol sulfate	Alupent
	Metaprel
metaraminol bitartrate	Aramine
Metaret	suramin
Metastron	strontium-89 chloride inj
metformin HCl	Glucophage
methadone HCl	Dolophine
methamphetamine HCl	Desoxyn
methazolamide	Neptazane
methenamine combination	Urised
methenamine hippurate	Hiprex
Methergine	methylergonovine maleate
methicillin sodium (W)	Staphcillin (W)
methimazole	Tapazole
methocarbamol	Robaxin
methohexital sodium	Brevital Sodium
methotrexate	Mexate
methotrexate, preservative-free inj	Folex PFS
methotrexate sodium tablets	Rheumatrex
methoxamine HCl	Vasoxyl
methoxsalen	Oxsoralen
methoxsalen extracorporeal administration	Uvadex
methscopolamine bromide	Pamine
methyclothiazide	Enduron
methyldopa	Aldomet
methyldopa; hydrochlorothiazide	Aldoril
methylergonovine maleate	Methergine
Methylin	methylphenidate HCl
Methylin ER	methylphenidate HCl SR
methylphenidate HCl	Methylin
	Ritalin
methylphenidate SR	Concerta
	Metadate ER
	Methylin ER
	Ritalin SR
methylprednisolone	Medrol
methylprednisolone acetate SR inj	Depo-Medrol
methylprednisolone sodium succinate inj	Solu-Medrol
methyltestosterone	Oreton Methyl
methysergide maleate	Sansert
Meticorten	prednisone
metoclopramide HCl	Reglan
metolazone	Diulo
	Zaroxolyn
Metopirone	metyrapone
metoprolol succinate SR	Toprol XL
metoprolol tartrate	Lopressor

MetroGel-Vaginal	metronidazole vaginal gel	Mirapex	pramipexole dihydrochloride
metronidazole	Flagyl	Mircette	desogestrel; ethinyl estradiol and ethinyl estradiol
metronidazole SR	Flagyl ER		
metronidazole vaginal gel	MetroGel-Vaginal		
metyrapone	Metopirone		
metyrosine	Demser	mirtazapine	Remeron
Mevacor	lovastatin	misoprostol	Cytotec
Mexate	methotrexate	Mithracin	plicamycin
mexiletine HCl	Mexitil	mitomycin	Mutamycin
Mexitil	mexiletine HCl	mitotane	Lysodren
Mezlin	mezlocillin	mitoxantrone HCl	Novantrone
mezlocillin	Mezlin		
Miacalcin	calcitonin-salmon	Mivacron	mivacurium chloride
mibefradil dihydrochloride (W)	Posicor (W)	mivacurium chloride	Mivacron
Micardis	telmisartan	M-M-R II	measles, mumps, rubella vaccines, combined
Micro K	potassium chloride SR		
miconazole nitrate	Monistat	Moban	molindone HCl
Micronase	glyburide	Mobic	meloxicam
Micronor	norethindrone	modafinil	Provigil
Microzide	hydrochlorothiazide	Moduretic	amiloride HCl; hydrochlorothiazide
Midamor	amiloride HCl		
midazolam HCl	Versed	moexipril HCl	Univasc
midodrine HCl	ProAmatine	moexipril HCl; hydrochlorothiazide	Uniretic
Mifeprex	mifepristone		
mifepristone	Mifeprex	molindone HCl	Moban
miglitol	Glyset	mometasone furoate topical	Elocon
Migranol	dihydroergotamine mesylate nasal spray	Mometasone furoate monohydrate nasal spray	Nasonex
milrinone lactate	Primacor		
Miltown	meprobamate		
Minipress	prazosin HCl		
Minocin	minocycline HCl	Monistat	miconazole nitrate
minocycline HCl	Minocin		
minoxidil tablets	Loniten	Monocid	cefonicid sodium
minoxidil topical	Rogaine	Monopril	fosinopril sodium
Mintezol	thiabendazole		
Miochol E	acetylcholine ophth	montelukast sodium	Singulair
MiraLax	polyethylene glycol 3350 powder	Monurol	fosfomycin tromethamine

moricizine	Ethmozine	Mylotarg	gemtuzumab ozogamicin
morphine sulfate	Roxanol	Myochrysine (WA)	gold sodium thiomalate
morphine sulfate, immediate release concentrated oral soln	Roxanol-T	Myoscint	imciromab pentetate
morphine sulfate inj	Duramorph	Mysoline	primidone
morphine sulfate SR	Kadian MS Contin Oramorph SR Roxanol SR		

N

Motrin	ibuprofen	NABI-HB	hepatitis B immune globulin (human)
moxifloxacin HCl	Avelox		
MS Contin	morphine sulfate SR	nabumetone	Relafen
Mucomyst	acetylcysteine	nadolol	Corgard
multivitamins for infusion	Cernevit-12	Nafcil (W)	nafcillin sodium
mupirocin nasal ointment	Bactroban	nafcillin sodium	Nafcil (W) Unipen
muromonab-CD3	Orthoclone OKT3	nalbuphine HCl	Nubain
Muse	alprostadil urethral suppository	Nalfon	fenoprofen calcium
Mustargen	mechlorethamine HCl	nalidixic acid	NegGram
		nalmefene HCl	Revex
Mutamycin	mitomycin	naloxone HCl	Narcan
M.V.I.-12	vitamin, multiple inj	naltrexone	ReVia
		nandrolone phenpropionate	Durabolin
Myambutol	ethambutol HCl		
Mycelex	clotrimazole	nandrolone decanoate	Deca-Durabolin
Mycifradin Sulfate	neomycin sulfate oral soln	naphazoline ophth soln	Vasocon
Myciguent	neomycin sulfate ointment and cream	Naprelan	naproxen sodium SR
		Naprosyn	naproxen
Mycolog Cream	nystatin; triamcinolone cream	naproxen	Naprosyn
		naproxen sodium	Anaprox
		naproxen sodium SR	Naprelan
mycophenolate mofetil	CellCept	naratriptan HCl	Amerge
		Narcan	naloxone HCl
Mycostatin	nystatin	Nardil	phenelzine sulfate
Mydriacyl	tropicamide	Naropin	ropivacaine HCl
Myleran	busulfan	Nasacort	triamcinolone acetonide nasal inhaler
Mylicon	simethicone		

N
R

nisoldipine SR	Sular	norepinephrine bitartrate	Levophed
Nitrek	nitroglycerin transdermal	norethindrone	Micronor
nitric oxide for inhalation	INOmax	norethindrone acetate; ethinyl estradiol	Estrostep Loestrin
Nitro-Bid	nitroglycerin SR		
Nitro-Dur	nitroglycerin transdermal	norethindrone; ethinyl estradiol (or mestranol)	Activella Femhrt Genora Ortho-Novum (products)
nitrofurantoin macrocrystals	Macrodantin		
nitrofurantoin macrocrystals and monohydrate	Macrobid	norethindrone acetate; estradiol transdermal	CombiPatch
nitrofurazone	Furacin		
nitroglycerin transdermal	Transderm-Nitro	Norflex	orphenadrine citrate
nitroglycerin inj	Tridil	norfloxacin	Noroxin
nitroglycerin ointment	Nitrol	Norgesic	orphenadrine citrate; aspirin; caffeine
nitroglycerin SR	Nitro-Bid		
nitroglycerin sublingual tablets	Nitrostat	norgestimate; ethinyl estradiol	Ortho Tri-Cyclen
nitroglycerin transdermal	Nitrek Nitro-Dur	norgestrel; ethinyl estradiol	Lo/Ovral Ovral
Nitrol	nitroglycerin ointment	Normiflo	ardeparin sodium
		Normodyne	labetalol HCl
nitroprusside sodium	Nipride	Noroxin	norfloxacin
		Norpace	disopyramide phosphate
Nitrostat	nitroglycerin sublingual tablets	Norplant	levonorgestrel implant
Nix	permethrin	Norpramin	desipramine HCl
nizatidine	Axid	nortriptyline HCl	Aventyl Pamelor
Nizoral	ketoconazole		
nofetumomab	Verluna	Norvasc	amlodipine besylate
Nolvadex	tamoxifen citrate		
Norco	hydrocodone bitartrate; acetaminophen	Norvir	ritonavir
		Novantrone	mitoxantrone HCl
Norcuron	vecuronium bromide	Novocain HCl	procaine HCl
		Novolin 70/30	isophane insulin suspension (NPH) 70%, insulin inj 30% (human)
Nordette	levonorgestrel; ethinyl estradiol		
Norditropin	somatropin inj		

Novolin L	insulin zinc suspension (Lente) (human)	olanzapine	Zyprexa
Novolin N	isophane insulin suspension (NPH) (human)	olopatadine HCl ophth soln	Patanol
		olsalazine sodium	Dipentum
Novolin R	insulin inj (human)	Olux	clobetasol foam
NovoLog	insulin aspart (rDNA origin)	omeprazole	Prilosec
		Omnicef	cefdinir
NovoSeven	coagulation factor VII a (recombinant)	Omnipaque	iohexol
		Oncaspar	pegaspargase
Nubain	nalbuphine HCl	OncoScint	satumomab pendetide
Numorphan	oxymorphone HCl	Oncovin	vincristine sulfate
Nupercainal	dibucaine	ondansetron	Zofran
Nuromax	doxacurium chloride	ondansetron orally disintegrating tab	Zofran ODT
Nuprin	ibuprofen		
Nutropin	somatropin for inj	Ontak	denileukin diftitox
Nutropin AQ	somatropin inj	Ophthaine (WA)	proparacaine
Nydrazid	isoniazid	Ophthalgan	glycerin ophth soln
nystatin	Mycostatin		
nystatin topical powder	Nystop	Ophthetic	proparacaine HCl
nystatin; triamcinolone cream	Mycolog Cream	opium; belladonna suppositories	B & O Supprettes
Nystop	nystatin topical powder	oprelvekin	Neumega
		Opticrom	cromolyn sodium
		OptiMark	gadoversetamide
		Optimine	azatadine maleate

O

		Optiray	ioversol
		Optivar	azelastine HCl ophth soln
OctreoScan	indium In-111 pentetreotide	Orabase	benzocaine
octreotide acetate	Sandostatin	Orajel	benzocaine
octreotide acetate susp for inj	Sandostatin LAR Depot	Oramorph SR	morphine sulfate SR
ofloxacin	Floxin	Orap	pimozide
ofloxacin otic soln	Floxin Otic	Oretic	hydrochlorothiazide
Ogen	estropipate	Oreton Methyl	methyltestosterone
		Organidin NR	guaifenesin
		Organan	danaparoid sodium

N
Rx

Orinase	tolbutamide	Oxilan	ioxilan
Orlaam	levomethadyl acetate HCl	Oxistat	oxiconazole nitrate cream
orlistat	Xenical	Oxsoralen	methoxsalen
Ornade Spansules	phenylpropanol- amine HCl; chlorphenir- amine maleate SR	oxtriphylline	Choledyl
		oxybutynin chloride	Ditropan
orphenadrine citrate	Norflex	oxychlorosene sodium	Clorpactin WCS-90
orphenadrine citrate; aspirin; caffeine	Norgesic	oxycodone HCl	Percolone Roxicodone
		oxycodone HCl SR	OxyContin
Ortho-Cept	desogestrel; ethinyl estradiol	oxycodone HCl; acetaminophen	Percocet 5/325; 7.5/500; 10/650 Endocet Roxicet
Orthoclone OKT3	muromonab-CD3		
Ortho-Novum (products)	norethindrone; ethinyl estradiol (or mestranol)	oxycodone HCl; aspirin	Percodan
		OxyContin	oxycodone HCl SR
Ortho-Prefest	17β-estradiol; norgestimate	oxymetazoline HCl	Afrin nasal spray Dristan Long Lasting
Ortho Tri-Cyclen	norgestimate; ethinyl estradiol (combinations)	oxymetholone	Anadrol-50
		oxymorphone HCl	Numorphan
Orudis	ketoprofen	oxytocin	Pitocin
Oruvail	ketoprofen SR		
Os-Cal 500	calcium carbonate		
oseltamivir phosphate	Tamiflu		**P**
Osmovist	iotrolan		
Otrivin	xylometazoline	Pacis	BCG intravesical
Ovidrel	choriogonado- tropin alfa	paclitaxel	Taxol
		palivizumab	Synagis
Ovral	norgestrel; ethinyl estradiol	Palladone XL	hydromorphone HCl SR
		Pamelor	nortriptyline HCl
Oxandrin	oxandrolone	pamidronate disodium	Aredia
oxandrolone	Oxandrin	Pamine	methscopolamine bromide
oxaprozin	Daypro		
oxazepam	Serax	Pancrease	pancrelipase EC
oxcarbazepine	Trileptal	pancrelipase	Cotazym
oxiconazole nitrate cream	Oxistat	pancrelipase EC	Cotazym-S Pancrease

pancuronium bromide	Pavulon	PedvaxHIB	haemophilus b vaccine
Pandel	hydrocortisone buteprate cream	pegaspargase	Oncaspar
Panretin	alitretinoin	pemirolast potassium ophth soln	Alamast
pantoprazole	Protonix		
papain; urea oint	Accuzyme Ethezyme	pemoline	Cylert
		penicillamine	Cuprimine
papaverine HCl SR	Pavabid	penciclovir cream	Denavir
paracetamol	acetaminophen	penicillin G benzathine	Bicillin L-A (for IM use only) Permapen (for IM use only)
Paradione	paramethadione		
Paraflex	chlorzoxazone 250 mg		
Parafon Forte DSC	chlorzoxazone 500 mg	penicillin G benzathine; penicillin G procaine	Bicillin C-R (for IM use only)
paramethadione	Paradione		
Paraplatin	carboplatin		
Parathar	teriparatide acetate	penicillin G procaine	Wycillin (for IM use only)
paregoric	camphorated tincture of opium	*penicillin V potassium*	Pen Vee K
		Penlac Nail Lacquer	ciclopirox soln
pargyline HCl	Eutonyl		
paricalcitol	Zemplar	pentaerythritol tetranitrate	Peritrate
Parlodel	bromocriptine mesylate	pentagastrin	Peptavlon
Parnate	tranylcypromine sulfate	Pentam 300	pentamidine isethionate inj
paromomycin sulfate	Humatin	pentamidine isethionate aerosol	NebuPent
paroxetine HCl	Paxil		
Parsidol	ethopropazine HCl	pentamidine isethionate inj	Pentam 300
Patanol	olopatadine HCl ophth soln		
Pavabid	papaverine HCl SR	Pentaspan	pentastarch
		pentastarch	Pentaspan
Pavulon	pancuronium bromide	pentazocine HCl	Talwin
		pentazocine HCl; naloxone HCl	Talwin Nx
Paxil	paroxetine HCl		
PBZ	tripelennamine HCl	pentobarbital sodium	Nembutal
PCE Dispertab	erythromycin base coated particles	pentosan polysulfate sodium	Elmiron
		pentostatin inj	Nipent
Pediazole	erythromycin ethylsuccinate; sulfisoxazole	Pentothal	thiopental sodium

pentoxifylline	Trental
Pen Vee K	penicillin V potassium
Pepcid	famotidine
Pepcid RPD	famotidine, oral disintegrating tablet
Peptavlon	pentagastrin
Percocet 5/325; 7.5/500; 10/650	oxycodone HCl; acetaminophen
Percodan	oxycodone HCl; aspirin
Percolone	oxycodone HCl
perflenapent emulsion	EchoGen
perflubron	Imagent GI
Pergonal	menotropins
Periactin	cyproheptadine HCl
Peri-Colace	docusate sodium; casanthranol
Peridex	chlorhexidine gluconate mouth rinse
perindopril erbumine	Aceon
PerioChip	chlorhexidine gluconate
Peritrate	pentaerythritol tetranitrate
Permapen	penicillin G benzathine (for IM use only)
permethrin	Nix
Permitil	fluphenazine HCl
perphenazine	Trilafon
perphenazine; amitriptyline HCl	Etrafon Triavil
Persantine	dipyridamole
petrolatum, white	Vaseline
Phenaphen with Codeine (#2, 3, and 4)	acetaminophen 300 mg with Codeine Phosphate (15, 30, and 60 mg)
phenazopyridine HCl	Pyridium
phendimetrazine tartrate	Plegine
phenelzine sulfate	Nardil
Phenergan	promethazine HCl
phenobarbital	phenobarbital
phenobarbital, ergotamine; belladonna	Bellergal-S
phenoxybenza-mine HCl	Dibenzyline
phentermine HCl	Fastin
phentermine resin	Ionamin
phentolamine mesylate	Regitine
phenylbutyrate sodium	Buphenyl
phenylephrine HCl	Neo-Synephrine
phenylpropanol-amine HCl; chlorphenir-amine maleate SR	Ornade
phenylpropanol-amine HCl; guaifenesin SR	Entex LA
phenytoin	Dilantin
Phospholine Iodide	echothiophate iodide
Photofrin	porfimer sodium
physostigmine ophth ointment	Eserine Sulfate
physostigmine salicylate	Antilirium
phytonadione	AquaMEPHY-TON
pilocarpine HCl ophth	Isopto Carpine
pilocarpine HCl tablet	Salagen
pimozide	Orap

pindolol	Visken	podofilox gel	Condylox
pioglitazone HCl	Actos	Polaramine	dexchlorphenir-
pipecuronium	Arduan	Repetabs	amine maleate
bromide			SR
piperacillin	Pipracil	poliovirus	Ipol
sodium		vaccine	
piperacillin	Zosyn	inactivated	
sodium;		polyethylene	CoLyte
tazobactam		glycolelectro-	GoLYTELY
sodium		lyte soln	
Pipracil	piperacillin	polyethylene	MiraLax
	sodium	glycol 3350	
piroxicam	Feldene	powder	
Pitocin	oxytocin	polymyxin B	Polytrim
Pitressin	vasopressin	sulfate;	
Placidyl	ethchlorvynol	trimethoprim	
Plan B	levonorgestrel	ophth soln	
Plaquenil	hydroxychloro-	polymyxin;	Neosporin
	quine sulfate	neomycin	Cream
Plasbumin	albumin human		Neosporin ophth
plasma protein	Plasma-Plex		soln
fraction	Plasmanate	polymyxin;	Neosporin
	Plasmatein	neomycin;	Ointment
	Protenate	bacitracin	Neosporin ophth
Plasma-Plex	plasma protein		Ointment
	fraction	polystyrene	Kayexalate
Plasmanate	plasma protein	sulfonate	
	fraction	sodium	
Plasmatein	plasma protein	polythiazide	Renese
	fraction	Polytrim	polymyxin B
Platinol AQ	cisplatin		sulfate;
Plavix	clopidogrel		trimethoprim
	bisulfate		ophth soln
Plegine	phendimetrazine	Pondimin (W)	fenfluramine
	tartrate		HCl (W)
Plendil	felodipine	Ponstel	mefenamic acid
Pletal	cilostazol	Pontocaine	tetracaine HCl
Plexion	sulfacetamide	poractant alpha	Curosurf
	sodium and	intratracheal	
	sulfur lotion	susp	
plicamycin	Mithracin	porfimer	Photofrin
pneumococcal	Pneumovax	sodium	
vaccine		Posicor (W)	mibefradil
pneumococcal	Prevnar		dihydro-
7-valent			chloride (W)
conjugate			
vaccine		potassium	K-Lyte
Pneumovax	pneumococcal	bicarbonate;	
	vaccine	potassium	
		citrate	
		effervescent	

potassium chloride; potassium bicarbonate effervescent	K-Lyte/Cl
potassium chloride SR	Kaon-Cl
	K-Dur
	Klor-Con 10
	Slow-K
	Micro K
potassium chloride; potassium gluconate	Kolyum
potassium citrate tab	Urocit-K
potassium gluconate	Kaon
povidone iodine	Betadine
pralidoxime chloride	Protopam
pramipexole dihydrochloride	Mirapex
pramoxine HCl	Tronothane HCl
Prandin	repaglinide
Pravachol	pravastatin sodium
pravastatin sodium	Pravachol
prazosin HCl	Minipress
Precedex	dexmedetomidine HCl inj
Precose	acarbose
prednisolone syrup	Prelone
prednisone	Deltasone
	Meticorten
Prelone	prednisolone syrup
Premarin	estrogens, conjugated
Premphase	estrogens, conjugated; medroxyprogesterone acetate
Prempro	
Prepidil	dinoprostone gel
Preven Emergency Contraceptive Kit	levonorgestrel; ethinyl estradiol
Prevacid	lansoprazole
Prevnar	pneumococcal 7-valent conjugate vaccine
Preveon	adefovir dipivoxil
Prevpac	lansoprazole; amoxicillin; clarithromycin
Priftin	rifapentine
Prilosec	omeprazole
Primacor	milrinone lactate
Primaxin	imipenemcilastatin sodium
primidone	Mysoline
Primsol	trimethoprim
Principen	ampicillin
Prinivil	lisinopril
Priscoline	tolazoline
ProAmatine	midodrine HCl
Pro-Banthine	propantheline bromide
probenecid	Benemid
probenecid; colchicine	ColBENEMID (W)
procainamide	Pronestyl
procainamide HCl SR	Procan SR
procaine HCl	Novocain HCl
Procan SR	procainamide HCl SR
Procanbid	procainamide HCl SR
procarbazine HCl	Matulane
Procardia	nifedipine
Procardia XL	nifedipine SR
prochlorperazine	Compazine
Procrit	epoetin alfa
procyclidine HCl	Kemadrin
progesterone gel	Crinone
progesterone micronized	Prometrium
Prograf	tacrolimus

ProHance	gadoteridol	Prostep	nicotine transdermal system
ProHIBiT	haemophilus b vaccine		
Prokine (WA)	sargramostim	Prostigmin	neostigmine methylsulfate
Prolastin	alpha$_1$-proteinase inhibitor (human)	Prostin E$_2$	dinoprostone vaginal suppositories
Proleukin	aldesleukin	Prostin VR	alprostadil
Prolixin	fluphenazine HCl	protamine sulfate	protamine sulfate
Proloid (W)	thyroglobulin (W)		
promazine HCl	Sparine	Protenate	plasma protein fraction
promethazine HCl	Phenergan	Protonix	pantoprazole
Prometrium	progesterone micronized	Protopam	pralidoxime chloride
Pronestyl	procainamide	protriptyline HCl	Vivactil
Propacet-100	propoxyphene napsylate; acetaminophen	Protropin	somatrem
		Protropin II	somatropin for inj
propafenone HCl	Rythmol	Proventil	albuterol
propantheline bromide	Pro-Banthine	Proventil HFA	albuterol sulfate inhalation aerosol
proparacaine HCl	Ophthaine (WA) Ophthetic	Proventil Repetabs	albuterol SR
Propecia	finasteride tablets 1 mg	Provera	medroxyproges- terone acetate
Propine	dipivefrin	Provigil	modafinil
propofol	Diprivan	Prozac	fluoxetine HCl
propoxyphene HCl	Darvon	Prudoxin	doxepin HCl cream
propoxyphene HCl; acetaminophen	Wygesic	pseudoephedrine HCl	Sudafed
propoxyphene HCl; aspirin; caffeine	Darvon Compound 65	pseudoephedrine HCl; bromphiramine maleate	Drixoral Syrup
propoxyphene napsylate; acetaminophen	Darvocet-N 100 Propacet-100	psyllium	Konsyl-D Metamucil
propranolol HCl	Inderal	Pulmicort Turbuhaler	budesonide inhalation powder
propranolol HCl; hydrochlorothi- azide	Inderide		
Propulsid (W)	cisapride (W)	Pulmozyme	dornase alfa
Proscar	finasteride tablets 5 mg	Purinethol	mercaptopurine
		Pyridium	phenazopyridine HCl
ProSom	estazolam		
ProstaScint	capromab pendetide	pyridostigmine bromide	Mestinon

pyrimethamine	Daraprim
pyrimethamine; sulfadoxine	Fansidar

Q

Quadramet	samarium SM 153 lexidronam
Quarzan	clidinium bromide
Questran	cholestyramine
quetiapine fumerate	Seroquel
Quinaglute	quinidine gluconate SR
quinapril HCl	Accupril
quinapril; hydrochloro-thiazide	Accuretic
quinethazone	Hydromox
Quinidex Extentabs	quinidine sulfate SR
quinidine gluconate SR	Quinaglute
quinidine sulfate	quinidine sulfate
quinidine sulfate SR	Quinidex Extentabs
quinupristin; dalfopristin	Synercid
Quixin	levofloxacin ophth soln
Qvar	beclomethasone diproprionate inhalation aerosol

R

RabAvert	rabies vaccine for human use
rabeprazole sodium	Aciphex

rabies immune globulin, human	Hyperab Imogam
rabies vaccine, adsorbed	rabies vaccine, adsorbed
rabies vaccine for human use	RabAvert
raloxifene HCl	Evista
ramipril	Altace
ranitidine bismuth citrate	Tritec
ranitidine HCl	Zantac
rapacuronium bromide	Raplon
Rapamune	sirolimus
Raplon	rapacuronium bromide
Raxar (W)	grepafloxacin HCl (W)
Rebetol	ribavirin
Rebetron	ribavirin; interferon alfa-2b
reboxetine mesylate	Vestra
Recombivax HB	hepatitis B vaccine
Redux (W)	dexfenfluramine HCl (W)
Refacto	antihemophilic factor (recombinant)
Refludan	lepirudin
Regitine	phentolamine mesylate
Reglan	metoclopramide HCl
Regranex	becaplermin gel
Regroton	chlorthalidone; reserpine
Relafen	nabumetone
Relenza	zanamivir for inhalation
Remeron	mirtazapine
Remicade	infliximab
remifentanil HCl	Ultiva
Reminyl	galanthamine HBr
Renagel	sevelamer HCl

Renese	polythiazide	ribavirin	Rebetol
Renova	tretinion topical		Virazole
Renovue 65	iodamide meglumine	ribavirin; interferon alfa-2b	Rebetron
ReoPro	abciximab		
repaglinide	Prandin	Ridaura	auranofin
Repronex	menotropins	Rifadin	rifampin
Requip	ropinirole HCl	Rifamate	isoniazid; rifampin
Rescriptor	delavirdine mesylate	rifampin	Rifadin Rimactane
Rescula	unoprostone isopropyl ophth soln	rifapentine	Priftin
		Rilutek	riluzole
reserpine	Serpasil	riluzole	Rilutek
RespiGam	respiratory syncytial virus immune globulin intravenous (human)	Rimactane	rifampin
		rimantadine	Flumadine
		rimexolone	Vexol
		Riopan	magaldrate
		risedronate sodium	Actonel
respiratory syncytial virus immune globulin intravenous (human)	RespiGam	Risperdal	risperidone
		risperidone	Risperdal
		Ritalin	methylphenidate HCl
		Ritalin SR	methylphenidate SR
Restasis	cyclosporine ophth emulsion	ritodrine HCl	Yutopar
		ritonavir	Norvir
Restoril	temazepam	Rituxan	rituximab
Retavase	reteplase	rituximab	Rituxan
reteplase	Retavase	rivastigmine tartrate	Exelon
Retin-A	tretinoin topical		
Retin-A Micro	tretinoin gel	rizatriptan benzoate	Maxalt
Retrovir	zidovudine		
Revex	nalmefene HCl	rizatriptan oral disintegrating tablet	Maxalt-MLT
ReVia	naltrexone		
Rezulin (W)	troglitazone (W)		
R-Gene	arginine HCl	Robaxin	methocarbamol
Rheumatrex	methotrexate sodium tablets	Robinul	glycopyrrolate
		Robitussin	guaifenesin
Rhinocort	budesonide nasal inhaler	Robitussin A-C	guaifenesin; codeine phosphate
RH$_O$ (D) immune globulin	RhoGAM		
		Robitussin-DM	guaifenesin; dextromethorphan
RH$_O$ (D) immune globulin IV (human)	WinRho SD		
		Rocaltrol	calcitriol
RhoGAM	RH$_O$ (D) immune globulin	Rocephin	ceftriaxone sodium

R
R/

407

rofecoxib	Vioxx	salsalate	Disalcid
Roferon-A	interferon alfa-2a	Sal-Tropine	atropine sulfate tablets
Rogaine	minoxidil topical		
Romazicon	flumazenil	Saluron	hydroflume-thiazide
ropinirole HCl	Requip		
ropivacaine HCl	Naropin	samarium SM 153 lexidronam	Quadramet
Rosiglitazone maleate	Avandia		
Rotashield (W)	rotavirus (W) vaccine, live, oral, tetravalent	Sandimmune	cyclosporine
		Sandoglobulin	immune globulin intravenous
rotavirus vaccine, live, oral, (W) tetravalent	Rotashield (W)	Sandostatin	octreotide acetate
		Sandostatin LAR Depot	octreotide acetate susp for inj
		Sanorex	mazindol
Rowasa	mesalamine	Sansert	methysergide maleate
Roxanol	morphine sulfate		
Roxanol SR	morphine sulfate SR	Santyl	collagenase
		saquinavir mesylate	Invirase
Roxanol-T	morphine sulfate, immediate release concentrated oral soln	saquinavir soft gel capsule	Fortovase
		Sarafem	fluoxetine
Roxicet	oxycodone HCl; acetaminophen	sargramostim	Leukine Prokine (WA)
Roxicodone	oxycodone HCl	satumomab pendetide	OncoScint
rubella virus vaccine live attenuated	Meruvax II	Sclerosol	talc, sterile aerosol
Rubex	doxorubicin HCl	scopolamine hydrobromide ophth	Isopto Hyoscine
Rythmol	propafenone HCl		
		scopolamine transdermal	Transderm Scop
		Sectral	acebutolol HCl
S		Seldane (W)	terfenadine (W)
		Seldane D (W)	terfenadine; pseudoephed-rine HCl (W)
sacrosidase	Sucraid		
Saizen	somatropin		
Salagen	pilocarpine HCl tablet	selegiline HCl	Carbex Eldepryl
salbutamol sulfate	albuterol sulfate	selenium sulfide	Selsun Blue
		Selsun Blue	selenium sulfide
salmeterol xinafoate	Serevent	sennosides	Ex Lax
		sennosides	Senokot
salmeterol xinafoate inhalation powder	Serevent Diskus	sennosides; docusate sodium	Senokot-S

Senokot	senna concentrates	simvastatin	Zocor
Senokot-S	sennosides; docusate sodium	Sinemet	levodopa; carbidopa
		Sinemet CR	levodopa; carbidopa SR
Septocaine	articaine; epinephrine	Sinequan	doxepin HCl
Septra	sulfamethox-azoletrimeth-oprim	Singulair	montelukast sodium
		sirolimus	Rapamune
		Skelid	tiludronate disodium
Ser-Ap-Es	hydralazine; hydrochloro-thiazide; reserpine	Slo-bid	theophylline SR
		Slo-Phyllin	theophylline SR
Serax	oxazepam	Slow Fe	ferrous sulfate SR
Serentil	mesoridazine		
Serevent	salmeterol xinafoate	Slow-K	potassium chloride SR
Serevent Diskus	salmeterol xinafoate inhalation powder	Slow-Mag	magnesium chloride SR
sermorelin acetate	Geref	sodium citrate; citric acid	Bicitra
Seromycin	cycloserine	sodium ferric gluconate complex in sucrose inj	Ferrlecit
Serpasil	*reserpine*		
Serlect	sertindole		
Seroquel	quetiapine fumerate	sodium fluoride	Luride
Serostim	somatropin (rDNA origin) for inj	sodium hyaluronate	Amvisc Healon Hyalgan
sertindole	Serlect	sodium phenylbutyrate	Buphenyl
sertraline HCl	Zoloft		
Serzone	nefazodone HCl	sodium phosphate tab	Visicol
sevelamer HCl	Renagel	sodium sulfacetamide lotion	Klaron
sevoflurane	Ultane		
short chain fatty acids enema	Colomed		
		sodium tetradecyl sulfate	Sotradecol
sibutramine HCl monohydrate	Meridia		
sildenafil citrate	Viagra	Solganal	aurothioglucose
Silvadene	silver sulfadiazine	Solu-Cortef	hydrocortisone sodium succinate
silver sulfadiazine	Silvadene		
simethicone	Mylicon	Solu-Medrol	methylpredniso-lone sodium succinate
Simulect	basiliximab		

Soma	carisoprodol	strontium-89	Metastron
somatostatin	Zecnil	chloride inj	
somatrem	Protropin	Sublimaze	fentanyl citrate
somatropin for inj	Genotropin	succinylcholine chloride	Anectine
	Humatrope	Sucraid	sacrosidase
	Norditropin	sucralfate	Carafate
	Nutropin	Sudafed	pseudoephedrine HCl
	Protropin II		
	Saizen	Sufenta	sufentanil citrate
somatropin inj	Nutropin AQ	sufentanil citrate	Sufenta
somatropin (rDNA origin) for inj	Serostim	Sulamyd sodium	sulfacetamide sodium ophth
Sonata	zaleplon	Sular	Nisoldipine SR
Soriatane	acitretin	sulfacetamide sodium and sulfur lotion	Plexion
sotalol	Betapace		
Sotradecol	sodium tetradecyl sulfate	sulfacetamide sodium ophth	Sulamyd sodium
sparfloxacin	Zagam	sulfadoxine; pyrimethamine	Fansidar
Sparine	promazine HCl	sulfamethoxazole	Gantanol
stavudine	Zerit	sulfamethoxazole-trimethoprim	Bactrim
spectinomycin HCl	Trobicin		Cotrim
			co-trimoxazole
spironolactone	Aldactone		Septra
spironolactone; hydrochloroth-iazide	Aldactazide	sulfasalazine	Azulfidine
		sulfinpyrazone	Anturane
		sulindac	Clinoril
Sporanox	itraconazole	Sultrin	triple sulfa vaginal cream
Stadol	butorphanol tartrate inj	sumatriptan	Imitrex
		Sumycin	tetracycline HCl
Stadol NS	butorphanol tartrate nasal spray	Suprane	desflurane
		Suprax	cefixime
		suramin	Metaret
stanozolol	Winstrol	Surfak	docusate calcium
Staphcillin	methicillin sodium	Surmontil	trimipramine maleate
Stelazine	trifluoperazine HCl	Survanta	beractant
		Sustiva	Efavirenz
Stilphostrol	diethylstilbestrol diphosphate	Symmetrel	amantadine HCl
		Synagis	palivizumab
Streptase	streptokinase	Synalar	fluocinolone acetonide
streptokinase	Streptase		
streptomycin sulfate	streptomycin sulfate	Synercid	quinupristin; dalfopristin
streptozocin	Zanosar	Synkayvite	menadiol sodium diphosphate
Stromectol	ivermectin		

S
R⋅

synthetic conjugated estrogens, A	Cenestin	technetium Tc99m sestamibi teboroxime kit	Cardiolite
Synthroid	levothyroxine sodium	Teczem	enalapril maleate; diltiazem malate
Synvisc	hylan G-F 20		
		tegaserod	Zelmac
		Tegretol	carbamazepine
T		Teldrin	chlorpheniramine maleate SR
		Telepaque	iopanoic acid
tacrine HCl	Cognex	telmisartan	Micardis
tacrolimus	Prograf	temazepam	Restoril
Tagamet	cimetidine HCl	Temodar	temozolomide
talc, sterile aerosol	Sclerosol	temozolomide	Temodar
Talwin	pentazocine HCl	tenecteplase	TNKase
Talwin Nx	pentazocine HCl; naloxone HCl	Tenex	guanfacine HCl
		teniposide	Vumon
Tambocor	flecainide acetate	Tenoretic	atenolol; chlorthalidone
Tamiflu	oseltamivir phosphate	Tenormin	atenolol
		Tensilon	edrophonium chloride
tamoxifen citrate	Nolvadex		
tamsulosin HCl	Flomax	Tenuate	diethylpropion HCl
Tapazole	methimazole		
Targretin	bexarotene gel	Tequin	gatifloxacin
Tarka	trandolapril; verapamil SR	Terazol	terconazole
		terazosin HCl	Hytrin
tarzarotene gel	Tazorac	terbinafine HCl	Lamisil
Tasmar	tolcapone	terbutaline sulfate aerosol	Brethaire
tasosartan	Verdia		
Tavist	clemastine fumarate	terbutaline sulfate tablets and inj	Brethine Bricanyl
Taxol	paclitaxel		
Taxotere	docetaxel	terconazole	Terazol
Tazicef	ceftazidime	terfenadine (W)	Seldane (W)
Tazidime	ceftazidime	terfenadine; pseudoephe- drine HCl (W)	Seldane D (W)
Tazorac	tarzarotene gel		
technetium Tc-99m bicisate kit	Neurolite	teriparatide acetate	Parathar
		Teslac	testolactone
technetium Tc-99m red blood cell kit	Ultratag	Teslascan	mangofodipir trisodium
		Testoderm	testosterone transdermal
technetium Tc-99m	Cardiotec	Testoderm TTS	testosterone transdermal

S R

testolactone	Teslac	Thrombate III	antithrombin III
testosterone	DEPO-		(human)
cypionate SR	Testosterone	thymalfasin	Zadaxin
testosterone gel	AndroGel	Thymoglobulin	anti-thymocyte
testosterone	Androderm		globulin,
transdermal	Testoderm		(rabbit)
	Testoderm TTS	thyroglobulin	Proloid (W)
tetanus immune	Hyper-Tet	(W)	
globulin (human)		thyroid	thyroid
tetracaine HCl	Pontocaine	Thyrogen	thyrotropin alpha
tetracycline HCl	Achromycin	Thyrolar	liotrix
	(WA)	thyrotropin	Thytropar
	Sumycin	thyrotropin	Thyrogen
tetrahydrozoline	Collyrium	alpha	
HCl ophth	Visine Extra	Thytropar	thyrotropin
Tetramune	diphtheria and	tiagabine HCl	Gabitril
	tetanus	Tiamate	diltiazem
	toxoids;		maleate SR
	pertussis	Tiazac	diltiazem HCl SR
	vaccine,	Ticar	ticarcillin
	adsorbed and		disodium
	haemophilus b	ticarcillin	Ticar
	conjugate	disodium	
	vaccine	ticarcillin;	Timentin
Teveten	eprosartan	clavulanic acid	
	mesylate	TICE BCG	BCG intravesical
thalidomide	Thalomid	Ticlid	ticlopidine
Thalomid	thalidomide	ticlopidine	Ticlid
Tham	tromethamine	Tigan	trimethobenz-
Theo-Dur	theophylline SR		amide HCl
theophylline	Elixophyllin	Tikosyn	dofetilide
	Slo-Phyllin	Tilade	nedocromil
theophylline SR	Slo-bid		inhalation
	Theo-Dur	tiludronate	Skelid
	Uniphyl	disodium	
TheraCys	BCG intravesical	Timentin	ticarcillin;
Theragran-M	vitamins;		clavulanic acid
	minerals	timolol maleate	Timoptic
thiabendazole	Mintezol	ophth soln	
thiethylperazine	Torecan	timolol maleate	Timoptic-XE
maleate		ophth soln, gel	
thioguanine	thioguanine	forming	
thiopental	Pentothal	timolol maleate	Blocadren
sodium		timolol maleate;	Cosopt
Thioplex	thiotepa	dorzolamide	
thioridazine HCl	Mellaril	HCl	
thiotepa	Thioplex	Timoptic-XE	timolol maleate
thiothixene	Navane		ophth soln, gel
Thorazine	chlorpromazine		forming

T
Rx

Timoptic	timolol maleate ophth soln	topiramate	Topamax
Tinactin	tolnaftate	topotecan HCl	Hycamtin
Tine Test Tuberculin Old	tuberculin, old	Toprol XL	metoprolol succinate SR
Tine Test PPD	tuberculin, purified protein derivative	Toradol	ketorolac tromethamine
		Torecan	thiethylperazine maleate
tinzaparin sodium	Innohep	toremifene citrate	Fareston
TNKase	tenecteplase	Tornalate	bitolterol mesylate
tioconazole	Vagistat-1		
tirofiban HCl	Aggrastat	torsemide	Demadex
tizanidine HCl	Zanaflex	Totacillin-N	ampicillin sodium
TOBI	tobramycin soln for inhalation	Tracrium	atracurium besylate
TobraDex	tobramycin; dexamethasone oint and susp	tramadol HCl	Ultram
		Trandate	labetalol HCl
tobramycin sulfate	Nebcin	trandolapril	Mavik
tobramycin sulfate ophth	Tobrex	trandolapril; verapamil SR	Tarka
tobramycin; dexamethasone oint and susp	TobraDex	Transderm Scop	scopolamine transdermal
		Transderm-Nitro	nitroglycerin transdermal
tobramycin soln for inhalation	TOBI	Tranxene	clorazepate dipotassium
Tobrex	tobramycin sulfate ophth	tranylcypromine sulfate	Parnate
tocainide HCl	Tonocard	trastuzumab	Herceptin
Tofranil	imipramine HCl	Trasylol	aprotinin
		Travasol	amino acid inj
tolazamide	Tolinase	trazodone HCl	Desyrel
tolazoline	Priscoline	Trecator-SC	ethionamide
tolbutamide	Orinase	Trelstar Depot	triptorelin pamoate
tolcapone	Tasmar		
Tolectin	tolmetin sodium	Trental	pentoxifylline
		tretinoin cream 0.025%	Avita
Tolinase	tolazamide	tretinoin gel	Retin-A Micro
tolmetin sodium	Tolectin	tretinion topical	Renova
tolnaftate	Tinactin		Retin-A
tolterodine tartrate	Detrol	tretinoin capsules	Vesanoid
Tonocard	tocainide HCl	triamcinolone acetonide	Aristocort Kenalog
Topamax	topiramate	triamcinolone acetonide aerosol	Azmacort
Topicort	desoximetasone		

T
R

triamcinolone acetonide nasal inhaler	Nasacort	trimethoprim	Primsol
		trimetrexate glucuronate	Neutrexin
triamcinolone acetonide nasal spray	Tri-Nasal	trimipramine maleate	Surmontil
triamterene	Dyrenium	Trimox	amoxicillin
triamterene 37.5 mg; hydro-chlorothiazide 25 mg	Maxzide -25MG Dyazide	Tri-Nasal	triamcinolone acetonide nasal spray
		Triostat	liothyronine sodium inj
triamterene 75 mg; hydro-chlorothiazide 50 mg	Maxzide	Tripedia	diphtheria & tetanus toxoids & acellular pertussis vaccine
Triavil	perphenazine; amitriptyline HCl		
		tripelennamine HCl	PBZ
triazolam	Halcion	Triphasil	levonorgestrel; ethinyl estradiol
Tricor	fenofibrate		
Tri-Cyclen	norgestimate; ethinyl estradiol	triple sulfa vaginal cream	Sultrin
		triprolidine HCl; pseudoephe-drine HCl	Actifed
Tridesilon	desonide		
Tridil	nitroglycerin inj		
Tridione	trimethadione	triptorelin pamoate	Trelstar Depot
trifluoperazine HCl	Stelazine		
		Trisenox	arsenic trioxide
trifluridine	Viroptic	Tritec	ranitidine bismuth citrate
trihexyphenidyl HCl	Artane		
Trileptal	oxcarbazepine	Tri-Vi-Flor	vitamins A, D, & C; fluoride
Tri-Immunol	diphtheria and tetanus toxoids and pertussis vaccine, adsorbed		
		Trobicin	spectinomycin HCl
Trilafon	perphenazine	troglitazone (W)	Rezulin (W)
Tri-Levlen	levonorgestrel; ethinyl estradiol	tromethamine	Tham
		Tronothane HCl	pramoxine HCl
		TrophAmine	amino acid inj
Trilisate	choline magnesium trisalicylate	Tropicacyl	tropicamide
		tropicamide	Mydriacyl Tropicacyl
trimethadione	Tridione	trovafloxacin	Trovan tablets
trimethaphan camsylate	Arfonad	Trovan tablet	trovafloxacin mesylate
trimethobenza-mide HCl	Tigan	Trovan inj	alatrovafloxacin mesylate IV

414

Trusopt	dorzolamide HCl
tuberculin, old	Tine Test, Tuberculin Old
tuberculin, purified protein derivative	Tine Test PPD
tuberculin skin test	Aplisol
tubocurarine	tubocurarine
Tucks	witch hazel pads
Tums	calcium carbonate
Tussi-Organidin NR	guaifenesin; codeine phosphate
Tussionex	hydrocodone polistirex; chlorpheniramine
Tylenol	acetaminophen
Tylenol with Codeine (#2, 3, and 4)	acetaminophen 300 mg with Codeine Phosphate (15, 30, and 60 mg)
Typhim Vi	typhoid vaccine
typhoid vaccine	Typhim Vi
tyropanoate sodium	Bilopaque

Ultravist	iopromide
Unasyn	ampicillin sodium; sulbactam sodium
Unipen (WA)	nafcillin sodium
Uniphyl	theophylline SR
Uniretic	moexipril HCl; hydrochlorothiazide
Univasc	moexipril HCl
Urecholine	bethanechol chloride
Urised	methenamine combination
Urispas	flavoxate HCl
urofollitropin for inj	Fertinex
urokinase	Abbokinase
unoprostone isopropyl ophth soln	Rescula
Uprima	apomorphine HCl
Urocit-K	potassium citrate tab
URSO	ursodiol
ursodiol	Actigall URSO
Uvadex	methoxsalen extracorporeal administration

T
Rx

U

UbiQGel	coenzyme Q10
Ultane	sevoflurane
Ultiva	remifentanil HCl
Ultralente U	insulin zinc suspension, extended (beef)
Ultram	tramadol HCl
Ultratag	technetium Tc-99m red blood cell kit

V

Vagifem	estradiol hemihydrate vaginal tab
Vagistat-1	tioconazole
valacyclovir	Valtrex
Valium	diazepam
valproate sodium inj	Depacon
valproic acid	Depakene
valrubicin, (for intravesical use)	Valstar

valsartan	Diovan	Ventolin	albuterol
Valstar	valrubicin, (for intravesical use)	VePesid	etoposide
		verapamil HCl	Isoptin
Valtrex	valacyclovir	verapamil HCl SR	Calan SR Verelan
Vancenase	beclomethasone dipropionate	verapamil HCl SR bedtime formulation	Covera HS Verelan PM
Vancenase AQ Nasal	beclomethasone dipropionate	Verdia	tasosartan
Vanceril	beclomethasone dipropionate	Verelan	verapamil HCl SR
Vancocin	vancomycin HCl	Verelan PM	verapamil HCl SR bedtime formulation
vancomycin HCl	Vancocin		
Vaniqa	eflornithine HCl cream	Verluna	nofetumomab
Vantin	cefpodoxime proxetil	Vermox	mebendazole
		Versed	midazolam HCl
Vaponefrin	epinephrine racemic	verteporfin inj	Visudyne
Vaqta	hepatitis A vaccine, inactivated	Vesanoid	tretinoin capsules
		Vestra	reboxetine mesylate
varicella virus vaccine	Varivax	Vexol	rimexolone
Varivax	varicella virus vaccine	Viactiv	calcium carbonate; vitamin D and K chewable
Vascor	bepridil	Viadur	leuprolide acetate implant
Vaseline	petrolatum, white		
Vaseretic	enalapril maleate; hydrochloro-thiazide	Viagra	sildenafil citrate
		Vibramycin	doxycycline hyclate
Vasocon	naphazoline ophth soln	Vicodin	hydrocodone bitartrate; acetaminophen
Vasodilan	isoxsuprine HCl	Vicoprofen	hydrocodone bitartrate 7.5 mg; ibuprofen 200 mg
vasopressin	Pitressin		
Vasotec	enalapril maleate		
Vasoxyl	methoxamine HCl	vidarabine monohydrate	Vira-A
vecuronium bromide	Norcuron	Videx	didanosine
Velban	vinblastine sulfate	vinblastine sulfate	Velban
Velosef	cephradine	vincristine sulfate	Oncovin
Velosulin Human	insulin inj (human)	vindesine sulfate	Eldisine
venlafaxine HCl	Effexor		
venlafaxine HCl SR	Effexor XR	vinorelbine tartrate	Navelbine

Vioform	clioquinol
Vioxx	rofecoxib
Vira-A	vidarabine monohydrate
Viracept	nelfinavir mesylate
Viramune	nevirapine
Virazole	ribavirin
Viroptic	trifluridine
Visicol	sodium phosphate tab
Visine Extra	tetrahydrozoline HCl ophth
Visipaque	iodixanol
Visken	pindolol
Vistaril	hydroxyzine pamoate
Vistide	cidofovir
Visudyne	verteporfin inj
Vitravene	fomivirsen sodium inj
Vivelle	estradiol trans-dermal system
Volmax	albuterol SR
Voltaren	diclofenac sodium
Voltaren-XR	diclofenac sodium SR
Vumon	teniposide

W

warfarin sodium	Coumadin
Welchol	colesevelam HCl
Wellbutrin	bupropion HCl
Wellbutrin SR	bupropion HCl SR
Wellcovorin	*leucovorin calcium*
Wellferon	interferon ALFA-n[1] lymphoblastoid
WinRho SD	RH$_O$ (D) immune globulin IV (human)

Winstrol	stanozolol
witch hazel pads	Tucks
Wyamine	mephentermine sulfate
Wycillin (for IM use only)	penicillin G procaine (for IM use only)
Wydase	hyaluronidase
Wygesic	propoxyphene HCl; acetaminophen
Wymox	amoxicillin
Wytensin	guanabenz acetate

XYZ

Xalatan	latanoprost
Xanax	alprazolam
Xeloda	capecitabine
Xenical	orlistat
Xopenex	levalbuterol HCl inhalation soln
Xylocaine HCl	lidocaine HCl
xylometazoline	Otrivin
Xyrem	gamma hydroxybutyrate
Yutopar	ritodrine HCl
Zadaxin	thymalfasin
Zaditor	ketotifen fumarate ophth soln
zafirlukast	Accolate
Zagam	sparfloxacin
zalcitabine	Hivid
zaleplon	Sonata
Zanaflex	tizanidine HCl
zanamivir for inhalation	Relenza
Zanosar	streptozocin
Zantac	ranitidine HCl
Zarontin	ethosuximide
Zaroxolyn	metolazone
Zecnil	somatostatin
Zelmac	tegaserod
Zemplar	paricalcitol
Zenapax	daclizumab

V
R

417

Zerit	stavudine	Zoladex	goserelin acetate implant
Zestoretic	lisinopril; hydrochloro- thiazide	zoledronic acid for inj	Zometa
Zestril	lisinopril	zolmitriptan	Zomig
Zetar	coal tar product	Zoloft	sertraline HCl
Ziac	bisoprolol fumarate; hydrochloro- thiazide	zolpidem tartrate	Ambien
		Zometa	zoledronic acid for inj
Ziagen	abacavir sulfate	Zomig	zolmitriptan
zidovudine	Retrovir	Zonegram	zonisamide
zidovudine; lamivudine	Combivir	zonisamide	Zonegram
		Zosyn	piperacillin so- dium; tazobac tam sodium
zileuton	Zyflo		
Zinacef	cefuroxime sodium	Zovirax	acyclovir
		Zyban	bupropion HCl SR
zinc acetate	Galzin		
Zinecard	dexrazoxane	Zydone 5/400, 7.5/400, 10/400	hydrocodone bitartrate; acetaminophen
Zithromax	azithromycin		
Zocor	simvastatin		
Zofran	ondansetron	Zyflo	zileuton
Zofran ODT	ondansetron orally disintegrating tab	Zyloprim	allopurinol
		Zyprexa	olanzapine
		Zyrtec	cetirizine HCl
		Zyvox	linezolid

References
1. Facts and Comparisons. St. Louis: Facts and Comparisons, Inc. (published monthly and online)
2. Billup NF, Billup SM. American drug index. St. Louis: Facts and Comparisons, Inc.yw (published yearly)
3. Physicians GenRx. St. Louis: Mosby. (published yearly)
4. Parfitt K. Ed. Martindale: 32nd edition. The Pharmaceutical Press. London, 1999.

Z
℞

Chapter 7

Normal Laboratory Values*

In the following tables, normal reference values for commonly requested laboratory tests are listed
in traditional units and in SI units. The tables are a guideline only. Values are method dependent
and "normal values" may vary between laboratories.

	Blood, Plasma or Serum	
	Reference Value	
Determination	**Conventional Units**	**SI Units**
Ammonia (NH₃) − diffusion	20–120 mcg/dl	12–70 mcmol/L
Ammonia Nitrogen	15–45 mcg/dl	11–32 μmol/L
Amylase	35–118 IU/L	0.58–1.97 mckat/L
Anion Gap (Na⁺ − [Cl⁻ + HCO₃⁻]) (P)	7–16 mEq/L	7–16 mmol/L
Antinuclear antibodies	negative at 1:10 dilution of serum	negative at 1:10 dilution of serum
Antithrombin III (AT III)	80–120 units/dl	800–1200 units/L
Bicarbonate: Arterial Venous	21–28 mEq/L 22–29 mEq/L	21–28 mmol/L 22–29 mmol/L
Bilirubin: Conjugated (direct) Total	≤0.2 mg/dl 0.1–1 mg/dl	≤4 mcmol/L 2–18 mcmol/L
Calcitonin	<100 pg/mL	<100 ng/L
Calcium: Total Ionized	8.6–10.3 mg/dl 4.4–5.1 mg/dl	2.2–2.74 mmol/L 1–1.3 mmol/L
Carbon dioxide content (plasma)	21–32 mmol/L	21–32 mmol/L
Carcinoembryonic antigen	<3 ng/mL	<3 mcg/L
Chloride	95–110 mEq/L	95–110 mmol/L
Coagulation screen: Bleeding time Prothrombin time Partial thromboplastin time (activated) Protein C Protein S	3–9.5 min 10–13 sec 22–37 sec 0.7–1.4 μ/mL 0.7–1.4 μ/mL	180–570 sec 10–13 sec 22–37 sec 700–1400 units/mL 700–1400 units/mL
Copper, total	70–160 mcg/dl	11–25 mcmol/L
Corticotropin (ACTH adrenocorticotropic hormone) − 0800 hr	<60 pg/mL	<13.2 pmol/L
Cortisol: 0800 hr 1800 hr 2000 hr	5–30 mcg/dl 2–15 mcg/dl ≤50% of 0800 hr	138–810 nmol/L 54–410 nmol/L ≤50% of 0800 hr
Creatine kinase: Female Male	20–170 IU/L 30–220 IU/L	0.33–2.83 mckat/L 0.5–3.67 mckat/L
Creatine kinase isoenzymes, MB fraction	0–12 IU/L	0–0.2 mckat/L

Blood, Plasma or Serum (Cont.)		
	Reference Value	
Determination	**Conventional Units**	**SI Units**
Creatinine	0.5–1.7 mg/dl	44–150 mcmol/L
Fibrinogen (coagulation factor I)	150–360 mg/dl	1.5–3.6 g/L
Follicle-stimulating hormone (FSH):		
Female	2–13 mIU/mL	2–13 IU/L
Midcycle	5–22 mIU/mL	5–22 IU/L
Male	1–8 mIU/mL	1–8 IU/L
Glucose, fasting	65–115 mg/dl	3.6–6.3 mmol/L
Glucose Tolerance Test (Oral)	mg/dL	mmol/L
	Normal	Normal
Fasting	70–105	3.9–5.8
60 min	120–170	6.7–9.4
90 min	100–140	5.6–7.8
120 min	70–120	3.9–6.7
	Diabetic	Diabetic
Fasting	>140	>7.8
60 min	≥200	≥11.1
90 min	≥200	≥11.1
120 min	≥140	≥7.8
(γ) – Glutamyltransferase (GGT):		
Male	9–50 units/L	9–50 units/L
Female	8–40 units/L	8–40 units/L
Haptoglobin	44–303 mg/dl	0.44–3.03 g/L
Hematologic tests:		
Fibrinogen	200–400 mg/dl	2–4 g/L
Hematocrit (Hct), female	36%–44.6%	0.36–0.446 fraction of 1
male	40.7%–50.3%	0.4–0.503 fraction of 1
Hemoglobin A_{1C}	5.3%–7.5% of total Hgb	0.053–0.075
Hemoglobin (Hb), female	12.1–15.3 g/dl	121–153 g/L
male	13.8–17.5 g/dl	138–175 g/L
Leukocyte count (WBC)	3800–9800/mcl	$3.8–9.8 \times 10^9$/L
Erythrocyte count (RBC), female	$3.5–5 \times 10^6$/mcl	$3.5–5 \times 10^{12}$/L
male	$4.3–5.9 \times 10^6$/mcl	$4.3–5.9 \times 10^{12}$/L
Mean corpuscular volume (MCV)	80–97.6 mcm^3	80–97.6 fl
Mean corpuscular hemoglobin (MCH)	27–33 pg/cell	1.66–2.09 fmol/cell
Mean corpuscular hemoglobin concentrate (MCHC)	33–36 g/dl	20.3–22 mmol/L
Erythrocyte sedimentation rate (sedrate, ESR)	≤30 mm/hr	≤30 mm/hr
Erythrocyte enzymes:		
Glucose-6-phosphate dehydrogenase (G-6-PD)	250–5000 units/10^6 cells	250–5000 mcunits/cell
Ferritin	10–383 ng/mL	23–862 pmol/L
Folic acid: normal	>3.1–12.4 ng/mL	7–28.1 nmol/L
Platelet count	$150–450 \times 10^3$/mcl	$150–450 \times 10^9$/L
Reticulocytes	0.5%–1.5% of erythrocytes	0.005–0.015
Vitamin B_{12}	223–1132 pg/mL	165–835 pmol/L
Iron: Female	30–160 mcg/dl	5.4–31.3 mcmol/L
Male	45–160 mcg/dl	8.1–31.3 mcmol/L
Iron binding capacity	220–420 mcg/dl	39.4–75.2 mcmol/L

Normal Laboratory Values (Cont.) Blood

Blood, Plasma or Serum (Cont.)		
	Reference Value	
Determination	**Conventional Units**	**SI Units**
Isocitrate Dehydrogenase	1.2–7 units/L	1.2–7 units/L
Isoenzymes		
Fraction 1	14%–26% of total	0.14–0.26 fraction of total
Fraction 2	29%–39% of total	0.29–0.39 fraction of total
Fraction 3	20%–26% of total	0.20–0.26 fraction of total
Fraction 4	8%–16% of total	0.08–0.16 fraction of total
Fraction 5	6%–16% of total	0.06–0.16 fraction of total
Lactate dehydrogenase	100–250 IU/L	1.67–4.17 mckat/L
Lactic acid (lactate)	6–19 mg/dl	0.7–2.1 mmol/L
Lead	≤50 mcg/dl	≤2.41 mcmol/L
Lipase	10–150 units/L	10–150 units/L
Lipids:		
Total Cholesterol		
Desirable	<200 mg/dl	<5.2 mmol/L
Borderline-high	200–239 mg/dl	<5.2–6.2 mmol/L
High	>239 mg/dl	>6.2 mmol/L
LDL		
Desirable	<130 mg/dl	<3.36 mmol/L
Borderline-high	130–159 mg/dl	3.36–4.11 mmol/L
High	>159 mg/dl	>4.11 mmol/L
HDL (low)	<35 mg/dl	<0.91 mmol/L
Triglycerides		
Desirable	<200 mg/dl	<2.26 mmol/L
Borderline-high	200–400 mg/dl	2.26–4.52 mmol/L
High	400–1000 mg/dl	4.52–11.3 mmol/L
Very high	>1000 mg/dl	>11.3 mmol/L
Magnesium	1.3–2.2 mEq/L	0.65–1.1 mmol/L
Osmolality	280–300 mOsm/kg	280–300 mmol/kg
Oxygen saturation (arterial)	94%–100%	0.94–1 fraction of 1
PCO_2, arterial	35–45 mm Hg	4.7–6 kPa
pH, arterial	7.35–7.45	7.35–7.45
PO_2, arterial: Breathing room air[1] On 100% O_2	80–105 mm Hg <500 mm Hg	10.6–14 kPa
Phosphatase (acid), total at 37°C	0.13–0.63 IU/L	2.2–10.5 IU/L or 2.2–10.5 mckat/L
Phosphatase alkaline[2]	20–130 IU/L	20–130 IU/L or 0.33–2.17 mckat/L
Phosphorus, inorganic,[3] (phosphate)	2.5–5 mg/dl	0.8–1.6 mmol/L
Potassium	3.5–5 mEq/L	3.5–5 mmol/L

[1] Age dependent
[2] Infants and adolescents up to 104 IU/L
[3] Infants in the first year up to 6 mg/dl

Normal Laboratory Values (Cont.) Blood

	Blood, Plasma or Serum (Cont.)	
	Reference Value	
Determination	**Conventional Units**	**SI Units**

Progesterone
Female
  Follicular phase
  Luteal phase
Male
	
	0.1–1.5 ng/mL
	0.1–1.5 ng/mL
	2.5–28 ng/mL
	<0.5 ng/mL
		
		0.32–4.8 nmol/L
		0.32–4.8 nmol/L
		8–89 nmol/L
		<1.6 nmol/L

Prolactin	1.4–24.2 ng/mL	1.4–24.2 mcg/L

Prostate specific antigen
Protein: Total
  Albumin
  Globulin
	0–4 ng/mL
	6–8 g/dl
	3.5–5 g/dl
	2.3–3.5 g/dl
		0–4 ng/mL
		60–80 g/L
		36–50 g/L
		23–35 g/L

Rheumatoid factor	<60 IU/mL	<60 kIU/L
Sodium	135–147 mEq/L	135–147 mmol/L
Testosterone: Female Male	6–86 ng/dl 270–1070 ng/dl	0.21–3 nmol/L 9.3–37 nmol/L

Thyroid Hormone Function Tests:
  Thyroid-stimulating hormone (TSH)
  Thyroxine-binding globulin capacity
  Total triiodothyronine (T_3)
  Total thyroxine by RIA (T_4)
  T_3 resin uptake
	
	0.35–6.2 mcU/mL
	10–26 mcg/dl
	75–220 ng/dl
	4–11 mcg/dl
	25%–38%
		
		0.35–6.2 mU/L
		100–260 mcg/L
		1.2–3.4 nmol/L
		51–142 nmol/L
		0.25–0.38 fraction of 1

Transaminase, AST (aspartate aminotransferase, SGOT)	11–47 IU/L	0.18–0.78 mckat/L
Transaminase, ALT (alanine aminotransferase, SGPT)	7–53 IU/L	0.12–0.88 mckat/L
Transferrin	220–400 mg/dL	2.20–4.00 g/L
Urea nitrogen (BUN)	8–25 mg/dl	2.9–8.9 mmol/L
Uric acid	3–8 mg/dl	179–476 mcmol/L
Vitamin A (retinol)	15–60 mcg/dl	0.52–2.09 mcmol/L
Zinc	50–150 mcg/dl	7.7–23 mcmol/L

Normal Laboratory Values—Urine

	Urine	
	Reference Value	
Determination	**Conventional Units**	**SI Units**
Calcium[1]	50–250 mcg/day	1.25–6.25 mmol/day
Catecholamines: Epinephrine Norepinephrine	<20 mcg/day <100 mcg/day	<109 nmol/day <590 nmol/day
Catecholamines, 24-hr	<110 mcg	<650 nmol
Copper[1]	15–60 mcg/day	0.24–0.95 mcmol/day

Creatinine: Child
    Adolescent
    Female
    Male
	8–22 mg/kg
	8–30 mg/kg
	0.6–1.5 g/day
	0.8–1.8 g/day
		71–195 μmol/kg
		71–265 μmol/kg
		5.3–13.3 mmol/day
		7.1–15.9 mmol/day

Normal Laboratory Values (Cont.) Urine

Urine		
	Reference Value	
Determination	**Conventional Units**	**SI Units**
pH	4.5–8	4.5–8
Phosphate[1]	0.9–1.3 g/day	29–42 mmol/day
Potassium[1]	25–100 mEq/day	25–100 mmol/day
Protein Total At rest	 1–14 mg/dL 50–80 mg/day	 10–140 mg/L 50–80 mg/day
Protein, quantitative	<150 mg/day	<0.15 g/day
Sodium[1]	100–250 mEq/day	100–250 mmol/day
Specific Gravity, random	1.002–1.030	1.002–1.030
Uric Acid, 24-hr	250–750 mg	1.48–4.43 mmol

[1]Diet dependent

Normal Laboratory Values—Drug Levels

Drug Levels†			
		Reference Value	
	Drug Determination	**Conventional Units**	**SI Units**
Aminoglycosides	Amikacin (trough) (peak) Gentamicin (trough) (peak) Kanamycin (trough) (peak) Netilmicin (trough) (peak) Streptomycin (trough) (peak) Tobramycin (trough) (peak)	 1–8 mcg/mL 20–30 mcg/mL 0.5–2 mcg/mL 6–10 mcg/mL 5–10 mcg/mL 20–25 mcg/mL 0.5–2 mcg/mL 6–10 mcg/mL <5 mcg/mL 5–20 mcg/mL 0.5–2 mcg/mL 5–20 mcg/mL	 1.7–13.7 mcmol/L 34–51 mcmol/L 1–4.2 mcmol/L 12.5–20.9 mcmol/L nd nd nd nd nd nd 1.1–4.3 mcmol/L 12.8–21.8 mcmol/L
Antiarrhythmics	Amiodarone Bretylium Digitoxin Digoxin Disopyramide Flecainide Lidocaine Mexiletine Procainamide Propranolol Quinidine Tocainide Verapamil	0.5–2.5 mcg/mL 0.5–1.5 mcg/mL 9–25 mcg/L 0.8–2 ng/mL 2–8 mcg/mL 0.2–1 mcg/mL 1.5–6 mcg/mL 0.5–2 mcg/mL 4–8 mcg/mL 50–200 ng/mL 2–6 mcg/mL 4–10 mcg/mL 0.08–0.3 mcg/mL	15.4 mcmol/L nd 11.8–32.8 nmol/L 0.9–2.5 nmol/L 6–18 mcmol/L nd 4.5–21.5 mcmol/L nd 17–34 mcmol/mL 190–770 nmol/L 4.6–9.2 mcmol/L nd nd

Normal Laboratory Values (Cont.) Drug Levels

	Drug Levels†		
		Reference Value	
	Drug Determination	**Conventional Units**	**SI Units**
Anti-convulsants	Carbamazepine	4–12 mcg/mL	17–51 mcmol/L
	Phenobarbital	10–40 mcg/mL	43–172 mcmol/L
	Phenytoin	10–20 mcg/mL	40–80 mcmol/L
	Primidone	4–12 mcg/mL	18–55 mcmol/L
	Valproic acid	40–100 mcg/mL	280–700 mcmol/L
Antidepressants	Amitriptyline	110–250 ng/mL[3]	500–900 nmol/L
	Amoxapine	200–500 ng/mL	nd
	Bupropion	25–100 ng/mL	nd
	Clomipramine	80–100 ng/mL	nd
	Desipramine	115–300 ng/mL	nd
	Doxepin	110–250 ng/mL[3]	nd
	Imipramine	225–350 ng/mL[3]	nd
	Maprotiline	200–300 ng/mL	nd
	Nortriptyline	50–150 ng/mL	nd
	Protriptyline	70–250 ng/mL	nd
	Trazodone	800–1600 ng/mL	nd
Antipsychotics	Chlorpromazine	50–300 ng/mL	150–950 nmol/L
	Fluphenazine	0.13–2.8 ng/mL	nd
	Haloperidol	5–20 ng/mL	nd
	Perphenazine	0.8–1.2 ng/mL	nd
	Thiothixene	2–57 ng/mL	nd
Miscellaneous	Amantadine	300 ng/mL	nd
	Amrinone	3.7 mcg/mL	nd
	Chloramphenicol	10–20 mcg/mL	31–62 mcmol/L
	Cyclosporine[1]	250–800 ng/mL (whole blood, RIA)	nd
		50–300 ng/mL (plasma, RIA)	nd
	Ethanol[2]	0 mg/dl	0 mmol/L
	Hydralazine	100 ng/mL	nd
	Lithium	0.6–1.2 mEq/L	0.6–1.2 mmol/L
	Salicylate	100–300 mg/L	724–2172 mcmol/L
	Sulfonamide	5–15 mg/dl	nd
	Terbutaline	0.5–4.1 ng/mL	nd
	Theophylline	10–20 mcg/mL	55–110 mcmol/L
	Vancomycin (trough)	5–15 ng/mL	nd
	(peak)	20–40 mcg/mL	nd

†The values given are generally accepted as desirable for treatment without toxicity for most patients. However, exceptions are not uncommon.
[1]24 hour trough values
[2]Toxic: 50–100 mg/dl (10.9–21.7 mmol/L)
[3]Parent drug plus N-desmethy7l metabolite
nd — No data available

Prices for the Tenth Edition

Medical Abbreviations: 15,000 Conveniences at the
Expense of Communications and Safety
by Neil M Davis
(ISBN 0-931431-10-7)

1–24 copies	$22.95 each plus S&H
25 or more copies	$16.25 each plus S&H

U.S. Shipping And Handling Charges

Number of Books Ordered	U.S. S&H charges to be added to each **order**
1–2	$5.00
3–6	$7.00
7–11	$10.00
12 or more	$14.00

Orders shipped to Pennsylvania must add 6% sales tax.
No sales tax for other states (subject to change).

Payable by–

Visa	MasterCard	Discover
American Exp.	Check	Money Order

Order from and make check payable to–

Neil M. Davis Associates
1143 Wright Drive
Huntingdon Valley PA 19006-2721

Orders may be mailed to above address or

Phone 215 947 1752
Fax 215 938 1937
Secure Web site http://www.neilmdavis.com
E-mail med@neilmdavis.com

Where applicable, please have ready credit card number and
expiration date, phone number, and mailing address. A PO
box address is not acceptable for orders for more than 2
books as they are shipped via UPS.

Price Information—continued

Outside of the United States

- Pay by credit card (VISA, MasterCard, Discover, American Express), or in U.S. dollars through a corresponding U.S. bank, or an International Money Order in U.S. currency.
- Prices as shown on the previous page plus shipping costs.
- To ascertain shipping cost, choose the method of shipment desired and calculate on the fact that each book weighs 350 grams.

Internet Access Dates

Each book purchased includes, at no extra cost, a single-use access license for the website version of the book, which is updated monthly. This license is valid for 24 months from the date of the initial log-in.

Order Form

```
PLEASE PRINT OR TYPE

Name _____

Address _____

_____

City _____ State _____ Zip Code _____

Phone ( ____ ) _____

Attention (If Applicable) _____

Number of copies ordered _____ PO # (If Applicable) _____

Method of payment:

_____ Check or money order enclosed

_____ Visa               _____ MasterCard

_____ Discover           _____ American Express

Card Number _____

Exp. Date _____

Signature _____
```